Global Perspectives on Interventions in Forensic Therapeutic Communities

Global Perspectives on Interventions in Forensic Therapeutic Communities: A Practitioner's Guide explores the validity and effectiveness of secure settings as therapeutic communities (TCs). Rooted in practice, this book examines the transferability of approaches within international TCs to other forensic settings, while considering how the environment contributes to effectiveness.

In this volume, Akerman and Shuker bring together leading clinicians from across the world to offer insight into critical topics, including the impact of gang membership on therapeutic process and the community, how core creative therapies are integrated and how the model is applied in international settings and across varied contexts. Leading clinicians draw on rare reports and papers to explain the therapeutic community model while keeping in mind the diverse contexts within which it is practiced. The book provides a much-needed global perspective on the diverse role TCs have across forensic services.

This groundbreaking book is valuable reading for forensic and clinical psychologists, counsellors, social workers and psychiatrists working in secure prison or rehabilitation settings, as well as students in these fields.

Geraldine Akerman is Chartered and Registered Forensic Psychologist and Principal Psychologist at HMP Grendon and Springhill. She is Chair of the Division of Forensic Psychology.

Richard Shuker is Chartered Forensic Psychologist and Head of Clinical Services at HMP Grendon, a therapeutic community prison for long-term prisoners with complex personality needs, where he leads the clinical provision and research programme.

Issues in Forensic Psychology

Series editors: Richard Shuker and Geraldine Akerman

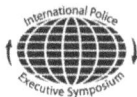

For more information about this series, please visit:
www.routledge.com/Issues-in-Forensic-Psychology/book-series/IFP

Global Perspectives on Interventions in Forensic Therapeutic Communities

A Practitioner's Guide

Edited by
Geraldine Akerman and Richard Shuker

Routledge
Taylor & Francis Group

LONDON AND NEW YORK

Cover image: © MirageC/Getty Images

First published 2022
by Routledge
2 Park Square, Milton Park, Abingdon, Oxon OX14 4RN

and by Routledge
605 Third Avenue, New York, NY 10158

Routledge is an imprint of the Taylor & Francis Group, an informa business

British Library Cataloguing-in-Publication Data
A catalogue record for this book is available from the British Library

Library of Congress Cataloging-in-Publication Data
Names: Shuker, Richard, editor. | Akerman, Geraldine, editor.
Title: Global perspectives on interventions in forensic therapeutic
communities: a practitioner's guide/edited by Geraldine Akerman and Richard Shuker.
Description: Abingdon, Oxon ; New York, NY: Routledge, 2022. |
Series: Issues in forensic psychology | Includes bibliographical references and index.
Identifiers: LCCN 2021033185 | ISBN 9780367322380 (hardback) |
ISBN 9780367322397 (paperback) | ISBN 9780367322397 (ebook)
Subjects: LCSH: Prisoners–Mental health services. |
Therapeutic communities. | Forensic psychology. | Criminals–Rehabilitation.
Classification: LCC RC451.4.P68 G56 2022 | DDC 365/.6672–dc23
LC record available at https://lccn.loc.gov/2021033185

ISBN: 978-0-367-32238-0 (hbk)
ISBN: 978-0-367-32239-7 (pbk)
ISBN: 978-0-429-31746-0 (ebk)

DOI: 10.4324/9780429317460

Typeset in Minion
by Newgen Publishing UK

To all of those who live and work in the TC environment.

Contents

Figures

Tables

Contributors

Geraldine Akerman is a principal chartered and registered forensic psychologist at HMP Grendon, chair of the Division of Forensic Psychology Executive Committee, founder and presenter of the Let's Talk Forensic Psychology YouTube channel, and director of the Forensic Psychology Network Ltd. Having worked at HMP Grendon for over 22 years, Geraldine has gained experience of the problems associated with integrating disparate groups of people into a democratic therapeutic community.

Naya Arbiter is Co-founder and Senior Vice President, Services and Training, of the Amity Foundation, where she began working in 1981. She has developed restorative paradigms for those marginalized through addiction, poverty, racism, sexism, trauma and violence. She has been recognized for the development of prosocial strategies for people who represent populations that have confounded the mainstream; her efforts in prisons have evidenced the highest recidivism reduction with the most criminogenic population ever studied. She authored 14 volumes of TC curriculum, which foster personal growth, emotional literacy and social responsibility. She has served on the Inter-American Commission for Drug Policy; as vice president of Therapeutic Communities of America; chair of the Standards and Goals Committee of the World Federation of Therapeutic Communities, and on numerous scientific committee advisory boards including that of the National Treatment Improvement Evaluation Study. She was also chosen by President Ronald Reagan as one of the conferees for the White House Conference for a Drug Free America. In 2013, Naya was the second American and the first woman to receive the prestigious Acknowledgment Award of the European Federation of Therapeutic Communities, given to those acknowledged to have made the greatest contribution to the ongoing development of the TC methodology. A native New Yorker, Naya Arbiter spent her adolescence between New York, Bolivia, and Mexico. She moved to the American Southwest and became involved in using and smuggling drugs over the Mexican/Arizona border. Arrested in Mexico, but released from jail before her eighteenth birthday, she was given a well-constructed chance by a courageous probation officer to go to the first American TC (Synanon). Her life's work has been to construct chances for those in seemingly impossible situations.

Jo Augustus is a qualified arts psychotherapist who has practised working within TCs for the past 22 years. She is currently the lead DTC Core Creative Psychotherapist at HMPPS Grendon and has worked there for the past 17 years. Previously she worked within an adolescent TC. Jo is currently responsible for development and management of the Core Creative Psychotherapies Department at Grendon, which comprises a team of nine Core Creative psychotherapists whose modalities are art therapy, music therapy and psychodrama. In addition, her clinical work at HMPPS Grendon is largely based working across two TCs, including the Enhanced Assessment Unit. Jo is also a qualified creative clinical supervisor and facilitates both group and individual supervision as well as reflective practice groups. Jo has also codeveloped functional evaluation and research methods concerning the efficacy of the arts psychotherapies within this TC custodial setting.

Natalie Bond is an HCPC-registered and BPS-chartered forensic psychologist with 16 years of experience in assessment and intervention work with high-risk and life-sentenced men within the prison service. She has worked predominantly in offender personality disorder services to include ten years as a wing psychologist at HMP Gartree Therapeutic Community (GTC) and a period at HMP Grendon assessment unit. Natalie has published research on the subject of offence paralleling in a TC, the impact on staff of working in a psychologically informed planned environment (PIPE) and work with offenders with intellectual difficulties.

Simone Bruschetta is a PhD researcher; freelance psychotherapist/group analyst/TC specialist; director of Quality Accreditation Program 'Visiting DTC Project', Catania (IT).

Virginie Debaere, PhD, works as a clinical psychologist/psychoanalytic psychotherapist in outpatient mental health care and as a researcher at Ghent University. For her PhD, she studied TC residents' processes of change from a psychoanalytic framework. She is board member at the Belgian TC for drug-addicted persons 'Trempoline' and works as an assessor for the Enabling Environments project at the Royal College for Psychiatrists in London.

Andrew Frost has been working, teaching and researching in offender rehabilitation since 1993. At the Ara Institute in Christchurch (NZ), he teaches in social work and professional supervision programmes. Prior to that he led a team of educators in the Domestic and Family Violence Practice programme at CQUniversity. His practice and award-winning research into group work with violent offenders, along with the establishment of a forensic TC, have spawned a range of publications across books and academic journals.

Theoretical models and other outcomes from this work have been used by state, NGO and independent service providers to inform practice. Andrew is co-author of a 2019 textbook on domestic and family violence for students and practitioners, published by Routledge UK.

Vicky Gavin's first career was in the arts, before training as a mental health nurse, and later a group analyst. Over the past 20 years she has been associated with three therapeutic community (TC) services: The Acorn programme at the Retreat Hospital in York, HMP Send DTC in Surrey, and TC+ at HMP Gartree in Leicestershire. She is co-author of 'Borderline Personality Disorder: Patterns of Self-Harm, Reported Childhood Trauma and Clinical Outcome', McFetridge, M., Milner, R., Gavin, V., and Levita, L. *BJPsych Open*. 2015 July 10, 1(1):18–20. https://doi.org/10.1192/bjpo.bp.115.000117. Vicky lives in Yorkshire, and currently works freelance and for Nottinghamshire Health Care NHS Foundation Trust teaching, advising and supervising TC practitioners in adult and custodial settings. She is a United Kingdom Council of Psychotherapy-accredited psychotherapist, a member of the Institute of Group Analysis and of Group Analysis International, the MB3 TC Elders group, and chair of trustees of a charity which aims to alleviate mental suffering through TC treatment, The Consortium for Therapeutic Communities (TCTC).

Hanne Holm Hage-Ali has been managing Opbygningsgården since 2006. She has over 25 years of experience of working in the field of drug treatment, first on a ship's project, before starting as a drug treatment facilitator at Opbygningsgården in 1993. She is a qualified gestalt therapist. Hanne has written several articles about Opbygningsgården's treatment method 'community as method'.

Ruslan Isaev, PhD, is a psychiatrist with 20 years' experience. He is CEO of 'Dr Isaev's Clinic', president of the Independent Narcological Guild, expert at the Civic Chamber of the Russian Federation and member of a group of editors of the *Therapeutic Communities* journal in the UK.

Jinnie Jefferies is a qualified UKCP-accredited psychodrama psychotherapist. She has headed up the Psychodrama Department since 1981 and is also the lead trainer for the TC-accredited training programme. The Butler Trust awarded her in 2008 the Terry Waite Award for her outstanding work with long-term prisoners. In addition to her work at Grendon, she is the founding director for The London Centre for Group and Individual Psychodrama and supervisor. In addition to her clinical work she has written widely and lectured internationally about her work and presented television programmes on psychodrama and collaborated on documentaries using action methods, *Gun 6* recently received a BAFTA award for single documentary category in 2019.

Kenneth Arctander Johansen is Communication Manager at the Norwegian Interest Organization for Substance Misusers (RIO). Since 2018, he has been a member of the Norwegian public drug policy reform committee that assessed and prepared the Norwegian government's decriminalization reform for use and possession of illicit substances. He is a PhD candidate at Ghent University where he studies contemporary drug policy discussions from historical perspectives. Kenneth is a former TC resident and a former TC staff member, and has been working clinically for years.

Jacqui Johnson is a registered social worker and is currently working as a family violence response specialist for Oranga Tamariki Ministry for Children in Christchurch (NZ). Prior to that, Jacqui's academic career saw her completing her masters of social work (applied) with Distinction at the University of Canterbury in 2010, and awarded the Fiona Leeves Memorial for leadership in social work. Jacqui went on to complete her doctoral thesis in 2020, documenting the stories of mothers during their time within the Mothers with Babies Units (MBU) in New Zealand women's prisons and their reintegration into their communities. Jacqui gained a wide range of insights into the life experiences of these women that could be used to further inform mother and child-centred programmes and policies in New Zealand and internationally. Throughout this time, Jacqui has attended and spoken at a number of national and international conferences in her field of expertise and is currently working on publishing work based on her research in this area.

George De Leon is an internationally recognized authority on treatment and research in TCs for addictions. He holds a PhD in psychology from Columbia University. He is a founding member and former president of the American Psychological Association's Division 50 on Addictions and clinical professor of psychiatry at New York University School of Medicine. He has published over 170 scientific papers and chapters, and authored and edited seven books and monographs.

Carine Minne has worked in National Health Service (NHS) mental health settings for over 30 years and in particular, forensic psychiatry settings due to her special interest in working with mentally disordered offender patients. She trained as a forensic psychiatrist and psychoanalyst and brings these two specialties together in her work at the Portman Clinic and the high-security hospital of Broadmoor, where she has been consultant psychiatrist in forensic psychotherapy for 20 years. One of her main interests is the provision of essential long-term therapeutic interventions for these patients due to the chronicity and deeply engrained nature of their damaged mental structures as a result of very early traumas, and how to convince policymakers and commissioners of this need. She is also committed to her work with Paul Kassman, designer of Changing the Game, a therapeutic intervention for gang members (90% Black and Minority Ethnic in London), and to the import- ance of knowledge of race and cultural issues in psychotherapy, an area of neglect in psychotherapy trainings and practice here. She is vice chair of the Loudoun Trust, a charity that works for the improvement of child protection from abuse. She is currently president-elect of the International Association for Forensic Psychotherapy (IAFP). Carine trains, teaches and supervises junior doctors and professionals from different disciplines within mental health organisations. She is also involved in training probation officers and is the mental health lecturer for the police chiefs' Strategic Command course. She has published papers and chapters in a number of books and lectures nationally and internationally.

Rod Mullen is Co-founder and President of the Amity Foundation. He is responsible for development, administration and management of a non-profit organization providing prevention, intervention and treatment, vocational training and housing services to men and women (and their children) who are substance abusers, mentally ill, homeless, veterans, under criminal justice supervision, or victims of trauma. In conjunction with the board of directors, Rod is responsible for developing and implementing the strategic goals of the organization and adhering to its mission. The Foundation operates TC programmes in Arizona, California and New Mexico – in both custody and community settings, residential and non-residential, and provides curricula and training for human services organizations.

Steve Pearce is a psychiatrist who specialises in the diagnosis and treatment of personality disorder and leads a nationally commissioned service in Oxfordshire. He has published extensively on the subject of efficacy of TCs and on working with those who have personality difficulties as well as designing and delivering training.

Johnny Lindblad Reinhardt has been working in the day treatment section of our prison project in Kragskovhede prison since 2015 and has been man- aging the prison project overall since 2017. He has over 25 years of experience working in the field of psychiatry and drug treatment. He has also worked on a freelance basis and is a qualified 'mindfulness' instructor. In addition, he is the author of two books.

Gareth Ross is an HCPC-registered and BPS-chartered forensic psychologist with 15 years of experience in assessment and intervention work with violent offenders. He currently works as the clinical lead for the Psychologically Informed Planned Environment (PIPE) at HMP Gartree and is an enabling environments assessor with the Royal College of Psychiatrists. Gareth is currently undertaking a PhD at the University of Huddersfield, exploring the relationship between prison social climate and criminal social identity.

Steve Shaw is Director of HMP Dovegate prison TC. He is a UKCP-registered psychoanalytic psychotherapist and Jungian practitioner.

Richard Shuker is a chartered forensic psychologist and head of Clinical Services at HMP Grendon, a TC prison for long-term prisoners with complex personality needs. Formerly lead psychologist within Grendon, he now leads the clinical and research provision within its TCs. He spent the early part of his career working with young offenders, and his special interests include working with those with complex needs and problematic behaviours associated with their offending. He is particularly interested in relationships and social climate within prisons and how these can provide the conditions for change. He is co-series editor for the book series *Issues in Forensic Psychology*. He has published widely in areas including risk assessment, treatment readiness, social climate and trauma, therapeutic outcome and clinical intervention. He is chair of TCTC research group and has co-edited a number of books and journals in the field of forensic psychology, social climate and TCs.

Apostolos Tsirgoulas has been working for KETHEA in Greece for more than a decade. Currently he is the manager of the first 24-hour TC for drug-addicted people, within a prison at Thessaloniki Detention Centre. He has a diploma and a bachelor's in psychology, has a master's in counselling and he is a trained group analyst and family therapist.

Claudia Vau is a creative action-methods practitioner and accredited psychodrama psychotherapist, trained by the London Centre for Psychodrama and the School of Playback Theatre UK. She has published a book and several articles on responsible communication and social accountability in Portugal, as well as articles on psychodrama, psychopathology and the TC environment in the UK. Claudia lives in Surrey and has been offering clinically supervised group and individual psychodrama psychotherapy since 2014, as honorary psychodramatist within Her Majesty's Prison and Probation Service (HMPPS), as volunteer counsellor in a bereavement service compliant with Improving Access to Psychological Therapies (IAPT), and as an independent practitioner working face to face and online. As a group facilitator, she has been working with women above all – women in prison, women living with learning dis-abilities and women recovering from eating disorders in the community. She has engaged in further creative action, in the non-custodial TC environment and community-based youth development, having been recognised by the British Psychodrama Association (BPA) for this latter type of work with an Anne Bannister Scholar Award, in 2014. Her academic qualifications include an advanced diploma in Group and Individual Psychodrama Psychotherapy, 2020; a master's in Communication Sciences – Communication and Arts, 2010; and a bachelor's (Honours) in Communication Sciences, 2004. Claudia Vau is a member of the BPA; the Humanist and Integrative Psychotherapy College of the UK Council for Psychotherapy (UKCP); The Consortium for Therapeutic Communities; and the International Playback Theatre Network.

Gary Winship is Associate Professor, University of Nottingham. He is editor of the *International Journal of Therapeutic Communities* and chair of Training Standards Universities Psychotherapy & Counselling Association.

Series foreword

From its origins as a *British Psychological Society* journal, the Issues in Forensic Psychology series has had two central aspirations. The first has been to promote novel, innovative and relevant ideas within forensic psychology into a wider academic and professional domain, beyond that inhibited by forensic psychologists themselves. The series has always intended to make forensic psychology open, accessible and available to practitioners in associated fields in other professional backgrounds. The second aspiration of the series has been to identify areas where gaps in research and practice were becoming apparent, and for editions within the series to identify and respond to areas of emerging need and interest. Issues in Forensic Psychology has also wanted to approach traditional themes in the field from fresh perspectives as developments in the field take new directions. This was evident from the first edition of the book series which took a critical view of some of the well-established and perhaps well-worn ideas in the risk assessment literature, revising and developing concepts within the field of risk management and clinical formulation. Later editions such as the edition on secure recovery came to be influential in establishing new directions in forensic service development. This examined the accepted concepts of patient 'illness', arguing how therapeutic arrangements enabling a patient's involvement and engagement were key in personal recovery. Some of these ideas became expanded and developed in the more recent edition on transformative environments and rehabilitation which made a powerful argument for an empowering social climate as the portal for personal and therapeutic change. Developing applied practice has been emphasised throughout the series. The edition on forensic research opened up a broad range of research methodologies to a wider audience, making a compelling case for their utility and value. A later volume on supervision skills and practice brought supervision to life, making a strong argument for its utility and value for all those working in the forensic field. A volume on forensic practice in the community was commissioned in response to literature being disproportionately weighted towards those working in closed conditions despite the reality that the vast majority of forensic service users are likely to be under supervision, risk management or treatment within the community. Further editions have provided in-depth focus on areas where understanding of offending needs to be improved. An edition on multi-perpetrator rape has expanded knowledge in a neglected area; a text exploring problematic sexual interests has given a thorough review of atypical sexual interests and ways through which they can be reliably assessed and managed; and most recently the contribution of psychological research to the prevention of miscarriages of justice and the development of effective investigative techniques has been documented in a work examining the psychology of criminal investigation.

In the current edition, the series editors wanted to develop a key theme which emerged in the previous edition on transformative environments; the importance of social relationships and the social context in which people live in enabling personal change and their move away from offending, abusive and harmful behaviour. The editors wanted to highlight the pioneering work of therapeutic communities, their growth and expansion, and their impact on and contribution to the delivery of forensic services across the world. They also wanted to capture the power and influence of their work, their potential and the struggles they have faced, and how they have provided an impetus for the development of relationally based practice within the wider forensic field.

In addition to the emphasis placed on highlighting the contribution that therapeutic communities have made placing relationally based therapeutic treatment at the centre of forensic practice, this latest edition of Issues in Forensic Psychology also has a number of other aims. Although therapeutic communities have sought to preserve their values and ethos since first emerging as a forensic service in the 1960s, they have also shown, despite criticisms to the contrary, the capacity to develop and enhance their practice. The editors wanted to demonstrate how they have provided the forum for other clinical developments. Section one of the book highlights new initiatives in drug rehabilitation services, their role within women's prisons, how they have developed a model for clinical supervision, and provides an illustration of how they have integrated within their work an intervention for residents previously involved in gang membership. Section two emphasises the importance of research within therapeutic communities and provides examples of current research within forensic settings, making a case for the effectiveness. An overview of the evidence base for therapeutic communities is provided in two chapters which explore the efficacy of democratic and hierarchical models. Differing approaches taken to measuring outcomes and effectiveness across services are presented. The final section of the book aims to highlight developments in practice within therapeutic communities in forensic settings and explore their further potential. A number of chapters describe how services have developed and been successfully integrated within wider forensic services. A range of international contributions are presented, recent initiatives discussed and a case is made for their expansion and relevance within other forensic settings. The book also provides an opportunity for practitioners to provide a narrative perspective on how their services have evolved over the years and how they have responded to threats, demands and struggles. In doing so, it becomes apparent that there is something enduring about the position therapeutic communities have come to adopt within forensic settings, illustrating their capacity to grow and their substantial impact on current developments within forensic services.

Geraldine Akerman and Richard Shuker
Series Editors

Foreword

As most people who have spent time in them realise, therapeutic communities are a largely hidden jewel in the panoply of modern interventions for complex mental health needs. As one of those people, with many hours of time inside, I know that extraordinary things can happen in them, that people's lives are often transformed (those of staff members as well as client members), and that there is a quality of relationship between the participants that simply does not exist in other settings. But this is not good enough for the modern thirst for a specific type of evidence: we must work harder. This book is part of that effort.

A major problem with therapeutic communities is that nobody really knows just what kind of animal they are, and there is no universally accepted definition. Perhaps this is one reason why they are largely hidden from wider understanding and acceptance. I believe it is entirely reasonable to describe them in at least seven different ways – all of which come from widely different frames of reference.

Most simply, they are *treatment units* – brick walls containing prison wings, custodial units, hospital wards, clinics, hospitals, day centres, schools or whatever. People go into them, something happens and they come out. There are several different histories and types of these; they have a great deal in common but so many differences that no single definition would fit them all. Secondly, they are a *theoretical model of care*, with explicit therapeutic principles based on established psychological and sociological theories. This is the main tradition from the British version of 'social psychiatry' following the wartime Northfield Experiments, which continues to this day in different sectors. Thirdly, they are an *intensive form of group psychotherapy* defined and recognised by democratically co-produced quality standards. The 'Community of Communities' network at the Royal College of Psychiatrists uses this approach. Fourthly, they constitute an *evidence-based treatment 'brand'* with an extensive qualitative evidence base going back many years, and at least one recent, modern, randomised controlled trial. This is a difficult area, particularly because their status as a recognised 'treatment' has recently been denied. Fifthly, they could be described as programmes which are *delivered by staff who have certain competencies*, gained through suitable selection, training, support and supervision. The systemic nature of the resultant team cohesion and common sense of purpose delivers a unique sort of therapy. Sixthly, they arise from a technology of *planned environmental engineering* which results in a milieu that is conducive to personal growth and self-actualisation or individuation. This is akin to the work of 'enabling environments' and what I have called the 'TC in the Head' or the 'TC without walls'. Finally, and somewhat related, they could be seen as a *radical and subversive ideology*: a social movement demanding a different and non-oppressive way for humans to relate to each other. This is beyond postmodernism, as there is a clear 'grand narrative' – of relationship. This means that relationality has priority over individuality, as with the 'foundation matrix' in group analytic psychotherapy – or waves and particles in physics. This way of thinking recognises the duality of individual minds and the relationship between them, but focuses on the waves. It is in tune with modern consciousness studies, and progressive ideas about how radical change is needed if humanity is to survive – particularly concerning the relationship we have to our natural environment.

Perhaps these could be called ontological (what are they?) and epistemological (how can you know what they do?) problems. But if the definition of therapeutic community does not include all these angles, and possibly others, we will be losing something of their essential, and edgy, nature. Similarly, if we irrefutably prove that one type of therapeutic community leads to a reliable change in one variable, we risk losing the breadth and depth of the approach, through standardisation and regulation. The wide scope of this book ensures that it does not make those reductive oversimplifications.

Then there is the problem of history, and what is usually called 'baggage' – and how it affects the political context of therapeutic community work. In some countries, different sorts of wildly diverse units, clinics and facilities all call themselves 'therapeutic communities'. Some do this proudly, with high clinical standards, transparent and accountable published processes, university collaborations and highly trained staff. Others have little understanding of the meaning of the name or the depth of history in therapeutic communities and simply think of the term as a useful name with which to market their services. In other countries, the name itself carries an unspoken stigma that conveys a whiff of disreputableness, tainted history and deliberate failure to face the reality of modern life. Here, only the most confident therapeutic communities can proudly assert their identity. The communities described in this book are amongst these, and can perhaps offer encouragement and support to those wanting to tread a similar path towards excellence – and membership of the extended family.

It is a paradox that the type of therapeutic communities that have always appeared to be most secure in their continued existence are those that are growing in what might be considered the stoniest and inhospitable soil – the criminal justice system. It is a paradox because it is extremely difficult to see how it is possible to give people in state custody a sense of openness, empowerment and personal dignity in settings which demand almost total social control and lack of freedom. Perhaps it is the very rigidity of the system – security over therapy – that ensures that, once therapeutic communities become part of the establishment, it is almost impossible to get rid of them all (though individual ones may have insurmountable local difficulties, of course), however counter-cultural they may appear. But it happens, and often in innovative and effective ways: this book gives a wide range of examples of what is possible.

Rex Haigh
Consultant Psychiatrist in Medical Psychotherapy, Berkshire;
Founder, Community of Communities, Royal College of Psychiatrists
Centre for Quality Improvement; Honorary Professor of Therapeutic
Environments and Relational Practice, Nottingham University.

Acknowledgements

To my loving family and friends who have always been there to form our own community. (Geri)

To Josie. (Richard)

Part I
Practice perspectives

Changing the game
An intervention addressing the impact of former gang members on the therapeutic process

Geraldine Akerman and Carine Minne

1

During years of studying the impact gang members had on the safety and management of prisons in general, it was noted (Griffin & Hepburn, 2006) that prison gangs can severely undermine the ability of prison staff to maintain a safe and orderly environment. This can result in staff and prisoners believing that officials are not in full control of prisons, and create fear and unrest (Wood & Adler, 2001; Wood, 2006; Wood, 2017). Camp and Camp (1985) and Fong (1990) described how prison gangs in adult institutions function on the acquisition of money and power, and how they use threats and violence to dominate staff and other prisoners, and such behaviour could clearly impact on relationships and the power balance within an establishment. Examples could be using illegal mobile phones to take photographs of staff and sending these to criminal associates outside and using this to threaten them. Smart phones enable users to find out information on other prisoners, which also empowers them. Wood (2017) noted that criminal activities can continue in custody, undermining the belief that once convicted a gang member will stop offending. Offences included car crime, burglaries, stolen goods and burglaries, as well as organising more serious assaults on those in the community or in other establishments.

Context for the intervention

HMP Grendon was opened in 1962 as a means of managing prisoners who were not responding to standard incarceration (for more details, see Shuker & Sullivan, 2010). The DTC model has subsequently been accredited by the Correctional Services and Advice Panel (CSAAP). Throughout its history HMP Grendon has housed men who have committed a wide range of offences and who have experienced events in their lives which have affected how they view the world, relationships and themselves. Many of those who participate

DOI: 10.4324/9780429317460-2

in therapy at HMP Grendon have reported adverse childhood experiences in their formative years and this has clearly impacted on how their personality developed and formed.

The DTC provides an opportunity for a corrective emotional experience and a safe space in which to develop its residents understanding of themselves and their interactions which led them to offend. The programme is explained extensively elsewhere (Akerman, 2019; Akerman & Mandikate, 2018; Brookes, 2010; Campling & Haigh, 1988; Genders & Player, 1995; Shine & Morris, 1999; Shuker & Sullivan, 2010; Stevens, 2010), but in brief is an intensive living-learning experience through which the residents are given an opportunity to explore their day-to-day living in custody and how that parallels their past. This involves them considering their thoughts, feelings and behaviour in the present day, making links to their past and gaining a chance to practise alternative ways of managing their responses. It is expected that in this environment a certain amount of behaviour from the past will be evident. Indeed this provides the work for therapy groups but at times this can be problematic. For instance, if alliances are formed which impact on groups and group work and communities, this can impede the work being undertaken by others. One such example is that of men who have been involved in gangs in the past (and sometimes in the present) and how this affects a culture which promotes an equal voice for all and a lack of hierarchy, one of the DTC core principles. The DTC principles will now be discussed briefly.

Democratic therapeutic community principles

In a DTC there are a number of principles (described fully by this volume) which guide the behaviour of those in it, for instance:

- Prisoners form positive relationships with staff and with each other, and are involved in planning and sharing in activities and making decisions. To be involved in the treatment of others and in all aspects of the day-to-day caring of the living environment. To abide by rules that have been agreed by the community (communalism).
- The environment is developed and maintained such that trust, safety and openness are promoted, and in which it is possible to challenge each other's inappropriate behaviour. To take responsibility for residents own behaviour, learning from instances when behaviour related to offending is shown in the community, and establishing links between current behaviour within treatment setting and offending patterns, for example, taking control, manipulating others, using aggression (known as offence paralleling) (reality confrontation).

- There is a certain level of tolerance so that behaviour similar to that which happened in the lead-up to offending is played out. Such behaviour is then explored, contained and challenged in a safe environment (permissiveness or more recently tolerance).
- All community structures are subject to influence by those who live and work in them (democratisation).
- There is the ability to question, inquire and explore reasons behind own and organisational decisions (culture of inquiry).
- To create an environment in which all interactions are seen as a learning opportunity. All aspects of the community are fed back to the wider community, and exclusive relationships are discouraged to avoid secrecy and collusion (living-learning environment).

Some of the principles may not align with previous beliefs and values of the community member, and so they may well feel uncomfortable and unconsciously seek to recreate what is familiar to them from their past.

Groups and gangs in a democratic therapeutic community

Groups

A group is defined by Forsyth (2006, p.3) as 'two or more individuals who are connected to one another by a social relationship', and larger groups tend to be comprised of smaller groups linked together for another common purpose. Within the DTC at HMP Grendon this is evident as the small (therapy) group is comprised of 8/9 people (in which all aspects of functioning are explored, including examining links between past and present behaviour, challenging anti-social beliefs, exploring attachment patterns, and discussing future relationships, etc). The large group (community) is comprised of approximately 45 residents and 16 staff members. The community meeting manages the business and organizational aspects of day-to-day living, along with conflict resolution, demonstrating the ability to manage emotions, dynamics within and between groups and so forth. There are other subgroups, for instance an art therapy or psychodrama group, groups of a particular religion, ethnicity, age, area of the country, interests, and these groups can have their own dynamics.

Yalom (1985) described the mechanisms of group psychotherapy, highlighting the catharsis gained from self-disclosure, gaining acceptance from others and seeing oneself as having similar problems/difficulties/ challenges as others do (universality); feeling good about oneself by helping others; gaining greater self-insight; being able to give constructive feedback to others; seeing others progress and make changes and that they can also achieve that (the instillation of hope); exploring how they are within relationships and how their behaviour impacts on others; and seeing themselves in others. It is also worth noting that within a group, individuals can behave in a way that they would not do alone, which can be either positive or negative. Groups can be a source of great reward, for example, providing common achievement and pro-social modelling, but also of conflict and aggression, and so the work of the therapy team in a DTC is to be attuned to the dynamics on a day-to-day and sometimes hour-by-hour basis, particularly in times of tension.

Gangs

The definition of what a gang is, and what its membership entails differs across research. For instance, Klein (1971, p.13) described it as 'any denotable adolescent group of youngsters who (a) are generally perceived as a distinct aggregation by others in their neighbourhood, (b) recognize themselves as a denotable group (almost invariably with a group name) and (c) have been involved in a sufficient number of delinquent incidents to call forth a consistent negative response from neighbourhood residents and/or enforcement agencies'. Weerman et al. (2009, p.20) describe a gang as 'any durable, street-orientated youth group whose involvement in illegal activity is part of its group identity'. The Home Office (2011, p.17) defined a street gang as 'A relatively durable, predominantly street-based group of young people who:

- See themselves (and are seen by others) as a discernible group;
- Engage in criminal activity and violence;
- Lay claim over territory (this is not necessarily geographical territory but can include an illegal economy territory);
- Have some form of identifying structural feature; and
- Are in conflict with other, similar gangs'.

Hallsworth (2013, p.102–3) commented, 'the term "gang" is now so nebulous, fluid and elastic that it is randomly applied to just about any group of young people "hanging around"'. This can make the term seem overused.

Within a custodial setting a gang has been defined (Wood, 2006) as a group of three or more prisoners whose behaviour had an adverse impact on the prison that holds them, which again is a very wide definition. In a DTC, having such a group could have an adverse impact on a community, such as carrying on a code of secrecy, not exposing any anti-social activities or challenging negative beliefs is in conflict with the values of a DTC. Further, their reputation from inside or outside of custody can impact on the power they hold. Moore and Vigil (1989) referred to an 'oppositional culture' and Lien (2002) reports that those who affiliate themselves with such a gang could view themselves as marginalised and oppressed by others, and targets of racism and inequality; what social psychology would call in-group out-group thinking. Nitsun (1996) described the 'anti-group' as the destructive aspect of groups that threaten integrity and therapeutic development. Therefore, a subgroup (gang) could have that function of undermining the larger group. This dynamic can see a bid made for who will be the most powerful. Just as those who are starved of love and affection can attack it when it is seen in others, so the anti-group can seek to destroy the therapeutic culture, albeit unconsciously.

Within a DTC the expectation is that new members will learn from those who have been there longer, known as culture carriers, and these senior members of the community will model appropriate behaviour to the newer residents. This will not be unfamiliar to a member of a gang who would also have 'elders' modelling to the 'youngers' what is expected of them, 'soldiers' to do the groundwork and 'wannabes' on the periphery. Gang members may abide by a set of values, expectations and 'codes' which new members learn as they progress in the ranks. In therapeutic terms, as a group forms it develops with conscious and unconscious rules, which again are learned through experience rather than made explicit prior to entering the group. In group analysis terms, a group forms a matrix between its members which is comprised of the collective idea of the expectations of its members. Weinberg (2008) discusses this as a 'social unconscious', in that members develop basic assumptions as to what is expected of them in relation to others and share memories of their past experiences. In a DTC, one of the main principles is that there is a flattened hierarchy in that each participant has an equal voice, staff and residents alike. This may feel unfamiliar to a former gang member, who may well be used to being the person who makes the decisions and tells others what to do. Other expectations could include that they side with each other, and they don't 'rat' or 'grass' on one another, whereas in DTC terms this would be a requirement, what would be viewed as reality confrontation, that is, pointing out inappropriate behaviour and challenging it.

Many of the men who apply for therapy at HMP Grendon have experienced traumatic events in their past, not least their own offending. Within the population of HMP Grendon, Akerman and Geraghty, (2015) noted that 50% reported having a self-harm history, 52% reported a history of physical abuse, 32% reported having been sexually abused and 69% reported loss of or separation from a primary caregiver. Research into those who have been involved in the gang culture indicates that gang membership was significantly associated with post-traumatic stress disorder (PTSD) and psychological distress, including anxiety, depression, numbing, suicidal ideation, paranoia and psychosis (Beresford & Wood, 2016). Those who join gangs may suffer with high levels of distress, which is largely unresolved. This may be why they joined or as a result of joining. In the *Diagnostic and Statistical Manual of Mental Disorders Version Five* (*DSM-V*; American Psychological Association, 2013), so-called personality disorders are categorized according to their emotional temperaments. Coid et al. (2013) found higher levels of self-reported anti-social personality disorder (ASPD) in those who were convicted of gang-related offences, rather than other violence. Kerig, Chaplo, Bennett and Modrowski (2016) suggested that involvement in street gangs could increase the risk of developing PTSD, due to exposure to violence.

A Public Health England report (2015) highlights that gang members are at increased risk of a range of mental health conditions, for instance conduct disorder, antisocial personality disorder (86%), anxiety (59%), psychosis (25%), drug (58%) and alcohol dependence (67%), and depression (20%), suggesting that the pre-existing factors could attract them to gangs and/or be a result of membership. An emotively titled review (Dying to Belong, Centre for Social Justice, 2009) presents statistics on the extent of involvement of young people in the gang lifestyle. Up to 6% of 10- to 19-year-olds self-report belonging to a gang (Sharp, Aldridge & Medina, 2006); police in London and Strathclyde have identified 171 and 170 gangs respectively; and there are between 600 and 700 young people estimated to be directly gang involved in the London Borough of Waltham Forest alone, with an additional 8,100 people affected by gangs. Gangs are most commonly found in areas of high deprivation, crime and family breakdown. In both Manchester and Liverpool around 60% of shootings are gang related, and at least half of the 27 murders of young people perpetrated by young people in London in 2007 were gang-related (Metropolitan Police Authority, 2009).

More recently the extent to which those affiliated to gangs are subject to sexual exploitation is coming to light, and it is noted that few report this or ask for help, either considering it normal, or out of fear, shame, lack of trust and so on. Berelowitz, Clifton, Firimin, Gulyurtlu and Edwards (2013) described how children as young as 11 were being serially raped. Phase 1 of the Inquiry reported that a total of 2,409 children were known to be victims of child sexual exploitation (CSE) by gangs and groups. In addition, the Inquiry identified 16,500 children and young people as being at risk of CSE.

So, whereas all those involved (in any way) with gangs may not have been victims, they would have heard of or witnessed such events. The Metropolitan Police Authority (2009) conducted research into and noted an increase in 'gang rape' (involving between three and eight assailants) from 73 in 2003/04 to 93 in 2008/09. They, like others (Centre for Social Justice, 2009; Smith, Rush & Burton, 2013) concluded that given the lack of consistent reporting and collating of evidence, it is difficult to have accurate data.

In recent years there has been an increase in so-called county lines drug dealing, which involves those who sell drugs exploiting young people to transport drugs across the country.

The Children's commissioner estimated that at least 46,000 children are involved in gang activity, with 6,000 in London alone being used for dealing drugs across county borders. Gang members identify children caught in poverty, or who are vulnerable in other ways and threaten, trick or groom them into carrying out the transportation of drugs. While these children can be viewed as criminals, the move is to recognise them as victims of trafficking and exploitation.

It appears clear that the trauma experienced is a contributory factor to the men joining gangs and/or a result of their membership. Fraser and Blishen (2007) highlight the unmet mental health needs of young people convicted of offences. Their behaviour is likely to include carrying weapons, selling and taking drugs, auto theft, extortion and so forth. The Greater London Authority (unpublished), which tracked asset risk assessments for 315 young people convicted of offences, found high-risk young offenders in London had 60% unmet psychological needs, 33% had been exposed to violence within the home, 30% had experience of bereavement, 30% physical/emotional/ sexual abuse, 15% parental drug misuse, 15% parental alcohol misuse, and 15% parental mental health issues. As teenagers, it is common for them to look outside of families and towards peers to form relationships, and if membership of a gang looks to offer a wide range of positive gains (such as a sense of belonging, money, girls, cars, status, protection, to name a few), they can viewed as a draw to young people (Harris, Turner, Garrett & Atkinson, 2011). However, at that stage they are unaware of the negative aspects of membership, such as the expectation that members will commit anti-social acts, feel apart from their families and live in constant fear of knives, guns or weapon-enabled violence. Some aspects of gang membership will feel familiar, such as sibling rivalry, and proving oneself, and wanting to live out teenage rebellion. However, the psychological cost can be a high price to pay. The expectation would be that once a member joins a gang, they take on a new identity, usually assigned by the use of a street name. This then develops a reputation with it and one which it can be difficult to maintain. There can be much peer pressure to uphold this image. Again, actions that they may never have undertaken alone can be enacted, such as the use of violence, criminal acts and so forth. In line with group psychology, the group can then be seen as responsible (as seen in conviction of joint enterprise) rather than an individual. So, having residents with this thinking and behavioural style can impact on the working of a DTC and this will now be discussed further.

The impact gang members can have on communities

Dawson (2008) described the impact that gangs have on communities outside of prison, for instance being a driving force of violent crime, and committing a large proportion of criminal acts. Such behaviour can be mirrored within a DTC. Therefore, one of the difficulties facing an ex-gang member in a DTC is the perceived dissonance between 'breaking the code' and exposing the aspects of themselves which have thus far remained hidden within the gang membership. The very reason they joined a gang may, for instance, be to gain a sense of belonging, and if they were to disclose information, they could fear being excluded. This can evoke powerful feelings of fear, guilt, shame and grief, emotions which thus far have been guarded against through the use of the macho gang mask. Within a DTC there can be a risk that rivals to be the alpha male in a community can come into conflict, and the need for dialogue as to the dynamics and the drive behind the behaviour is vital. Short and Strodtbeck (1965) commented that it is not clear how the original hierarchy of status is established, but that the leader does not tend to be aggressive or dominance seeking generally, unless their status is directly challenged. Likewise, in custody the leader is less likely to be evident, instead giving instructions to others, who will trade contraband, carry out assaults and collect debts. In a TC, it may be that the leader is not challenged by others and could be voted into more trusted jobs, which is mirrored in mainstream prisons with dominant prisoners being given jobs on the servery. If they are moved, there can be an unsettled period while a replacement is sought.

Within a DTC, when anti-social behaviour, such as drug-dealing and taking, use of phones, and increased debt, increases the community becomes very compromised, with little or no challenge occurring. This can escalate to the use of violence, which can again go unchallenged or reported. Until this stranglehold is addressed, there can be little progress made in challenging offence-paralleling behaviour.

How can a DTC help?

A DTC can offer the opportunity to develop understanding of the risk factors associated with gang offending, including: having loyalty to anti-social peers, relationships difficulties; distorted attitudes towards women; difficulties relating to authority; use of violence and weapons; emotional management difficulties; and substance misuse. Young, Fitzgibbon and Silverstone (2013) suggest the use of a multi-agency approach to help encourage gang members to leave the gang and so the Changing the Game programme being based within a DTC may well serve that purpose.

The Changing the Game Programme The TC environment brings together a diverse set of prisoners to create a democratic and therapeutic environment. For example, TC members are expected to break the established prison code by accepting the presence of those with sexual convictions in the community and groups, listening to their experiences and providing constructive support and challenge. In contrast, the Changing the Game programme targets urban gang members, whose shared experiences provide the group with a distinct identity. Whilst the often Black, Asian and minority ethnic (BAME) group members may have experienced marginalisation or discrimination both in society and even the prison system (i.e. Lammy report), Changing the Game develops a space where group members present a shared set of experiences within their contexts as gang members, as well as share a broader narrative as members of our larger cities' poorer, hard-to-reach communities. Within this context it is possible to develop a culturally competent approach which understands gang culture, as well as the cultures of the communities where gang culture is located and enacted. The values, rules and expectations of life in a gang are implicitly recognised and understood by members and facilitators, without anything getting lost in literal or conceptual translation, allowing members to explore their experiences, acknowledging the damaging emotional impact of exposure to serious violence, and the severe costs of adherence to gang codes and loyalties. Developing a therapy environment in which the experiences described by members are shared and resonate so strongly across the group, develops not only a shared sense of understanding but also a strong sense of empathy, as members' shared feelings emerge.

In addition to a psychoanalytically anchored group psychotherapy approach, this intervention emphasises the importance of cultural awareness, building upon an understanding of gang life and culture as it is lived and acted out by gang members. It is crucial for the group therapists to have credibility and hence, legitimacy and the possibility of being trusted, by having a knowledge of gangs and the broader social and community experiences of gang members.

The programme also utilises the narratives of the communities in which many gangs are located and explores broader issues with regard to identity and a deviation from the original sense of identity and values of these communities (i.e. the Windrush generation). If gangs provide members with a sense of identity, what deficit in their personal or broader social identity does this meet? As with many immigrant communities, issues around identity, culture, belonging and 'fitting in' become problematic. Schouler-Oak et al. (2015) describe how immigrants and their children can experience physical and mental health issues following their migration and this can be further exacerbated by their feeling isolated from their family and culture and, the extent to which illness can be discussed. For instance, the notion of depression does not exist in all cultures, even though aspects of it, such as sadness and unhappiness, do. This is accentuated if there is little social support. Schouler-Oak (2015) report results from a meta-analysis which finds that interventions adapted for individual needs are effective. The value of the Changing the Game programme is that it takes account of the individual cultures and prejudices and the psychological impact this could have on those involved. The importance of cultural knowledge and skills is highlighted.

Working through and sharing their experiences generates a collective sense of reflection among participants, developing their thinking, emotional regulation skills and positive self-image. Addressing the dynamics of the 'group' (such as sense of belonging and identity), and how individual members experience feelings of fear, shame, regret or even individual personal objectives and priorities, can aid in understanding what needs were being met and constructing alternative strategies. In the evaluation interviews (described below) the residents at Grendon describe being involved in group violence despite not wanting to be. Therefore, gang culture and violence can become a serious management issue.

Efficacy of the programme

In order to evaluate the efficacy of the programme, data was collected from former participants in a focus group (Geraghty & Akerman, 2017). Participants spoke of how mainstream prisons can provide perfect conditions for recruiting new gang members. Pressure is applied to those who do not wish to comply, including threats being made against their families, not unlike communities outside (Geraghty & Akerman, 2017). The vulnerability of, and difficulties faced by, young people in custody in particular was acknowledged, and the ways in which gang membership (girls, money, fast cars) is glamorized, and its negative aspects (emotional trauma, fear, anxiety) are downplayed, is acknowledged. Residents suggested ways to try to prevent their involvement in gang activities, including the provision of subjects of interest to them (such as music, art, meaningful employment) to draw them away from this lifestyle but also ensure that they gained a sense of purpose by having to work for it. Each resident in HMP Grendon has a six-monthly assessment of progress and works towards treatment targets, and each has a target relating to resettlement.

Much attention is given to ambitions and plans for the future. Events such as conferences, Visits with a Difference (where family members learn about the therapeutic community and residents speak about their progress), and leaving meals provide the opportunity for residents to speak of their hopes and aspirations for the future in a public manner, thus affirming their internal hopes. Maruna (2000) explained that understanding the past and public declaration of future plans helped internalize these. Both the therapy in a DTC and the Changing the Game programme provide such an understanding and in that way, complement each other.

The Changing the Game programme has been evaluated at HMP Isis and had a significant impact in Incentives and Earned Privileges[1] entries, finding 65% improvement in positive entries and 40% reduction in negative entries (3 months pre-and post-delivery).

Conversely, prison can also provide a place of refuge for gang members. Some residents spoke of how time spent in prison was a 'rest' and allowed them 'time to breathe' as it was safer than living life in a gang in the community. The process of 'elders' grooming 'youngers' through offering money, illegal employment, accommodation and protection both outside and in custody was also discussed. The residents highlighted that this might not always be a conscious process by elder gang members (Geraghty & Akerman, 2017). In fact, they expressed their regret that they had done to others what had been done to themselves in that regard.

The DTC environment may create anxiety and paranoia initially for those who have been part of a gang, as they tend to question the motives of those offering them support, both staff and more experienced residents. As Nitsun (1996) explains, the anti-group, which is the destructive aspect of groups, impacts on the cohesion and integrity of the TC processes. The group can be seen as a threat. In the case of gang members, there may be fear that its members will reveal information or change in their views. Thus, when the anti-group operates, there can be hostility and derision shown to group processes. This is undermining, particularly to new, less confident members. Such processes need to be exposed, explored and understood. Residents who have participated on the Changing the Game programme report how they value the opportunity to tell their story without feeling judged. They developed their own understanding of why they joined a gang, and the negative impact it had on them. They explained that the negative influence of a punitive prison environment can reinforce the 'gang mentality', whereas providing a safe, boundaried therapeutic space can help ex-gang members develop trust and dismantle barriers to disclosure. Those involved in the Changing the Game programme described how they found it helpful to have that shared experience and help educate their own therapy group and wing about the processes involved in gang membership. This work could be continued further within the TC environment. Those involved in the programme, albeit a small sample, indicated that they thought there was a need to be more creative in the approach to tackling gang crime and the importance of adopting a holistic approach which can address both psychological and societal issues (Akerman & Geraghty, 2016; Geraghty & Akerman, 2017).

Conclusion

This chapter discussed how those who have been in a gang can respond in a DTC and the impact of engaging in the Changing the Game programme. It also helped them understand why they joined a gang and the impact membership had on them. While other TC members have committed acts of violence, these may have different motivation, for instance poor emotional control or financial gain. Former gang members describe how they became enmeshed in the culture and committed acts of violence as a way of belonging or out of fear of retribution if they did not. While the gang mentality can have an impact on how a DTC works at a given time, once it is identified and discussed, the reasons for it can be explored and alternatives sought. There are times when the balance can go too far such that a community is compromised, and it is not possible to challenge others or speak out. This can result in offending behaviour (such as use of mobile phones, drugs, aggression and violence) becoming rife, thus damaging the integrity and safety a community. This may lead to the need for residents to be removed for the good of the community. Such a decision is never taken lightly. The Changing the Game programme has allowed the discussion to be had in a more open forum and enabled the participants to feel like they are talking to others who understand how they feel, and the particular context of their behaviour and or values they may have subscribed to as gang members. This has been fed back into their group and community and so helped others there to understand. The Public Health England report (2015) emphasises that novel approaches are required, including the provision of holistic support in young peoples' own environments and the use of key workers or mentors who can build trusting relationships with young people involved with gangs. Anecdotal feedback, and the research undertaken, supports that the Changing the Game programme achieves this aim.

Research has found that the typical gang member is aged 20 years and that the upper age limit tends to be around 25 years (Dawson, 2008; Marshall, Webb & Tilley, 2005), and so it has been viewed as a maturational process between adolescence and adulthood. Those seeing a way out of that lifestyle, as stated previously (by getting a job, going into education, becoming a father or even going to prison), may want to leave that life behind them. Maruna

(2000) describes how in order for a person to change, it is important that they change their view of themselves and can see themselves as a person who lives a prosocial life. Having redemptive scripts that they voice helps this process and this is actively encouraged within a DTC. Treatment targets focus on resettlement and what each resident wants for their future. Maruna (2000) found that the more those who could understand and explain their past in a way that they could save face, the more likely they were to succeed in the future, so for instance seeing their past behaviour as part of their journey, or a lesson learned. Both the therapy in a DTC and the Changing the Game programme provide such an understanding and, in that way, complement each other. When residents falter in their confidence to change, others will encourage them through their own experience and so they can access positive role models. Furthermore, previous residents are welcomed back to visit and speak of their struggles and success, which in turn instils further hope. Just as with others who want to change their previous lifestyle, for instance due to drug-taking and or offending, residents are helped to develop positive and realistic plans for the future, with consideration given to any possible hurdles and how these can be overcome. A range of options are considered and back-up plans developed to help the resident feel more confident. Residents report how they value the opportunity to tell their story without feeling judged. They explained that the negative influence of a punitive prison environment can reinforce the 'gang mentality', whereas providing a safe, boundaried therapeutic space can help ex-gang members develop trust and dismantle barriers to disclosure. One of the aims of a DTC is to provide an emotionally corrective experience. The residents stressed the importance of not taking a soft approach to the impact of gang violence on communities but encouraged professionals to 'keep it real'. Those involved in the Changing the Game programme found it helpful to have that shared experience and help educate their own therapy group and wing about the processes involved in gang membership. They note similarities to how other youths have managed their emotions, while also recognising differences too.

It is always important that those involved in the DTC and in the Changing the Game programme relay their perspective of how they experienced working on the two interventions.

Acknowledgements

Special thanks to Paul Kassman, who developed the Changing the Game programme, which recently received a special mention in Her Majesty's *Inspection of Prisons* report as an important intervention in prisons, and was a runner-up in the Criminal Justice Alliance Awards. Also, to all those who took part in the research discussed in the chapter and for being so frank in their thoughts and feelings.

Note

1 The Incentives and Earned Privileges (IEP) scheme works with the expectation that prisoners would earn additional privileges through demonstrating responsible behaviour and participation in work or other constructive activity. On 30 April 2013 Ministers announced the outcome of a review of the IEP scheme and made it clear that, in order to earn privileges, prisoners will now have to work towards their own rehabilitation, behave well and help others. The absence of bad behaviour alone will no longer be sufficient to progress through the scheme.

References

Akerman, G. (2019). Communal living as the agent of change. In D. Polaschek, A. Day & C. Hollin (Eds.). *The Wiley International Handbook of Correctional Psychology* (chap. 37). Wiley Blackwell.

Akerman, G., & Geraghty, K.A. (2016). An exploration of clients' experiences of group therapy, *Therapeutic Communities: The International Journal of Therapeutic Communities, 37*, 101–8. http://dx.doi.org/10.1108/TC-12-2015-0026

Akerman, G., & Mandikate, P. (2018). Creating a therapeutic community from scratch: Where do we start? In R. Shuker and G. Akerman (Series Editor). G. Akerman, A. Needs and C. Bainbridge (Eds.). *Transforming environments and rehabilitation. A guide for practitioners in forensic and criminal justice* (pp.163–79). Taylor & Francis Group.

American Psychiatric Society (2013). *Diagnostic and statistical manual of mental disorders, 5th edition: DSM-5.* APA Publishing.

Berelowitz, S., Clifton, J., Firimin, C., Gulyurtlu, S., & Edwards, G. (2013). *'If only someone had listened'.* Office of the Children's Commissioner's Inquiry into Child Sexual Exploitation in Gangs and Group.

Beresford, H., & Wood, J. (2016). Through the trauma lens: Internalizing and externalizing symptoms in at-risk and gang-involved males. Presentation given at the 25th Annual conference of the Division of Forensic Psychology. 14–16 June 2016. Hilton Brighton Metropole Hotel.

Brookes, M. (2010). Putting principles into practice: The therapeutic community regime at HMP Grendon and its relationship with the 'Good Lives' model. In R. Shuker, and E. Sullivan (Eds.). *Grendon and the emergence of forensic therapeutic communities: Developments in research and practice* (pp.99–113). John Wiley and Sons.

Camp, G.M., & Camp, C.G. (1985). *Prison gangs: Their extent, nature and impact on prisons.* Criminal Justice Institute.

Campling, P., & Haigh, R. (Eds.) (1988). *Therapeutic communities past present and future.* Jessica Kingsley.

The Centre for Social Justice. (2009). *Breakthrough Britain: Dying to belong.* Centre for Social Justice, www.centreforsocialjustice.org.uk/core/wp-content/uploads/2016/08/Dyingto BelongFullReport.pdf

Coid, J.W., Ullrich, S., Keers, R., Bebbington, P., DeStavola, B.L., Kallis, C., & Donnelly, P. (2013). Gang membership, violence, and psychiatric morbidity. *American Journal of Psychiatry, 170*(9), 985–93. https://doi.org/10.1176/appi.ajp.2013.12091188

Dawson, P. (2008). *Monitoring data from the Tackling Gangs Action Programme.* Home Office Crime Reduction Website. Home Office. http://safecolleges.org.uk/sites/default/files/Home_ Office_2008_TGAP_data.pdf

Fong, R.S. (1990). The organizational structure of prison gangs: A Texas case study. *Federal Probation, 54*(1), 36–43.

Forsyth, D.R. (2006). *Group dynamics* (4th ed.). Thomson-Wadsworth.

Fraser, M., & Blishen, S. (2007). *Supporting young people's mental health. Eight points for action: A policy briefing from the mental health foundation.* www.mentalhealth.org.uk/sites/ default/files/supporting_young_people.pdf

Genders, E. & Player, E. (1995). *Grendon: A study of a therapeutic prison.* OUP.

Geraghty, K.A., & Akerman, G. (2017). 'Changing the Game': An evaluation of a pilot intervention for former gang members engaged in group therapy. Paper presented at the 26th Division of Forensic Psychology Conference. 13–15 June 2017. Mercure Bristol Grand Hotel.

Griffin, M.L., & Hepburn, J.R. (2006). The effect of gang affiliation on violence misconduct among inmates during the early years of confinement. *Criminal Justice and Behavior, 33,* 419–48. https://doi.org/10.1177/0093854806288038

Hallsworth, S. (2013). *The gang and beyond: Interpreting violent street worlds.* Palgrave Macmillan.

Harris, D., Turner, R., Garrett, I., & Atkinson, S. (2011). Understanding the psychology of gang violence: Implications for designing effective violence interventions. *Ministry of Justice Research Series 2/11.* www.justice.gov.uk/publications/research.htm

Home Office. (2011). *Ending gang and youth violence: A cross-government report including further evidence and good practice case studies.* Home Office.

Kerig, P.K., Chaplo, S.D., Bennett, D.C., & Modrowski, C.A. (2016). 'Harm as harm': Gang membership, perpetration trauma, and posttraumatic stress symptoms among youth in the juvenile justice system. *Criminal Justice and Behavior, 43,* 635–52. https://doi.org/10.1177/ 0093854815607307

Klein, M.W. (1971). *Street gangs and street workers.* Prentice Hall.

Lien, I. (2002). The pain of crime and gang mentality. Unpublished paper.

Marshall, B., Webb, B., & Tilley, N. (2005) *Rationalisation of current research on guns, gangs and other weapons: Phase 1.* University College London Jill Dando Institute of Crime Science.

Maruna, S. (2000). *Making good: How ex-convicts reform and rebuild their lives.* American Psychological Society.

Metropolitan Police Authority. (2009). *Multi perpetrator rapes and youth violence.* MPA, www. policeauthority.org/Metropolitan/committees/sop/2009/091105/07/index.html

Moore, J., & Vigil, J.D. (1989). Chicano gangs: Group norms and individual factors related to adult criminality. *Aztlan, 18,* 31–42.

MPA Youth Scrutiny (Metropolitan Police Authority, 29 May 2008), MPA: Committees: MPA reports - 29-05-08 (05) (policeauthority.org) pp.4–5.

Nitsun, M. (1996). *The anti-group. Destructive forces in the group and their creative potential.* Routledge.

Public Health England. (2015). *The mental health needs of gang affiliated young people.* Commissioned from the WHO Collaborating Centre for Violence Prevention based at the Centre for Public Health, Liverpool John Moores University. A briefing produced as part of the Ending Gang and Youth Violence programme.

Schouler-Ocak, S., Graef-Calliess, I.T., Tarricone, I., Qureshi, A., Kastrup, M/C., & Bhugra, D. (2015). EPA guidance on cultural competence training. *European Psychiatry, 30,* 431–40.

Sharp, C., Aldridge, J., & Medina, J. (2006). *Delinquent youth groups and offending behaviour: Findings from the 2004 Offending, Crime and Justice Survey.* Home Office.

Shine, J., & Morris, M. (1999). *Regulating anarchy. The Grendon programme.* Leyhill Press.

Short, J.F., & Strodtbeck, F.L. (1965). *Group process and gang delinquency.* University of Chicago Press.

Shuker, R., & Sullivan, E. (Eds.) (2010). *Grendon and the emergence of forensic therapeutic communities: Developments in research and practice.* John Wiley and Sons.

Smith, C.F., Rush, J., & Burton, C.E. (2013) Street gangs, organized crime groups, and terrorists: Differentiating criminal organizations. *Sciences Journal, 5,* 1–18.

Stevens, A. (2010). Introducing forensic democratic therapeutic communities. In R. Shuker, & E. Sullivan (Eds.). *Grendon and the emergence of forensic therapeutic communities: Developments in research and practice* (pp.7–24). John Wiley and Sons.

Weerman, F.M., Maxson, C.L., Esbensen, F., Aldridge, J., Medina, J., & van Gemert, F. (2009). Eurogang program manual background, development, and use of the Eurogang instruments in multi-site, multi-method comparative research. Eurogang program manual - Citation formats | Research Explorer | The University of Manchester

Weinberg, H. (2008). So, what is this social unconscious anyway? *Group Analysis: The International Journal of Group-Analytic Psychotherapy, 40,* 307–21.

Wood, J. (2006). Gang activity in English prisons: The prisoners' perspective. *Psychology, Crime & Law, 12,* 605–17.

Wood, J. (2017). The psychology of gangs: What do we know and where does this leave us? Presented at The Innovations in Forensic Psychology Conference, Centre of Research and Education in Forensic Psychology. University of Kent, 13 April 2017.

Wood, J.L., & Adler J.R. (2001). Gang activity in English prisons: The staff perspective. *Psychology Crime and Law, 7,* 167–92. https://doi.org/10.1080/10683160108401793

Yalom, I.D. (1985). *The theory and practice of group psychotherapy.* (3rd ed.). Basic Books.

Young, T., Fitzgibbon, W., & Silverstone, D. (2013). *The role of the family in facilitating gang membership, criminality and exit. A report prepared for Catch22.* London Metropolitan University.

A community of women in prison

More than a voice – therapeutic use of visual and psychodramatic arts

2

Vicky Gavin and Claudia Vau[1]

This chapter explains the context of the only women's democratic therapeutic community (DTC) in the English prison estate, at Her Majesty's Prison
(HMP) Send. Following a brief history, the chapter highlights the importance of recognising distinctive contextual factors reflected in the experience
of women – as residents, visitors and staff – by contributions in their own
words. We provide a rationale that links the various interventions described
as affirmative adaptive experiences. These particular experiences expand the
potential for healthy choices and development for DTC residents. While the
interventions were open to all residents, some chose to engage, whilst others
were free not to. The very introduction of choice, aside from the value of the
experience or intervention, is in itself safeguarding against the development
of institutionalised behaviours in a prison context, where residents' lives are
subject to a high level of environmental control. This environmental control
is linked to a societal requirement to contain and punish serious crime. It is
epitomised by hierarchical authority, barred windows and barbed wire-topped
fences, yet crucial to the function of the secure prison estate.

Physical boundaries are acknowledged as essential to the very meaning,
purpose and safety of the setting. In this chapter about HMP Send, we relate a
model of healthy permeable boundaries, in terms of openness to innovation,
new ideas and the thwarting of the ill effects of isolation from family and
society that prisoners can be prone to. We suggest this is important in DTCs,
where the accredited manual provides a quality standard for audit, based on
evidence. Over time, it is essential we continue to create new evidence and
train new practitioners, so we can continue to effectively support the criminal
justice aim of reducing reoffending by way of facilitating affirmative adaptive
experiences. In the longest running of these experiences, Vau, Shepal and
Amaal describe how psychodrama has developed as a core creative therapy
(CCT) and has been integrated into the DTC programme. Vau also describes
an innovative art-based psychodrama group, which held the frame of the art

DOI: 10.4324/9780429317460-3

therapy group in the interim between two qualified art therapists, and enabled the DTC residents to have a novel time-limited CCT experience.

The women's DTC began at West Hill in 2003. At that time, West Hill was a small women's prison adjacent to HMP Winchester. Research indicating that the links between adverse life events and the development of crimino-genic needs in women required a holistic treatment approach and further study were a key factor in setting up the women's DTC (Stewart & Parker, 2007). However, the "Hope and Idealization" (Stewart &Parker, 2007, p. 72) which characterised this innovation was severely tested when, a year after being founded, it was rehomed to HMP Send, in a parallel process echoing the disrupted attachments of many of its residents. Apart from three clinical staff, including the then full-time director of therapy, the DTC suffered the loss of a staff team that had midwifed the community into existence. Subsequently, five women left treatment prematurely, and the original plan for a community of 40 women was never realised.

More recently, since 2013, the number of residents in therapy at one time has tended to be just below 20. From 1 April 2016 to 31 March 2017, 44 women were referred to the DTC, most of whom had convictions for ser-ious violent crimes. Every resident's story is different. However, Shepal's story demonstrates the societal failures and personal tragedy that Murray, Cheliotis and Maruna (2007) associate with criminal activity. Shepal volunteered her personal narrative as a self-reflection exercise, to support case-study evi-dence of how a resident's life is like, before DTC; another resident's testimony is presented further ahead, to evidence self-reported outcomes of the DTC experience, based on personal reflection.

Shepal's story

I am an Asian woman in my late thirties from a Bangladeshi background. I was born in Bangladesh and came over to London when I was young. I spent much of my upbringing in both countries. This led to difficulties trying to pick up the English language. School was not an enjoyable place for me either in Bangladesh or London, as I was bullied in both places. Bangladesh schools had strict discipline and physical punishment was commonplace, although that wasn't the case in London. I was still bullied for my shy, timid ways, and children would pick and make fun of my name. School became a place of intimidation for me and home was not much better.

I have a large family and I am the eldest daughter, which placed me under a lot of pressure of responsibility. As I reached adolescence, I lost my younger sister and then a year later, my dad also tragically passed away. Losing both of them at a young age had a massive impact on me and my family members. The family dynamics changed and I struggled with my grief. After losing both my family members, my mother began to play a more dominant role and became stricter and angrier towards me and my siblings. I wasn't given the opportunity to grieve and nor did I understand how to, as in my culture feelings don't get talked about; you are expected to just get on with it. Life at home had rules that I had to follow. Not having a social life outside of home was non-existent, and boyfriends were something that our culture is totally against, so when I was seen talking to a boy while I was walking back home from school one day, it brought severe consequences. My brother-in-law had seen me and reported to my mother. My mother was furious and, along with my brother-in-law, they gave me a beating to warn me off this boy.

For my mother, she saw what I had done as bringing shame and disrespect to my father. She felt humiliated that my brother-in-law had bought this to her attention. I had always been brought up to keep secrets and told it was shameful to discuss things with outsiders, and that's something we don't do in her eyes. As the boy became my boyfriend, the beating at home got worse, to the point that I nearly took my own life. My brother-in-law and mother began to make plans to take me back home. I became desperate and my boyfriend persuaded me to leave home and live with him. I was only 15 at the time. My family disowned me for a number of years until after I had my son at 18. Initially after leaving home, I lived with my boyfriend's parents. I was used as a domestic slave and as someone his parents could receive financial gain from by claiming benefits for. His parents made sure we had an Islamic marriage and then legally registered us when I turned 16. Once I and my husband then, moved away, and after our son was born, the marriage began to break down. I would be told by the people in our neighbourhood that my husband was being unfaithful, and from seeing his own actions and behaviour change, I knew this to be true. I was pressured into having three terminations by my husband, and trying to voice my concerns about his infidelity fell on deaf ears. The only way I felt I could get any form of control or expression of how I was feeling was to withhold sex from him. This led to physical and sexual abuse from him. He decided to leave one day after I wouldn't consent to him taking another wife. He abandoned me and my son; in my culture women living without husbands are looked down upon. I became vulnerable and a target to be preyed upon, someone to take advantage of as I didn't have a male figure to protect me. It was then that someone reached out and thought to help me: my victim. At first he represented as a father figure type to me as he assisted me in making benefit claims and paid for things such as a phone credit and Arabic classes for my son. Little did I realise that these were ways of trying to manipulate me and make me more vulnerable to him. He paid for my phone credit so that I would have no excuse not to call him when he demanded, and he paid for my son's classes so that he could be alone with me.

He pressured and forced me into having sex with him and then continued to make threats whenever I would decline. His threats were to endanger my younger sister. Having already lost one sister, this threat heightened my fear and made me more compliant. He began to harass my neighbour, who was also my closest friend at the time. I felt trapped and unable to cope or speak out about the situation.

Affirmative adaptive experiences in the context of the prison democratic therapeutic community for women

Considering the life experiences described above, Shepal's dispirited response to being advised to join the DTC treatment in the last years of her sentence illuminates the cognitive and affective style she had developed:

> Where do I even start, I was suggested to do TC by my Offender Supervisor just before my first parole in 2015. It felt like a big disappointment which caused me to see nothing but negativity in my future, I felt the helplessness, I refused to take any risk and complained about the unfairness of life and said 'nothing I do will make a difference'.

When we refer to interventions as affirmative adaptive experiences, we mean that these aim to disconfirm beliefs pertaining to the patterns of affect and cognition that drive risk-related behaviours, developed over a lifetime, which Shepal describes.

The rationale for these interventions weaves together a behaviour explanation hypothesis within the fabric of a therapeutic community (TC) environment, and clinical findings in neurobiology and personality disorder research.

Chris Holman, a Quaker psychiatrist and group analyst who founded a service which later became the first accredited TC for women (with severe self-injurious behaviours at The Retreat Hospital in York, mid-1990s–2018), made an important clinical observation in simple language that staff and residents could appreciate: 'the treatment for bad experiences is good experiences'. Asked to elaborate on this recently, Holman wrote:

> My idea was 'the treatment for bad experiences is good experiences', the point being that people who have had adverse experiences have of course become adapted to expecting and predicting them. It is only through having good experiences that they can learn that this is maladaptive. The problem, of course, is that they don't pay attention to, or actively invalidate, the good experiences, which don't match their expectations: one element of the therapy is both to acknowledge the experience, and drawing attention to the affective response

they have and encouraging/enabling them to modulate it in a more adaptive manner.

(Holman, 2018)

When it comes to negative risk-taking, the expectation that negative experiences will be repeated and the patterns of affect and cognition that drive repetition compulsion (Freud, 1920), are linked to mental health diagnosis, that tend to prevail in the DTC. Montgomery (2013) provides a scientific explanation for the psychobiological dysfunction that is characteristic of post-traumatic responses, borderline personality organisation and dissociative conditions, while Dolan and Völlm (2009) report that 50% of female offenders meet criteria for a personality disorder. A personality disorder diagnosis is not required for admission to the DTC programme at HMP Send, but the service is integrated into the Women Offenders Personality Disorder pathway, and does attract women with traits consistent with personality disorder and complex trauma.

History of the need for an intervention

Up until 2011, women in treatment on the DTC had limited opportunity to engage in non-verbal CCTs. Some of the residents were able to benefit from exploring creative and destructive processes in art therapy; however, with only a sessional art therapist, places in the art therapy group were very limited, and did not often become available for new residents. The non-verbal nature of a CCT is viewed by staff and residents as particularly beneficial for women whose first language is not English, or who have no words for the traumata they have experienced. Furthermore, beyond providing a much-needed 'embodied' form of psychotherapy for women in treatment on the DTC, providing a training placement for a senior trainee of the London Centre of Psychodrama (LCP) enabled the Service to influence clinical practice and promote TC practice and values.

For any DTC providing a training placement, there are obligations to the trainee and training organisation, which need to be planned for. This includes developing a good working relationship and communication with a liaison tutor, from the training organisation. Secondly, it is necessary to provide resources for additional supervision, focusing on TC theory and practice, and the trainee's needs pertaining to the development of group work skills, as well as the ability to perform and communicate effectively, as a team member. To ensure the personal safety and access to necessary facilities for the trainee, who may not work in the establishment for sufficient hours to hold keys, and ensure optimal communication about therapy sessions with the team

as a whole, at HMP Send we always provide an officer as co-facilitator with
trainees. This chapter refers to specific CCT groups: *a long-term psychodrama
group* and a *brief, art-based psychodrama group*, offered to DTC residents from
January 2016 to September 2018, and from May to October 2017, respectively.

Sixteen DCT residents in total joined the psychodrama group throughout
its duration; seven were part of the art-based psychodrama group. All these
women had committed violent crimes and were motivated to engage with
therapeutic work creatively, either through visual or dramatic arts, to heal
from past traumas, forgive themselves, take responsibility for repairing meaningful relationships and discover healthier ways of being, within themselves
and in community.

General psychodramatic frame

Mirroring the co-creative nature of psychodrama itself, the interventions
described in this chapter indicate how both structured psychodrama and an
integrative creative approach, combining visual arts, role analysis and dramatic
action, promote, hold and contain deeply therapeutic group work, giving the
unheard and the unseen not only a voice but healthy, fully functional, inner
and relational creative expression.

Psychodrama was founded by Jacob Levy Moreno (1889–1974) as the
original form of group psychotherapy, involving a collective dramatisation
of an individual's 'memories […], unfinished situations, inner dramas, fantasies, dreams, preparation for future risk-taking situations, or unrehearsed
expressions of mental states in the here and now' (Kellermann, 1992, p. 20).

Role theory is based on Moreno's teaching practice and written word
about a relational concept of *role*, which bridges psychiatry and sociology –
he defined role as 'the actual tangible forms which the self takes' (Moreno,
1961, republished by Fox, 1987, p. 62). Moreno distinguished three types of
roles: (1) *psychosomatic* roles, such as the role of the 'eater' and the 'sleeper'
(which one develops in early life, for survival purposes); (2) *social* roles, such
as the 'mother' and the 'friend' (born out of attachment and socialisation);
and (3) *psychodramatic* or intrapsychic roles (born in one's relationship with
parts of one's *self*), such as the 'self-critic'. This concept and these types of
roles constitute the essential theory behind the practice of psychodrama and
sociodrama, as well as a theory of personality and child development, whereby
phenomena otherwise explained in different therapeutic modalities and psychological theories are viewed in terms of role relations, that is, as the impact
relationships have on one's sense of *self* and in one's development (Dayton,
1994). In this sense, role theory and psychodrama are as relevant today as they

ever were – neuroscientists such as Allan Schore and Daniel Siegel recognise that 'initial relationships shape the very structure of our brains, and the constant sea of interpersonal encounters in which we swim continues to modify our brain wiring' (as cited in Badenoch & Cox, 2013, p. 1).

The LCP's approach is a classically structured dramatic method of working through intra- and interpersonal issues in action, aiming to fulfil a *session contract* that is agreed upon before the re-enactment; creative psychotherapeutic work is oriented by *role analysis* (Jefferies, 2019), gradually deepened, held, and safely closed within a session, ideally lasting two hours and 30 minutes. This happens throughout three sequential phases: (1) a *warm-up* with protagonist selection; (2) *action*; and (3) *sharing*, often including de-roling and grounding exercises (Karp, 1998, p. 3).

As Figure 2.1 suggests, the action phase can assume one of two forms in classical psychodrama – that is, according to Moreno's words and practice (Bradshaw-Tauvon, 1998; Bustos, 1994):

- 'Full psychodrama': starting with the re-enactment of a recent situation, often going to another recent situation (further back in time,

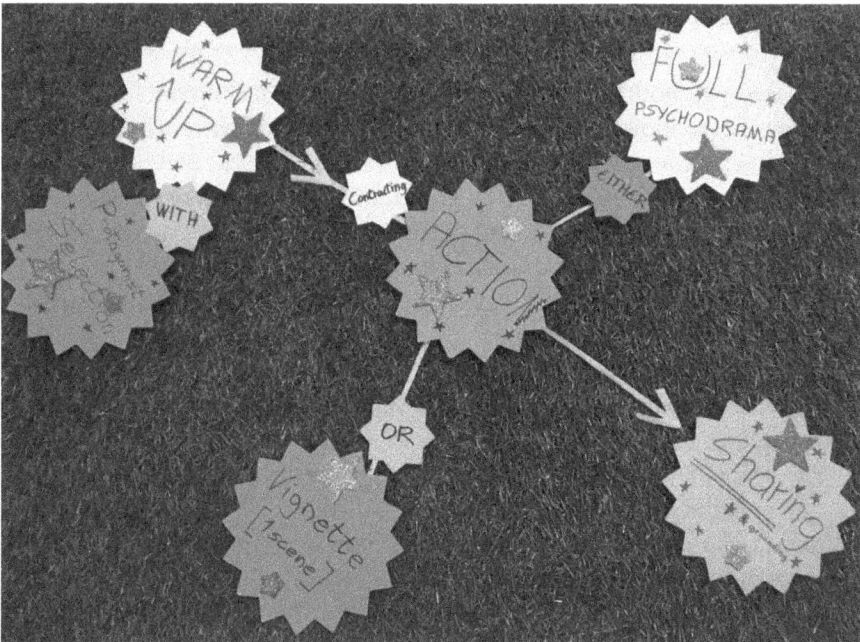

Figure 2.1 Star-shaped labels used in an open psychodrama session at HMP Send's DTC, representing the classical structure of psychodrama.

but still in the recent past), and then to a scene in the distant past, where (*locus*) and when (*status nascendi*) the protagonist's problem, as experienced in the present originated (*matrix*), so that reparative work can be done. Once freed from past scripts, the protagonist is brought back to the first *scene* (now re-named *role training*) to attempt more functional behaviours – different, more adequate, new, in a word, spontaneous (*re-matrixisation*). Each scene is de-roled, the stage is cleared before the next scene is set and, again, cleared at the end of the role training scene.

- 'Vignette': one-scene psychodrama, usually focused on a present-day situation or a vision of the future, and occasionally a dream, although full dream re-enactments follow a specific structure (in vignettes, all present, past, reality and dream elements are kept on stage until the end of the action phase).

After an initial check-in and once established as a working group, a typical DTC psychodrama group follows this structure in its two-hour sessions.

Art-based psychodrama group

The art-based psychodrama group on the other hand (lasting only one hour and 30 minutes), allowed for one hour of engagement with art materials, where group members produced individual pieces of work, and 30 minutes for these pieces to be presented to the group, with application of role analysis to the content of the pieces of art, and the option to work through some of this content with the use of psychodrama techniques.

Blatner (1996) and Williams (1991) describe the action techniques that were applied in this group, namely:

- the *empty chair* (use of chairs to vent unexpressed feelings and thoughts),
- *role reversal* (changing roles with other people or parts of self to share and gain insight on those roles),
- and *doubling* (offering statements as if you were the protagonist, to tease out what is difficult to express).

At the end of the art-based psychodrama sessions, group members were invited to engage in grounding exercises and share what they would like to take away, and leave behind.

Development of the interventions

To design and develop specialised therapy groups such as the long-term psychodrama group and brief art-based psychodrama group this chapter refers to, Yalom (1995, p. 451) suggests 'three steps: (1) assess the clinical situation; (2) formulate appropriate clinical goals; and (3) modify traditional technique to be responsive to these 2 steps – the new clinical situation and the new set of goals'.

Considering each group as a whole, the *clinical situation* in the DTC reflects a complex psychosocial reality, where voluntary yet intensive psychotherapy is undertaken by individuals in legally enforced custody (for punishment, public safety and rehabilitation purposes), under relatively flexible conditions for a prison setting (i.e. under therapeutically informed, living-learning conditions). The physical setting and wider container of such groups incorporates strict control systems, involuntary routines and imposed power structures, while the actual therapeutic work is a discretionary possibility for those who choose to join DTC.

Generic, *prosocial clinical goals* aimed at risk reduction and rehabilitation are translated into individual therapeutic targets, for prisoners whose lives (including family background, past traumas, psychopathology and offence history) are poured into clinical formulations that help recognise and work therapeutically towards changing ingrained antisocial beliefs and behaviours.

The above-mentioned *clinical formulations* of each TC member are elaborated at their intake or assessment stage by the clinical team of the DTC (usually, the clinical lead, a group psychotherapist and/or a forensic psychologist). The formulation culminates in a set of *therapeutic targets* for each individual, which influence the themes group members identify for potential pieces of work and psychodrama contracting. Because therapeutic targets are periodically reviewed and updated, according to DTC members' progress in therapy, residents are expected to work on such targets and indeed use all the groups they take part in to do so.

Modifying traditional techniques to accommodate the clinical situation and the goals of specific groups is a constant task, and different stages of group development reveal specific needs in terms of technique modification: some sessions cannot follow a classical psychodrama structure, and at least one psychodramatic concept requires reframing. Still, all group psychodrama has to offer is within reach for DTC residents – they can bring forward and re-enact intra- and interpersonal difficulties they currently face; they can trace beliefs driving dysfunctional ways of behaving and acting out; they can experience catharsis, containment and reparation; and they can attempt more adequate, new behaviours.

Developed by Jefferies (2019), the LCP's 'role analysis' guides the psychodrama director to track the critical components of problematic situations, where actions are driven by dysfunctional beliefs that keep individuals from fully accessing adequate, innovative *spontaneity* and healing, potential-fulfilling *creativity*, which are considered innate. The role analysis components investigated in the action phase of a psychodrama are: context, behaviours, feelings, beliefs and consequences. These are discovered and fed back to the protagonist at crucial moments of the drama, with particular relevance in the locus as a catalyst for reparative work.

Role analysis provides a consistent clinical guidance for the CCT work described in this chapter, but the classic psychodrama structure taught by the LCP (i.e. role analysis in itself) does not formally apply to the forming stage nor to the storming periods of the long-term psychodrama group (Tuckman, 1965). As for the art-based psychodrama group, it follows a particular structure, previously described, with art taking the lead as expressive means and psychodrama being used complementarily and non-prescriptively, to deepen the work.

Without a proper definition, for individuals with poor self-control, 'spontaneity' can sound intimidating, in its association to (negative) risk-taking, if and when the concept is erroneously equated with 'disorderly conduct, emotionalism, or impulsivity, [in] an escape from discomfort' (White, 2011, p. 13). To prevent this, the concept was introduced in a written text made available to the DTC residents who were assessed for psychodrama, where it was defined in Moreno's terms, as 'adequate responses to new situations and new responses to old situations' (White, 2011, p. 13).

The idea of 'role training' – that is, the idea of experimenting with different, more functional behavioural responses to given situations – seemed quite appealing in the context of the women's prison DTC, where residents develop living-learning skills, are keen on acquiring more functional behaviours and value practicing them with the support of doubles and 'feedback' from their groups. In the DTC, psychodrama group members are encouraged to build on their psychodramatic work, by exercising new behaviours in the community, and referring back to their own psychodramas in their small therapy groups.

Assessment, inclusion and exclusion criteria

General DTC inclusion and exclusion criteria are applied to CCTs, but the individual assessments for these groups ultimately dictated the suitability of the applicants to join them. The residents who applied to join either of the CCT groups were individually assessed and signed contracts to attend one of these groups for either a minimum of six months (in the case of the psychodrama group), or the entire duration of the group (20 sessions, in the case of the art-based psychodrama group). Exceptions to this rule were made, with the community's agreement, to enable highly motivated DTC residents to engage with a CCT of their choice, when they had less than the desirable minimum DCT time left to complete.

Once selected for the CCT groups, residents could remain beyond their initial contracts if they so wished, as long as they remained in the DTC. Disruptive behaviour and lack of engagement due resistance or defences would be worked through in action, rather than framed as an exclusion criterion.

Assessments for the psychodrama group were structured to comprise focused exercises, adapted and applied to fulfil three objectives: (1) to evaluate the willingness or readiness of potential group members to work in action; (2) to inquire about their therapeutic goals; (3) and to investigate their cultural, social and family backgrounds, including significant transgenerational patterns. These individual sessions lasted 30 to 45 minutes and were mandatorily conducted in the presence of an officer who acted as auxiliary and helped maintain the frame of co-facilitated sessions (followed in small therapy groups), which meant explorations had to be conducted with clarity and concisely in order to reduce awkwardness, contain anxiety, avoid wasting precious time and obtain as much relevant information as possible, within the frame and circumstances of these sessions.

The first part of these sessions was designed to meet assessment objectives 1 and 2 (as stated earlier), and it was inspired by the *Janus Gate* exercise (White, 2011):

> The god Janus was the Roman god of doors, gates and windows. He is always pictured on Roman coins with back-to-back profiles: looking forward and looking back. January is named after him, as it is the gateway from the old year to the new.

> The 'Janus Gate' is an exercise that is both simple and powerful. In it, we stop, take stock, and look ahead. It is brief and carefully focused, going to the core of our changes [...] It facilitates discovering and articulating changes that have taken place within our healing process, and helps anchor a readiness for a richer perspective.

> (White, 2011, p. 116)

White's original exercise is as group practice, whereby different group members hold different roles (protagonist, protagonist looking back, protagonist looking forward, supporter or witness, and director). The protagonist – or the person whose drama is being played – finds answers to crucial questions through role reversal and role-taking, experiencing insight from the mirror position, when in role as witness.

In the individual assessments of DTC residents, each woman was prompted to hold the roles of 'leaving behind' and 'carrying forward', one after the other, by sitting on chairs placed back to back. Mindful breathing was used to facilitate the transition from one role to the other.

These individual assessment sessions were Vau's introduction as psychodrama director to the women who would later join the group – role predictability and stability were important, so the director did not role-reverse with the women; keeping the director in the role of director and the women in their own roles also helped manage time in these sessions, which included the second exercise. The director was proactive when words did not come easily to the women in this first exercise, and either invited doubling statements from the officer in the room, or offered them herself, to obtain a response and introduce the psychodramatic technique of the double experientially, sometimes as a development of reflecting back.

The second part of these sessions consisted of elaborating a *genosociogram* (Schützenberger, 1998, pp. 10–16) – a sociometric family tree covering three generations, constructed with symbols and lines representing family relations – to satisfy assessment objective 3.

Sitting around a table after the first exercise, the psychodramatist introduced Schützenberger's genosociogram methodology and conventional symbols (Schützenberger, 1998, pp. 70–2). Then, Vau asked the woman being assessed to draw a circle framed by a square in the lower centre of a piece of paper, write her age inside the circle, and her initial just below. The process continued with parents and being represented above the framed circle, grandparents above these, siblings (in each generation) at the same level, and children underneath, all connected by lines.

This methodology offered structure and guidance to the second part of the assessment, but still permitted co-creative allowances in the design of each piece of work – the woman was invited to draw the piece (as opposed to it being conventionally drawn by the director, with information she provided) and was given permission to create different symbols to adorn each family member represented in her piece of work, to indicate health conditions and other characteristics not included in the list of symbols provided in the sheet pictured bellow (Figure 2.2).

To promote empowerment and ownership, all women were given the option of either drawing their *genosociogram* under the trainee psychodramatist's guidance or having her do it for them, based on their answers to her questions. Throughout Vau's clinical placement, all but one woman, with prominent blanks in her family background, chose to draw their own pieces.

The genosociogram was not used at the individual assessment stage of the brief art-based psychodrama group; rather, it was introduced at the first

➡ GENOSOCIOGRAM

Type of family tree drawn from memory, and annotated with important life events, dates, links and emotional context of frame work (sociometric links, marked with arrows or colored lines).

O	Female person	△○ Parents	
△	Male person	Children (number indicate sibling order)	
▢	Unknow sex	△○ Twins	
○△▢	Miscarriage or abortion		
▣◉	Person for whom the genosociogram was built	△↔△ Two people that got along	
△○	Marriage	△⤬△ The person has died; date and age at death are added	
△○	Unmarried couple	O+	
△○	Intimate relationship	People living under the same roof (circle)	
	Divorce or separation	△○ A slash indicates broken off relations	
△¹○²△	Multiple marriages are numbered	△⌇○ Zigzag indicates conflict	
Ä	Homosexual of bisexual	\ Dominating individual	
Ä(	Unmarried at 45	* Emigrant	
▤	Brother/sister born 12 to 20 maths apart (near twins)	% Mental problems	
▤	or near triplets		

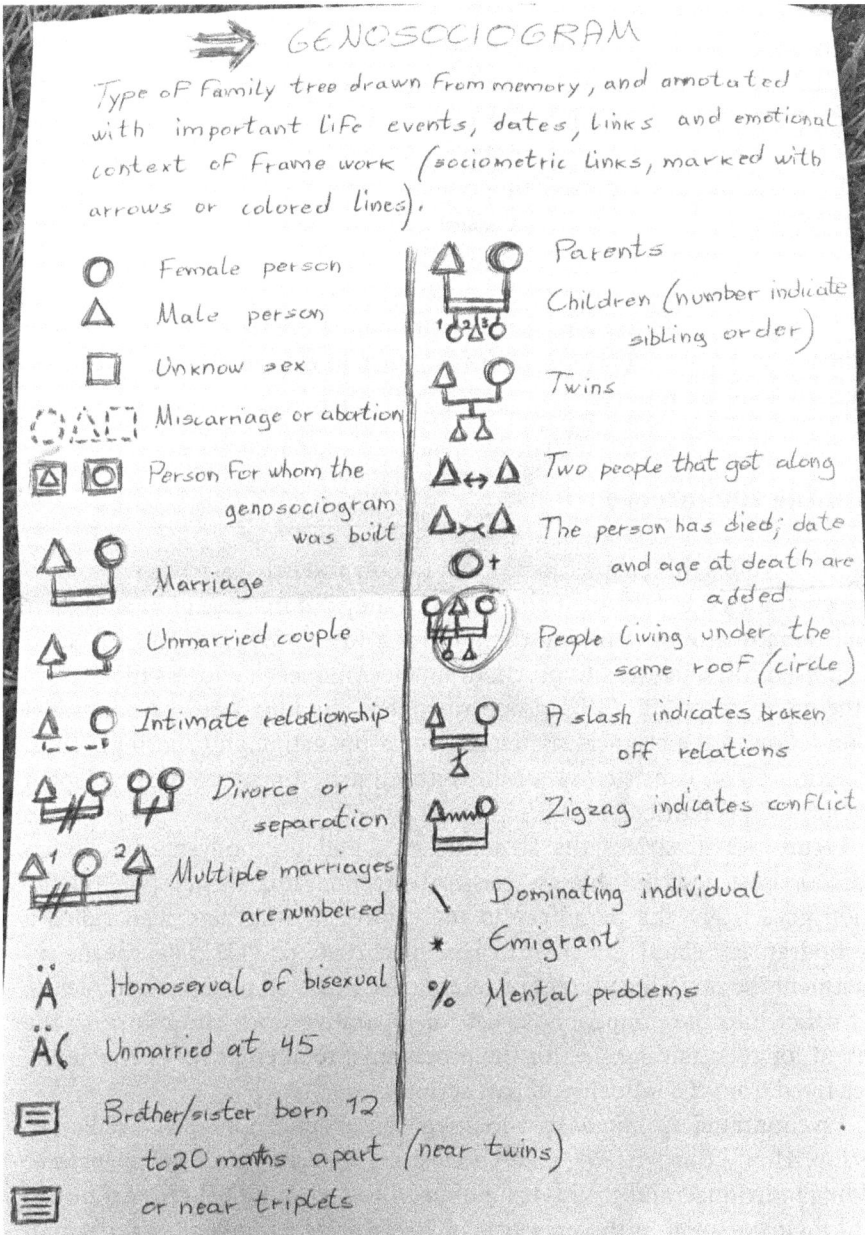

Figure 2.2 List of genosociogram symbols used in individual assessment sessions.

group session, where all group members were invited and supported to engage with the methodology and draw their genosociogram as their first piece of art. Assessments for this group consisted of verbal discussion of the Janus Gate themes (what the women wished to 'carry forward', and what they wanted to 'leave behind'), and inquiry of the applicants' willingness to engage with psychodrama techniques to unpack the content of some pieces of art work, during their presentation and group discussion. Because this brief group replaced art therapy interventions, where residents were not required to work in (dramatic) action and could feel overexposed by this offer, initial openness to role analysis and potential engagement with psychodramatic techniques were an inclusion criterion, but refusal or resistance to engage did not determine exclusion from the group.

Running the interventions

The CCT groups this chapter focuses on ran on a weekly basis, and members were encouraged to take the personal work they did in these groups to their small therapy groups (running three times a week). Whereas the art-based group used role analysis and psychodrama techniques to address the themes of the art work produced by group members, the long-term psychodrama group followed the classical structure (warm-up, action and sharing). Thus, the action phase consisted of a full psychodrama, a vignette or an adapted exploration of a particular action model.

Figure 2.3 illustrates the structure of a full psychodrama. Goldman and Morrison describe this as: 'classical psychodrama theory [where] the action goes from "the periphery to the centre" in what has been called a psychodramatic spiral' (as cited in Hudgins, 2000, p. 232). This means re-enactments begin in the present or recent past, move on to connected scenes, go further into the protagonist's past for reparative work and return to the present for role training (i.e. for the protagonist to attempt new behaviours, once freed from the influence of past scripts).

Psychodrama is not a past-focused therapeutic approach (Williams, 1991, p. 41 and Bustos, 1994, p. 49). Revisiting the past serves the purpose of ridding individuals and groups from unhelpful scripts and beliefs, so they can fulfil their potential in the present. For this reason, protagonists and group members are always brought back to the present at the end of a psychodrama, to co-create positive change and reconnect with others in the here and now.

In addition, 'bearing in mind the exigencies of working within the criminal justice system and, by extension, within the broader framework of public protection' as Baim (2000, p. 157) points out, psychodramatic work around

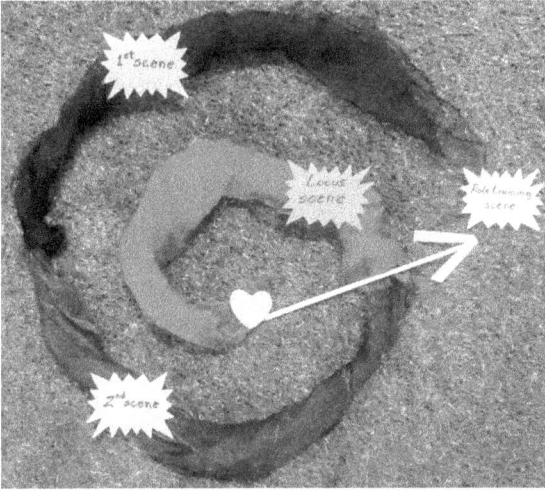

Figure 2.3 Concretisation of the Psychodrama Spiral, representing the structure of the action phase of a full psychodrama, as practiced at the LCP.

the prisoners' trauma history is never undertaken to justify crimes or absolve individuals from culpability.

When these intentions were present in the psychodrama group, and/ or when there was risk of vicarious traumatisation of other group members and the director, scenes were played as static sculpts rather than in action, sometimes with objects rather than group members holding potentially traumatic roles. Particular action models were also used in the DTC psychodrama group, to allow for heavily charged themes to be addressed in a safe, contained manner.

In this sense:

- Addiction was addressed using Chesner's addictions compass (Chesner, 2019);
- Trauma was sometimes addressed using aspects of the therapeutic spiral model (TSM) (Hudgins, 2000).

Chesner's model is a way of working in action that is useful for tackling addiction at any stage, from active addiction to sustained recovery, as deeply or as lightly as individuals wish to, and always with impact in terms of action-insight and connection to others. As taught at the LCP, the addictions compass is based on role-taking in a circular configuration, including the roles of the *protection* that an addictive substance or behaviour provides, its *cost*, its *promise* and the *wise(r) self* of the addict. In the simplest application of the addictions compass, individuals take on each of these roles, one after the other, and access messages to self that originate from them. Once a message is accessed and voiced, the protagonist steps out of the role and reverses roles with another group member, who takes on the role and repeats the message back to the protagonist, as she stands in the mirror position.

In terms of psychodramatic technique, TSM also uses role-taking, role reversal and mirror, with practitioners becoming certified is its application through specialised training. It provides 'clinical guidelines and action intervention structures for Psychodrama with trauma survivors [so that] the pace and intensity of experiential therapy can be clinically controlled [and] regression is chosen, conscious, and always in the service of the ego' (Hudgins, 2000, pp. 229–30). It provides *experiential self-organisation*; clear *clinical structures for safe psychodrama psychotherapy* (preventing retraumatisation); and *advanced action intervention modules* (for containment, expression, reparation and integration of unprocessed trauma material), aiming to build and sustain an *integrated state of spontaneous learning*. This model covers the roles that compose the 'trauma survivor's intrapsychic role atom' (Hudgins, 2000, p. 236), but in the context of the clinical placement contextualising the CCT interventions that are described in this chapter, group members experienced very specifically, adaptations of the module pertaining to the *trauma triangle* (victim, perpetrator and abandoning authority/witness/rescuer), which serve expression or communication functions.

Trauma recovery is 'based upon the empowerment of the survivor and the creation of new connections' (Herman, 1997, p. 133), which renders therapeutic/healing relationship(s) fundamental. In such a relationship, it is possible to gradually cover the essential stages of recovery: 'establishing safety, reconstructing the trauma story, and restoring the connection between survivors and their community' (Herman, 1997, p. 3). In the context of psychodramatic work, relationships between group members, and between these and the director evolve in an authentic fashion, with non-judgemental group support and increasing empathy contributing to the gradual engagement of all group members, even those who start their journeys in a resistant or defensive position.

Evaluation of interventions

The evaluation of CCT interventions is based on self-reporting by current as well as former group members and on clinical observation, translated into qualitative reports concerning progress with regards to individual targets, which are produced for interim and final case reviews. Ethics, safeguarding and security issues limit what can be published, but further thoughts of Amaal, a former DTC resident, exemplify how self-reporting evaluates psychodrama as a CCT intervention. In her own words, Amaal points out the themes psychodrama allowed her to work on, and achieve progress with: namely, in her case, relationships and communication, self-confidence and problem-solving, offence and trauma.

Amaal's self-reported outcomes

As part of the TC, I was encouraged to take part in a CCT. I knew I needed something that would push me out of my comfort zone and challenge me a little further. This led to me applying for psychodrama. I was a little nervous, as I had heard/seen many previous members crying after sessions and was told that psychodrama made you re-enact your offence and past traumas! I was almost put off and then I met Claudia, the psychodramatist who put me at ease straightaway. She could see the work that I needed to do on myself and encouraged me by telling me that I would see the benefits over time. Initially, when I saw the intensity of the work, I stepped away from the role of the protagonist as I didn't feel I had the courage and was afraid of the emotional impact it would have on me. When I stayed in supporting roles, I soon realised that it had an impact on me regardless and at times felt like I had been in the role of the protagonist due to the effect it had on me. Seeing the benefits it had on other members made me challenge myself a bit more by putting myself in the role of protagonist a number of times. Psychodrama enabled me to work on exploring relationships with others, to develop my communication skills so that I could assert myself better, problem-solve and the see impact of my offence on my direct/indirect victims. I was also able to work on past traumas and the effect that they had left on me. My confidence and self-esteem were lacking when I first joined psychodrama, but over time I developed my self-worth. I never would have undertaken the opportunity to try something as different as psychodrama before, but have gained invaluable skills and it has now given me the confidence to try different things.

Conclusion

Based on staff reports and self-reporting by women like Amaal, the introduction of psychodrama as a CCT and its short-term use to support the art therapy frame opened up new therapeutic possibilities for women who feel drawn to drama and embodied ways of working, and also for those to whom this implies a step out of the comfort zone. Psychodrama and art therapy enabled past maladaptive life experiences to be adaptively revisited, through creative experiences with a positive impact on the present and future of DTC residents.

Creative warm-up for therapy was deemed important: contained spontaneity was enhanced by these, and potential protagonists were encouraged to take back to their small talking groups the themes they named in the initial part of the psychodrama sessions, or depicted in their art work. Whether these themes were worked through in action or not, art and psychodramatic warm-up exercises, as well as both protagonist and auxiliary role-taking seemed to warm up the women for further therapeutic work in talking groups, enhancing their self-confidence, self-reflection and prosocial relating. CCTs seemed to allow for affirmative adaptive experiences, which reinforced new adaptive ways of thinking, managing emotions and behaving.

Adequate support and supervision of the psychodramatist and her participation in staff meetings was deemed crucial for creative group work to flourish in a safe, contained, sustained way, built on and built by the DCT living-learning experience as a whole.

The CCT model presented in this chapter is neither static nor prescriptive. The combination and format of the CCTs offered to women in prison have been evolving. The approach adopted, incorporating practice-based evidence and residents' experiences and reflections, adds to the existing work from male DTCs demonstrating the role of CCTs in enhancing practice and improving outcomes.

Note

1 Shepal and Amaal are pseudonyms used by two DTC residents who write in the first person about their difficult past and their CCT experience in the wider DTC context, where community-based processes and activities, meetings and group sessions (small and large) all contribute to – and constitute – affirmative adaptive experiences.

References

Badenoch, B., & Cox, P. (2013). Integrating interpersonal neurobiology with group psychotherapy. In S.P. Gantt and B. Badenoch (Eds.). *The interpersonal neurobiology of group psychotherapy and group process*. Karnac Books.

Baim, C. (2000). Time's distorted mirror – trauma work with adult male sex offenders. In P.F. Kellermann and M.K. Hudgins (Eds.). In *Psychodrama with trauma survivors. Acting out your pain*. Jessica Kingsley, 155–75.

Blatner, H.A. (1996). *Acting in: Practical applications of psychodramatic methods*. Springer, 6–126.

Bradshaw-Tauvon, K., 1998. Principles of psychodrama. In M. Karp, P. Holmes and K. Bradshaw-Tauvon (Eds.). *The handbook of psychodrama*. Routledge, 29–46.

Bustos, D.M., 1994. Wings and roots. In P. Holmes, M. Karp and M. Watson (Eds.). Locus, matrix, status nascendi and the concept of clusters. *Psychodrama since Moreno: Innovations in theory and practice*. Routledge, 46–55.

Chesner, A. (2019). Working with Addictions. In A. Chesner (Ed.). *One-to-one psychodrama psychotherapy: Applications and technique*. Taylor & Francis, 68–79.

Dayton, T. (1994). *The drama within: Psychodrama and experiential therapy*. Health Communications.

Dolan, M., & Völlm, B. (2009). Antisocial personality disorder and psychopathy in women: A literature review on the reliability and validity of assessment instruments. *International Journal of Law and Psychiatry, 32*, 2–9.

Freud, S. (1920). Beyond the Pleasure Principle. In *The standard edition of the complete psychological works of Sigmund Freud* (Vol. 18, *1920–1922: Beyond the pleasure principle, group psychology and other works*, 1–64). [Translated from the German under General Editorship of J. Strachey in collaboration with A. Freud, and published in 2001]. Vintage.

Herman, J. (1997). *Trauma and recovery. The aftermath of violence – from domestic abuse to political terror*. Basic Books.

Holman, C. (2018). *Email to Victoria Gavin*, 18 Dec.

Hudgins, M.K. (2000). The therapeutic spiral model: Treating PTSD in action. In P.F. Kellermann and M.K. Hudgins (Eds.). *Psychodrama with trauma survivors. Acting out your pain*. Jessica Kingsley, 229–54.

Jefferies, J. (2019). Role theory and role analysis. In A. Chesner (Ed.). *One-to-one psychodrama psychotherapy: Applications and technique*. Taylor & Francis, 19–30.

Karp, M. (1998). An introduction to psychodrama. In M. Karp, P. Holmes, and K. Bradshaw-Tauvon (Eds.). *The handbook of psychodrama*. Routledge, 3–14.

Kellermann, P.F. (1992). *Focus on psychodrama – the therapeutic aspects of psychodrama*. Jessica Kingsley.

Montgomery, A. (2013). *Neurobiology essentials for clinicians*. W.W. Norton.

Moreno, J.L. (1961). The role concept. A bridge between psychiatry and sociology. In J. Fox (Ed.). 1987. *The essential Moreno: Writings on psychodrama, group method, and spontaneity by J.L. Moreno MD*. Springer, 60–5.

Murray, J., Cheliotis, L., & Maruna, S. (2007). Social factors and crime. In M. Parker (Ed.). *Dynamic security: The democratic therapeutic community in prison*. Jessica Kingsley, 23–36.

Schützenberger, A.A. (1998). *The ancestor syndrome – transgenerational psychotherapy and the hidden links in the family tree*. [Translated from the 1993 French edition, by A. Trager]. Routledge.

Stewart, C., & Parker, M. (2007). Send: the women's democratic therapeutic community in prison. In M. Parker (Ed.). *Dynamic security: The democratic therapeutic community in prison*. Jessica Kingsley, 69–82.

Tuckman, B.W. (1965). Developmental sequence in small groups. *Psychological Bulletin, 63*, 384–99.

White, L. (2011). *Still life. A therapist's responses to the challenge of change*. Liz White in Action.

Williams, A. (1991). *Forbidden agendas: Strategic action groups*. Routledge.

Yalom, I.D. (1995). *The theory and practice of group psychotherapy*. (4th ed.). Basic Books.

Group supervision for prison officers (POs)

An orthopedagogical approach to emotional management[1]

Steve Shaw and Gary Winship

3

Background: Prison officers (POs) are on the front line of managing everyday encounters which can often be emotionally charged. POs ordinarily are not trained with a psychological mindedness to manage these encounters. **Objective:** The challenge is to develop a model of education and practice (orthopedagogy) that offers a level of psychological mindedness for POs which can in turn yield a safer prison wing milieu. A framework of reflective practice, which provides opportunities for POs to learn and apply the concept of projective identification (PI) is outlined. **Data:** Drawn from reflective practice, the conducting of supervision groups for POs is described and attention is drawn to the dual roles of supervision and education as well as a structured process that offers a containing space. **Conclusions:** The focus on PI as the central tenet of supervision for POs represents an innovation in education in the prison sector. Implications for practice are considered, both in terms of practice in secure forensic therapeutic communities and psychologically informed planned environments (PIPEs), as well as the case is made for a more general level of application of psychoeducation across the prison estate, where a working knowledge of PI could improve transactions between prisoners and prison staff.

Context

The current crisis in prisons in terms of rising levels of violence, substance misuse, self-harm and attacks on prison officers (POs) is well known to us (*Safety in Custody*, Ministry of Justice, 2016). It has been estimated that during an average day in UK prisons there will have been 350 assaults, 90 assaults on staff and 600 incidents of self-harm (Ministry of Justice, 2016; HMIP, 2016). POs face considerable strain, and many prisons suffer chronic staff shortages where poor staff retention leads to a self-defeating cycle of inexperience. There

DOI: 10.4324/9780429317460-4

are, however, some prisons operating under the rubric of a therapeutic community (TC) approach which are bucking this trend (Aslan, 2018; Magor-Blatch, Bhullar, Thomson, & Thorsteinsson, 2014) with an approach tallied to partial democratic engagement, with ingredients fostering everyday conditions more conducive to a restorative environment for both staff and prisoners. The efficacy of this democratic approach to helping people with personality disorder has been demonstrated by Pearce et al. (2017) in a randomised control trial. Psychologically informed planned environments (PIPEs) are also an organisational attempt to provide a pathway facility for offenders with complex needs, such as personality disorder (MoJ & DOH, UK, 2012), where the staff are upskilled with a base of psychological knowledge which informs practice.

Staff working in prisons, and especially prison officers, will encounter a range of distressing textures of emotion in prisoners, from feelings of frustration to an amplification of strong sometimes violent emotions (Crawley, 2004). Staff can become the target of intolerable feelings such as hostility and neediness, which are projected onto them, and these emotions have the potential to lead to burnout (Cooke, Stephenson, & Rose, 2017). The challenge for prison officers is considerable and requires a knowledge and skill set that merits serious consideration (Liebling, Price, & Shefer, 2011). Walker et al. (2017) have drawn attention to evidence pointing to a range of potential hazards for frontline prison staff, from low levels of distress to enduring disabling traumatic disorders. They highlight strategies employed by prison staff which present a facade of coping, but note that these patterns of coping can lead to staff being desensitised and less effective in their everyday contact with prisoners, and in the long run these ineffective coping strategies can lead to damaging psychological distress.

The work can be considered a hazardous occupation. Clinically trained staff have at their disposal the training and the resources to monitor their subjective responses to prisoners, whereas POs by comparison, generally lack training and support (Cooke et al., 2017). Familiarising POs with psychological models of emotional management does not generally feature as an introduction to working in prisons, although the offender personality disorder pathway (OPDP) outlined an ambition to upskill staff with an agenda for education, practice and progressive environments (Joseph & Benefield, 2012). The idea of considering the optimal conditions for a wider delivery of environments for prisoners conducive to the reduction of levels of violence and self-harm moves the agenda on from the idea of targeted mental health (Brooker, Repper, Sirdifield, & Gojkovic, 2009), to a more holistic vision of service provision.

It has been argued that POs, with their sustained everyday interactions with prisoners, are an untapped resource for deepening and elaborating our psychological understanding of the way in which offending behaviours are paralleled in the milieu of the prison wing (Atkinson & Mann, 2012). Cooke et al. (2017) have identified a model for psychological co-working where clinical staff and custodial officers can build a workforce synergy which can yield informative accounts of the life and challenges of mental health for the prisoner. Importantly, they note that there is a clear and present need to develop a training and education agenda for the custodial staff. As yet, a clear pedagogical framework for a wider system approach, for instance the way in which prison officers might be educated with an agenda for emotional management in situations of encounters with self-harm, has not yet cohered (Walker et al., 2017).

In some parts of the prison estate, most notably in TCs and PIPEs, at the core of the development of the PO's skills and knowledge is the process of supervision. Supervision is a tripod of i) reflection on practice; ii) pastoral support and iii) education (Pedder, 2011). For new POs, supervision is primarily an educative encounter resembling the sort of orthopedagogy conceptualised by TC colleagues, especially the late Eric Broekaert in Ghent. Orthopedagogy springs from a concern with matters of social justice and education for well-being (Broekaert, Vandevelde, & Briggs, 2011; Vanderplassen, Vandevelde, Van Damme, & Yates, 2017), where there is an explicit agenda concerned with identifying living-learning opportunities for all community members. The 'ortho' frame here is commensurate with the focal mission of the prison TC as a corrective experience which seeks to engender rehabilitation. For new POs, the learning in the supervision group is not necessarily down to the supervisor; rather, the learning comes from listening and sharing ideas with peers (Yerushalmi, 1999), that is, learning from other POs and other members of the multidisciplinary team, ideally, including the participation of psychologists, counsellors, art therapists and psychotherapists. There are also similarities here with various models of staff reflection, supervision and support groups (Haigh, 2000), perhaps the best known being the 'Balint group' model which has proved effective and enduring in helping general practitioners develop psychological mindedness about their patients and prevent burnout (Benson & Magraith, 2005). In this sense, supervision is not necessarily the preserve of clinical practitioners but rather something that can be more widely applicable to a range of practitioners.

For clinicians, it is the case that demonstrable ongoing supervision is a requirement of maintaining registration. The potential impact of inadequate supervision systems has been brought into focus in a case before the High Court in the UK, where damages were awarded to a prison officer who delivered a sexual offender programme without adequate preparation or supervision (Johnston, 2003). Although practice in relation to such offender treatment has changed significantly since this case, the prospect of being found to be neglectful of supervision is a salient reminder of the value we should attach to supervision generally. Clarke (2012) has argued that practitioners in forensic settings can be regarded as working in a critical and hazardous occupation, and this is especially the case for POs, who are exposed on a day-to-day basis to individuals who may are hostile and challenging with histories of trauma and trauma perpetration.

There is a particular challenge for POs to become comfortable with a new process of learning which is not based on a didactic exchange, but rather one based on reflective experiential engagement. It is likely that new POs will feel de-skilled by the unfamiliar territory that is the space of the supervision group, feeling ill-equipped to handle to new language of the idea of psychological and emotional mindedness. As Baudry (1993) noted: 'the supervisory relationship requires on the part of the supervisee a considerable amount of personal involvement and degree of revelation of the workings of his or her mind and sharing emotions. This process creates intimacy and is also quite threatening' (Baudry, 1993, p.597).

There is a wide set of knowledges that inform PO work in the prison TC, so the challenge is to make knowledge available in a way which is programmatic and easy to digest for POs. Concepts like transference and counter-transference are essential, but arguably the concept of projective identification (PI) offers the greatest potential for explaining the elements of emotional transaction. As a concept, PI is often contested and considered to be one of the more intricate psychodynamic knowledges. In the following section we provide a synthesis of the model, followed by illustrations of how the concept is threaded into supervision practice.

Projective identification – a working concept in practice

Colleagues who have worked in the field of treating serious offenders have found it necessary and helpful to consider what we might call the 'primitive' aspects of human nature (Doctor, 2003; Gordon, 2004; Welldon, 1993, 1997). The idea of 'primitive' here pertains to those aspects of psychic functioning which are on the one hand the atavistic animalistic urges that are part of the human condition, and on the other hand, characteristic of thwarted development where prisoners can present with needy urges and demands which are hungrily aggressive or at other times woefully despairing and anxious. In understanding the mechanisms of primitive communications Klein's (1946) theory of PI continues to offer a formative account of how feelings, and often difficult feelings, can be transmitted between people, and how some of these primitive states can be understood. Although the theory of PI has been critiqued and modified over time (Fountain, 2000), Klein's original conceptual formulation remains extant. Klein's (1946) thesis for PI was a speculation that the infant was able to 'split off' emotions, particularly those experiences which were felt to be injurious, and then project these outwards. The 'identification' part of the emotional enactment was then the subsequent introjection of the feeling by the concerned other, usually the mother in the first place. Klein argued that PI was a necessary ordinary mechanism of communication between infant and mother whereby the mother would able to receive communications from the infant, long before there was a capacity for words.

The idea of PI was developed by Klein's followers, especially Bion and Rosenfeld, who noted that PI was particularly helpful when the usual mechanisms of conscious communication were defeated by distress acuity, for instance when working with seriously psychotic patients (Bion, 1962; Rosenfeld, 1965). The challenge for the therapist when working with patients who were either unable to communicate or were communicating in a way that one would think of as pre-verbal, was to be receptive to the messages the client was projecting.

Whereas the process of projection might describe the way affective states are attributed to others – for example, we may feel low in mood and then view others around us likewise – PI was conceived as offering a model for the cyclical dynamic of emotional interaction between people. PI might be a case of feeling oneself to be depressed for no good reason in the presence of another person, but this might well be because the other person has split off their unpalatable emotions and projected them onto the other person. PI therefore is a mechanism of communication, and understanding how it works is a helpful tool for practitioners. PI is predicated on the fact that at least one of the interacting individuals has the capacity to receive emotional communications.

Segal (1997) elucidated that PI might take the form of a destructive attack whereby 'nasty or unbearable or mad parts of the self are evoked in other people in order to destroy their comfort, their piece of mind or their happiness' (Segal, 1997, p.36). It has been argued that understanding PI is fundamental to making sense of violent offences and the interpersonal relations between offender and victim (Meloy, 1988), and that this same principle can be applied to the prison system as a whole (Hinshelwood, 1993). PI has been considered 'an unconscious inducement of another to undertake a reciprocal role, for example, the victim role or the inducing of a partner into a nurturing role through self-injury by a borderline personality disordered patient' (Pollock & Belshaw, 1998, p.637). The concept has been variously applied in forensic practice, including adapted use in cognitive analytic therapy (Pollock & Belshaw, 1998) and as a vital resource for making sense of challenging encounters. For example, in her work with an adolescent sentenced for murder Marriot (2007) was able to draw on PI theory in order to make sense of her subjective response to the client: 'During the sessions when he refused to engage I felt confused and powerless, which could be understood as a projective identification of his experience. It was important for me to contain him and tolerate the difficulties' (Marriot, 2007, p.258). We might think of PI as a communication event whereby one person is able to make another person feel what it is that they are feeling, and there are occasions when this brings with it the element of suffering on the part of the person receiving the projection. But knowing the potential of this communication as having the potential for distress, one might build-in mechanisms for pastoral support for staff who are working in environments where pernicious PI is likely to present (Kurtz, 2005).

More recently, Welldon (2015) has considered the following application of an understanding of PI in prison practice as follows:

> The common retaliatory responses to violence are characterized by splitting and projective mechanisms that see people as 'good' or 'bad' in a black and white way, which is itself similar to the non-thinking, acting-out way of the perpetrators. 'Good' people need to safeguard their own goodness by locating badness in others. This is the universally employed mechanism of defense known as projective identification.
>
> (p.98)

And McGauley (2015) similarly applied the concept to working with females in secure settings: 'All too often the primitive defence mechanisms of splitting, projection and projective identification become mobilised both in violence and in the commonly evoked blaming and retaliatory responses to violence or sexual abuse' (p.205).

To summarise, it is apparent from the literature that an understanding of the process of PI seeks to throw light on the transactions in the prison environment, especially where those transactions are characterised by levels of violence and hostility. Understanding PI, at least according to the wisdom of colleagues, offers the promise of situational thoughtfulness, an understanding of actions and therefore reactions, ultimately pointing to a way of managing and de-escalating distress and violence.

Orthopedagogical practice – prison officer supervision

The following data is drawn from reflection on practice (Schön, 1983, 1987) or as Barton (2008) calls it, 'practitioner ethnography'. The data here was generated retrospectively and drawn together on the merits of case reflection which were considered to be relevant examples that might illustrate theoretical and practice application of the concept of PI. The distinction between prospective narrative-based case study research and reflective data capture is important, and arguably there are clear ethical benefits when naturalistic everyday practice is not sullied by intentional data capture (Winship, 2007). The setting for the case accounts pertains to prisoners held under the security class of category B. All identifying details in the illustrative vignettes here have been removed, and some elements of the data altered to render 'thick disguise' (Gabbard, 2000). The illustrative vignettes selected here have been drawn from recurring themes shared in group supervision encounters collected by qualified clinical supervisors.

Supervision groups on TCs are commonly held once weekly for an hour. The space is established to offer an opportunity for POs to reflect on the range of encounters during the week, and there is evidence that clinical supervision is integral to a successful therapeutic community prison regime operated (Bennet & Shuker, 2017, 2018). As well as the formal group work, the focus of the supervision group may also look across encounters in the everyday milieu of the prison wing. The TC model considers all events to be living-learning opportunities, for example, through shared responsibility such as cleaning, managing food and other domestic duties, as well as leisure and play on the wing. The interpersonal demands of working in a therapeutic forensic setting are complex and emotionally challenging, and the aim of supervision is to seek to understand the dynamics of the offender–PO interaction (Atkinson & Mann, 2012; Mothersole, 2000), where there is the likelihood of re-enactment (Carpy, 1989; Joseph, 1985, 1988) in which relationships between prisoners and staff can come to resemble previous offending patterns and part of what we call offending paralleling behaviour sequences (Daffern, Jones, & Shine, 2010).

The following vignettes provide illustrations of how the theory of PI was made manifest in the course of reflecting on challenging encounters.

Vignette 1

PO members in the supervision group were talking about Peter, a prisoner who had been angry for a number of days after a catalogue of frustrations related to various issues of prison procedure and administration. These procedural frustrations might be ordinarily considered unsurprising, the sort of situations that one would think of as reality confrontation that one would usually face, and work through, but Peter had a short fuse. He had taken to playing music too loudly, and this had created a level of antagonism on the wing that had been escalating in recent days. PO John said that he thought that the music might have been a way of communicating the anger that Peter was not able to do ordinarily through talking, Peter didn't find it easy to speak in groups, and was isolated on the wing generally. There was some discussion about 'attention seeking'. Peter would take to coming into the office and talking to staff, who then often felt cornered by him. While there was a clear and present feeling of irritation among the POs, links were made between Peter's experience of growing up where his mother was often absent through drug misuse. Two of the POs said they often felt that Peter sought them out for attention, because he was needy, and they were concerned that Peter might make the other prisoners resentful because he received more attention from the staff. But they felt resigned, if still somewhat uncomfortable, about having to give Peter attention. In terms of PI, the supervisor was able to draw attention to the way in which Peter was able to elucidate feelings in the POs that seemed to point towards his unmet needs, and that the POs were appreciating Peter's need for a parent figure. And the supervisor wondered if the feeling of being cornered by Peter might also be something of a PI. In other words, as the staff felt cornered, this was a clue to how Peter was feeling. It was at this point in the group that Peter went into the communal group room which was next to the staff office (where group supervision was happening) and turned on the music on the television (the room could be seen through the window of the staff office). One of the POs noticed this, and said: 'here we go'. Sure enough, Peter turned the TV up so loud that it soon became intrusive. One of the POs said: 'he really knows how to press my buttons', and it was apparent that conversation in the group was impacted by the noise. The supervisor said: 'it is quite difficult to think', and one of the POs volunteered to go and turn the music down. The supervisor said that it wasn't his intention or suggestion that the PO should act; rather, it was an observation of what the music was communicating – perhaps Peter did not want to think, and he wanted the group to know what that was like. A short debate ensued as to whether Peter should be asked to turn the music down, and the consensus was that at least for the moment the staff should not act. It was, after all, time when the staff were not to be interrupted and the residents on the wing knew this. The supervision group continued and tolerated the noise as best it could. Then, after about five minutes, two other prisoners (one of whom was the wing chairman) went into the room asked Peter to turn the music down, which he did.

In another supervision session:

Vignette 2

PO David was discussing a community meeting in the morning where two residents had been talking about their harrowing offences involving violence towards others. David said he was struck by a strong feeling that the prisoners were talking without compassion, in way that seemed to numb the seriousness and tragedy of the events. In the small group later, David said that he had felt 'cut-off', and hadn't been able to work out what he should say. Later in supervision his sense of feeling cut-off had turned to anger, and he wanted to know why none of the other group members spoke up. The other staff in the supervision group were likewise angry, and this seemed to offer a level of reasonable outrage that reassured David that he wasn't on his own in holding a moral compass. The supervisor said he wondered if David was feeling the outrage that had otherwise been absent from the group, that this had been split off and perhaps projected into him. Or maybe the group members also felt frozen and numbed, unsure what to do. This feeling of being numb and cut-off seemed important to explore more generally, not just in relation to David's experience but also a more general level of reflection on offending behaviours. The supervision group talked about whether or not the two residents did in fact have any compassion, and whether their lack of compassion was actually the fuel for their offences. David and the supervision group reflected on these ideas, building some thoughtful hypotheses on the criminal mind, and what it takes to commit an offence in terms of switching off feelings, also exploring their own reactions, even on their own capacity to shed compassion and cut themselves off from feelings sometimes at work.

A third and final vignette:

Vignette 3

PO Grace was visibly shaken when she talked about an encounter during the week with Alec, one of the residents who was in prison for a violent sexual assault. Grace had confronted Alex about his behaviour and the fact he seemed to hold scant regard for others. He would come into the office and interrupt his peers when they were speaking to the staff, he would push in the queue at meal times, and so on. When Grace had pointed this out to him he became angry, and he had said to her: 'you keep pushing me and you know what you will get'. The supervision group was able to reflect on the offending parallels: the fact that Grace was a female; Alec's aggressive occupation of spaces that were not his to occupy. The supervisor wondered if the feelings that Grace had experienced were at some level feelings that Alec himself experienced. That is, Grace had been coerced into feeling Alex's own sense of powerlessness and fear through PI. This idea was not easily received at first, and one of the POs thought this line of inquiry was unhelpful, and instead they should be talking about what action should be taken. The supervisor concurred that action should be taken, but wondered where this feeling of fear and powerlessness featured for Alec. A few weeks later, Alec was once again the subject of discussion in the supervision group after Alec had been talking about growing up in a house where his father would be beat his mother and also him and his siblings. The possibility opened up that the staff could consider two sides of Alec, on the one hand the part of him that had a capacity for terrible violence, but on the other hand the part of Alec which had been subject to fear and abuse of power.

Orthopedagogical reflections

Part of the challenge for practitioners working in an intense forensic thera-peutic milieu is to recognise the potential for re-enactments of offending behaviours, but also patterns of re-enactment from earlier developmental stages. In the vignette above, PO David had encountered a re-enactment that had been difficult for him to talk about. David felt uncomfortable at first and then angry later. His reaction was to some extent an intuition. PI was posited as the process by which David had come to be the recipient of disturbing emotions. The group supervision process offered David a chance to share how he was feeling. We know that in the process of PI the recipient needs to have their own 'hooks', that is to say some personal reference points from which to identify the projection (Ogden, 1989), and in the supervision group, the staff were able to consider their own capacity to shut-off feelings. The supervision process served a dual function: there was some awareness about the prisoners and how they functioned, but also some self-awareness for the POs about how the work made them feel.

In the vignette concerning prisoner Alec, understanding the process of PI offered a key to unlocking some new hypotheses about the transactions between Alec and the POs. It is not easy to hold boundaries in the treatment of offenders with severe disturbances and personality disorders who have a proclivity to act out aggressively and sometimes violently (Gilligan, 1999). Group supervision become a space which installed a pause for reflection. The idea that the group might consider where it was that Alec himself had felt intimidated and violated was not a welcome thought. The POs were rightly concerned that boundaries were set and that Alec's intimidating behaviour be challenged. But the supervisor's focus on the emotional exchange arguably created a space for curiosity, and the subsequent receptivity to new knowledge about what lay behind Alec's abusive behaviour. In this case Alec was repeating an experience where he too had suffered.

In the above vignettes, the group supervision process happened weekly for an hour. This is custom and practice. The aim for supervision is for it to be an experience which can stay in the minds of the staff in between supervision groups. This is Casement's (1985) idea that the supervisor becomes an internalised agent in the mind of the supervisee. The supervision therefore offers a containing mental space not just during the time of supervision but also in between supervision sessions. The containment here is thereupon both the physical space of the prison, the bricks, mortar and security of locked doors and fences, as well as the psychical space where the group supervision encounter can hold and contain emotions, as well as offer a space for learning about them. It is beyond the remit of this chapter to unfold the concept of containment in more detail, but in brief Bion (1961) builds on Klein's notion of PI by introducing the concept of the container and the contained. Bion says that the recipient of a projection acts as a container of feelings. The concept of containment here is an act of thoughtfulness, and if the emotions that have been projected can be understood, then the outcome is a sense of being emotionally contained. The task of containment might mean that a PO need not respond initially to a behaviour, request or demand, but sit with trying to understand what is being communicated. This was the case in the vignette above with Peter who was playing his music loudly. The containment process was such that the POs waited until the negative emotional state was understood before taking action. Of course this does not mean that action is always deferred, and of course POs need often to act swiftly, but a capacity to reflect on experience and consider PI offers an extra capability in the armoury of PO skills. The supervisor needs to recognise the dual role of a PO in terms of the task of being actively alert to the necessity of maintaining clear security boundaries, alongside the task of facilitating and educating psychological mindedness.

In the group, the supervisor is exposed to the projective processes and in turn tries to make sense of these projective processes in the group. The projection of the disturbing and frightening work associated with the contact, which has such an intrusive quality with offenders, has a bearing on the supervisor's experience. The supervisor's role is to try and raise to a level of consciousness that which is felt in the group but not easily immediately understood. The task for the supervisor is to recognise the subtle but compound enactments in the supervision group and to try and differentiate that which belongs to the prisoners, and that which is the province of the staff dynamics. Especially in the high-intensity milieu of a prison, there may be a plethora of staff relationships which are in a dynamic flux, sometimes conflictual, sometimes affectionate. POs might well have differences of opinion with each other, and also with the supervisor. The task is to harness this discussion, to create a group milieu where POs can agree to disagree while acceding to democratic intent and always attempting to see how these conflicts are closely tied to the psychic and interpersonal disturbance of the offenders for whom they are responsible (Tucker, Bau, Wagner, Harlem, & Sher, 1992).

The supervisor in this way operates as a thoughtful emotional container for the staff, at the same time ensuring that the task of the supervision group remains focused on the offenders rather than drifts too far into personal 'therapy' for the staff. That is not to say the group supervision should not feel therapeutic for those attending. Main's (1957) paper 'The Ailment', was an effort to understand how the staff relationships in a TC could be disentangled in order that the patient could be seen more lucidly. We might say that in the prison milieu, the challenge of understanding and gauging the staff relationship has similarities. For the supervisor, it is necessary to recognise the dynamic flux of the staff group relationship and the inherent anxieties this might bring and to get engaged with this, but also the supervisor needs to stay one step removed from the flux in order to keep a clear head. The supervisor becomes a sort of external gatekeeper, ensuring that the task of supervising the group remains focused on the clients rather than drifting too far into personal therapy or becoming a staff group sensitivity session (Winship & Hardy, 1999). Hinshelwood (1994) talks about the satellite function of the supervisor as being both present enough to facilitate engagement but separate enough to keep a clear head. Sedlak (1997) highlights that for untrained practitioners, the emotional strain of the work is often hard to manage, especially for new staff. Supervision offers a gradual and sustained education where POs can learn about the idea of PI and how this knowledge can be applied in practice. The group offers a space for looking into the offender's inner world and discovering mental states which are characterised by despair, anger, trauma, neglect, frustration and so on, but also space for imaginative inquiry where POs can be curious about themselves and how they tick. As Driver (2008) states: 'The aim of supervision is to engage the supervisee's internal world and stimulate dialogue between the conscious and unconscious in an internal dialectic that generates insight' (p.17).

We believe there is a case for a more ubiquitous application of the orthopedagogical potential of group supervision for POs across the prison estate, and also where not ordinarily practiced in other secure settings. The idea that there is an educative potential which can bring about a greater level of social cohesion is in keeping with the orthopedagogical philosophy of colleagues like Eric Broekaert and others (Broekaert, Vandevelde, & Briggs, 2011; Vanderplassen, Vandevelde, Van Damme, & Yates, 2017) where the aim is to develop an education approach with the express purpose of fostering social justice for communities of stakeholders, including those who might be otherwise marginalised with particular educational needs (Maeyer, Vandenbussche, Claes, & Reynaert, 2017). Prisons are such environments which face particular challenges to learning, where the values of prisoners are the subject of corrective intentions. The 'ortho' in this case applies to the corrective aspiration, where the aim for the prison milieu is to help prisoners develop prosocial ways of interacting and the task for the staff is to identify the living–learning situations where this can take place. The 'pedagogy' in this instance is the social science of that education process. As far as we are aware, an orthopedagoical perspective has not been so clearly applied to prison settings. There is scope to deepen our understanding of the ways in which regular supervision for prison officers could improve prison outcomes.

The benefits of supervision, if rolled out more widely, will go some way to meeting the agenda for 'prison safety and reform' in regard to supporting staff and building capability. In the current climate, the stress that POs face is substantial, and the result is that it is a significant challenge to retain staff. Many prisons suffer chronic staffing shortages, and this leads to a cycle of inexperience where there is an absence of senior staff who can provide a secure base for new staff to learn. The establishment of supervision for POs more widely across the prison estate may go some way to providing a therapeutically informed environment which not only alleviates stress but also provides a solid and sustained foundation for staff education, encouraging retention in the long run to the benefit of the whole prison.

Note

1 This chapter is based on the paper: Winship, G., Shaw, S., & Haigh, R. (2019). Group supervision for prison officers: An orthopedagogical approach to emotional management. *The Journal of Forensic Psychiatry & Psychology, 30* (6), 1006–20, https://doi.org/10.1080/14789949.2019.1673794

References

Aslan, L. (2018). Doing time on a TC: How effective are drug-free therapeutic communities in prison? A review of the literature. *Therapeutic Communities: The International Journal of Therapeutic Communities, 39* (1), 26–34.

Atkinson, D.F., & Mann, R.E. (2012). Prison officers as observers of offence paralleling behaviours: An untapped resource? *The Journal of Forensic Psychiatry & Psychology, 23* (2), 139–55.

Barton, T.D. (2008). Understanding practitioner ethnography. *Nurse Researcher, 15* (2), 7–18.

Baudry, F.D. (1993). The personal dimension and management of the supervisory situation with a special note to the parallel process. *Psychoanalytic Quarterly, 62*, 588–614.

Bennett, J., & Shuker, R. (2017). The potential of prison-based democratic therapeutic communities. *International Journal of Prisoner Health, 13*, (1), 19–24.

Bennett, J., & Shuker, R. (2018). Hope, harmony and humanity: Creating a positive social climate in a democratic therapeutic community prison and the implications for penal practice. *Journal of Criminal Psychology, 8*, (1), 44–57.

Benson, J., & Magraith, K. (2005). Compassion fatigue and burnout: The role of Balint groups. *Australian Family Physician, 34*, (6), 497–502.

Bion, W. (1961). *Experiences in groups.* Basic Books.

Bion, W.R. (1962).. *Learning from experience.* Heinemann.

Broekaert, E., Vandevelde, S., & Briggs, D. (2011) The postmodern application of holistic education. *Therapeutic Communities, 32* (1) 18–34.

Brooker, C., Repper, J., Sirdifield, C., & Gojkovic, D. (2009). Review of service delivery and organisational research focused on prisoners with mental disorders. *The Journal of Forensic Psychiatry & Psychology, 20* (1), 102–23.

Carpy, D.V. (1989). Tolerating the countertransference: A mutative process. *International Journal of Psychoanalysis, 70*, 287–94.

Casement, P (1985) *Learning from the patient.* Routledge.

Clarke, J. (2012). *The resilient practitioner. Forensic psychology in practice: a practitioners handbook.* Palgrave Macmillan.

Cooke, E., Stephenson, Z., & Rose, J. (2017). How do professionals experience working with offenders diagnosed with personality disorder within a prison environment? *The Journal of Forensic Psychiatry & Psychology, 28* (6), 841–62.

Crawley, E. (2004). *Doing prison work: The public and private lives of prison officers.* Willan.

Daffern, M., Jones, L., & Shine, J. (2010). *Offence paralleling behaviour: A case formulation approach to offender assessment and intervention.* Wiley.

Doctor, R. (2003). *Dangerous patients. A psychodynamic approach to risk assessment and management.* Karnac Books.

Driver, C. (2008). Assessment in supervision: An analytic perspective. *British Journal of Psychotherapy, 24* (3), 328–42.

Fountain, G. (2000). A critical review of the concept of projective identification and its clinical applications. *Psychoanalytic Quarterly, 69* (1), 189–90.

Gabbard, G.O. (2000). Disguise or consent: Problems and recommendations concerning the publication and presentation of clinical material. *International Journal of Psychoanalysis, 81*, 1071–86.

Gilligan, J. (1999). *Violence: Reflections on our deadliest epidemic.* Jessica Kingsley.

Gordon, J. (2004). Review of dangerous patients. *Psychoanalytic Psychotherapy, 18*, 347–51.

Haigh, R. (2000). Support systems. 2. Staff sensitivity groups. *Advances in Psychiatric Treatment, 6* (4), 312–19.

Hinshelwood, R. (1993). Locked in role: A psychotherapist within the social defence system of a prison. *The Journal of Forensic Psychiatry, 4* (3), 427–40.

Hinshelwood, R.D. (1994). The relevance of psychotherapy. *Psychoanalytic Psychotherapy, 8*, 283–94.

HMIP. (2016). *HM Chief Inspector of Prisons for England and Wales Annual Report 2015–16.* www.gov.uk/government/uploads/system/uploads/attachment_data/file/538854/hmip-annual-report.pdf

Johnston, P. (2003). £150,00 award for prison officer on sex wing. *The Telegraph*, 1 April.

Joseph, B. (1985). Transference: The total situation. *International Journal of Psychoanalysis, 66*, 447–54.

Joseph, N., & Benefield, N. (2012). A joint offender personality disorder pathway strategy: An outline summary. *Criminal Behaviour and Mental Health, 22*, 210–17.

Klein, M. (1946). Notes on some schizoid mechanisms. *International Journal of Psychoanalysis, 27*, 99–110.

Kurtz, A. (2005). The needs of staff who care for people with a diagnosis of personality disorder who are considered a risk to others. *The Journal of Forensic Psychiatry & Psychology, 16* (2), 399–422.

Liebling, A., Price, D., & Shefer, G. (2011). *The prison officer*. Willan.

Maeyer, J. D, Vandenbussche, H., Claes, C., & Reynaert, D. (2017). Human rights, the capability approach and quality of life: An integrated paradigm of support in the quest for social justice. *Therapeutic Communities, 38* (3), 156–62.

Magor-Blatch, L., Bhullar, N., Thomson, B., and Thorsteinsson, E. (2014). A systematic review of studies examining effectiveness of therapeutic communities. *The International Journal of Therapeutic Communities, 35* (4), 168–84.

Main, T.F. (1957). The ailment. *Psychology and Psychotherapy: Theory, Research and Practice, 30* (3), 129–45.

Marriott, S. (2007). Applying a psychodynamic treatment model to support an adolescent sentenced for murder to confront and manage feelings of shame and remorse. *The Journal of Forensic Psychiatry & Psychology, 18* (2), 248–60.

McGauley, G. (2015). Increasing the pro-social and decreasing risk: An overarching aim of forensic psychotherapy. *Psychoanalytic Psychotherapy, 29* (3), 205–10.

Meloy, J.R. (1988). *The psychopathic mind: Origins, dynamics and treatment.* Jason Aronson.

Ministry of Justice. (2016). *Safety in Custody Statistics Bulletin England and Wales.* www.gov.uk/governmentuploadssystem/uploads/attachment_data/file/543284/safety-in-custody-bulletin.pdf

Ministry of Justice & Department of Health. (2012). *A Guide to Psychologically Informed Planned Environments (PIPEs).* Ministry of Justice and Department of Health.

Mothersole, G. (2000). Clinical supervision and forensic work. *Journal of Sexual Aggression, 5*, 45–58.

Ogden, T. (1989). *The primitive edge of experience.* Jason Aronson.

Pearce, S., Scott, L., Attwood, G., Saunders, K., Dean, M., De Ridder, R., & Crawford, M. (2017) Democratic therapeutic community treatment for personality disorder: Randomised controlled trial. *British Journal of Psychiatry, 210* (2), 149–56.

Pedder, J.R. (2011). *Attachment and new beginnings.* (G. Winship, Ed.). Karnac Books.

Pollock, P., & Belshaw, T. (1998). Cognitive analytic therapy for offenders. *The Journal of Forensic Psychiatry, 9* (3), 629–42.

Rosenfeld, H.A. (1965). *Psychotic states.* Hogarth Press.

Schön, D.A. (1983). *The reflective practitioner.* Basic Books.

Schön, D.A. (1987). *Educating the reflective practitioner.* Jossey-Bass.

Sedlak, V. (1997). Psychoanalytic supervision of untrained therapists. In B. Martindale, M. Morner, M.E.C. Rodriguez, & J.P. Vidit (Eds.). *Supervision and its vicissistudes* (pp.25–38). Karnac.

Segal, H. (1997). The uses and abuses of countertransference. *Psychoanalysis, literature and war: Papers 1972–1995* (J. Steiner, Ed.). Routledge.

Tucker, L., Bau, S., Wagner, S., Harlem, D., & Sher, I. (1992). Specialised extended hospital treatment for borderline patient. *Bulletin of the Menninger Clinic, 56,* 465–78.

Vanderplasschen, W., Vandevelde, S., Van Damme, L., & Yates, R. (2017). A search for integrating science, arts and practice: The legacy of Prof. Eric Broekaert. *Therapeutic Communities, 38* (3), 121–24.

Walker, T., Shaw, J., Hamilton, L., Turpin, C., Reid, C., & Abel, K. (2017). Coping with the job: Prison staff responding to self-harm in three English female prisons: a qualitative study. *The Journal of Forensic Psychiatry & Psychology, 28* (6), 811–24.

Welldon, E.V. (1993). Forensic psychotherapy and group analysis. *Group Analysis, 26,* 487–502.

Welldon, E.V. (1997). Let the treatment fit the crime: Forensic group psychotherapy. *Group Analysis, 30,* 9–26.

Welldon, E.V. (2015). Definition of forensic psychotherapy and its aims. *International Journal of Applied Psychoanalytic Studies, 12* (2), 96–105.

Winship, G. (2007). The ethics of reflective research in single case study inquiry. *Perspectives in Psychiatric Care, 43* (4), 174–82.

Winship, G., & Hardy, S. (1999). Disentangling group dynamics: Staff group sensitivity and supervision. *Journal of Psychiatric and Mental Health Nursing, 6,* 307–12.

Yerushalmi, H. (1999). The roles of group supervision of supervision. *Psychoanalytic Psychology, 16* (3), 426–47.

Opbygningsgården's drug rehabilitation programme at Kragskovhede Prison in Denmark

4

Hanne Holm Hage-Ali and
Johnny Lindblad Reinhardt

Prologue

Both the therapeutic process and the presence of the therapist help the person undergoing treatment in reaching his goals over time. This happens as a result of the direct impact of two people meeting, the phenomenological approach and not least the reciprocity between the two parties. Two people meeting, with all their attention focussed on the here and now, absorbing the key moments of the meeting - these are all essential components. Meeting the person in treatment makes demands on the therapist, first and foremost on a personal level, but also on a professional level, as the skills of the therapist are put to the test in the context of that meeting. Change occurs reciprocally yet differently, when the person and the therapist meet in an atmosphere, where appreciation, equality, acceptance and humanity are all characteristic of the approach the therapist uses at the meeting. The person undergoing treatment needs an environment where he can feel calm and safe, so that he can get to know himself and slowly build his confidence, with the result that he emerges into a reality where experience, realisation and consciousness about values and choices gradually manifest themselves during the process, with the therapist acting as the facilitator of that process.

In treatment terms, giving the person the opportunity to learn more about himself is seen as critical. Being aware of yourself and the world around you is the best way to learn to navigate all the demands placed on you as regards family, work, and society in general. The recovery process is about becoming aware of what it means to be a person, coming to terms with the circumstances of your life, and making that life as meaningful as possible.

US
Until I can see myself in you,
I cannot acknowledge myself.
I want to meet you in a spirit of mutuality and respect.

DOI: 10.4324/9780429317460-5

When I recognise myself in you and in others
I understand without words
Love for everything that grows.

(M.T. Ness)

From "Glimpses and echoes from Nothing" by M.T. Ness

Opbygningsgården has been providing residential drug treatment since 1977. Located in the north-west of Denmark near Thisted, it was originally a farm but was then rebuilt and turned into a drug treatment unit, with both therapists and residents living there – hence the name 'Opbygningsgården', which literally means 'build up farm' in Danish. It lies in very homely surroundings, and until 1991 it was a treatment commune. It became a therapeutic community (TC) in 1991, when two therapists from a TC in Norway called 'Veksthuset' ('hot house') introduced the TC treatment model to Opbygningsgården. They spent the next few years implementing the TC model at Opbygningsgården. It is the only drug treatment unit in Denmark using the TC method, which has caused us some problems over the years, for example, the lack of professional sparring with other Danish TCs. It is essential that our treatment model continues to develop and evolve over time, in the same way as society, culture and legislation in Denmark evolves. Sparring with other Danish TC's, for example, discussing and sharing ideas on how to adapt the TC treatment model in Denmark, would have been of great benefit, but as stated this has not been possible. Attending international TC conferences and reading literature about other TCs is therefore an important part of our work. It has also been important for us to visit TCs in other countries. Every time we visit a TC in another country, we always feel at home, in spite of the cultural and linguistic differences, because the TC treatment method's elements, the weekly schedule and the physical environment (e.g. 'the bench' and the 'slip box') are the same at TCs all over the world. We have also discovered that our TC in Denmark has evolved in a very similarl way to TCs in other countries over the past few years.

Opbygningsgården has experienced many changes since it started as a TC in 1991, and our TC has a less hierarchical and more democratic approach to drug treatment now than when it started. Our aim is to provide an environment where each resident is the main agent in his/her own treatment programme, and the 'community' is the framework in which the treatment takes place. Many of the TC elements have been adjusted over the years, so they are appropriate for the people coming to Opbygningsgården for treatment nowadays. We have had to discard some elements, because they no longer make sense in the world we live in today. TCs are about change on an individual level. On an organisational level, the process of change can be just as cumbersome and difficult for the staff as it is for the individual residents. Throughout the process of change, our focus has been on our desire to continue being a

TC. Every time we have wanted to implement a change to our treatment programme, we have had to ask ourselves what the essence of the TC is, and how we can go about implementing the change in question without losing that essence. Community as method, help through helping yourself and the daily structure of activities are three essential elements of the TC treatment model which we will never discard.

The Danish government implemented a new system of regional inspectorates in 2014, whose remit is inspecting and monitoring all forms of social institutions, including drug rehabilitation treatment centres such as Opbygningsgården. The five regional inspectorates supervise the quality of the services provided by social institutions such as ours. The inspectorate's monitoring of our services involves checking that we do not infringe the legal rights of our residents. This is in line with our own commitment to upholding the ethical guidelines and Bill of Rights for Members and Clients, issued by the European Federation of Therapeutic Communities (EFTC), in the way we treat the residents in our treatment programme. It is very important that the residents enter the treatment programme voluntarily and take part in all aspects of the programme voluntarily. The residents have the fundamental right not to be subjected to the use of force in any shape or form.

The Danish Prison and Probation Service approached Opbygningsgården in 2011 to ask if we might be interested in setting up a drug treatment unit using the TC treatment model in a prison in Denmark called Kragskovhede Statsfængsel. We submitted a tender for the contract, in which we explained how the TC treatment method works. We won the contract, and the TC treatment unit opened at the prison in 2012, with 14 residents. Before the new unit opened, we visited a prison near Liverpool in the United Kingdom with a large well-run TC treatment unit. The visit inspired us, and the feeling of being in well-known surroundings struck us when we visited the prison, as we saw how the daily routine operated in the prison TC, with its daily morning meeting and all the other routines from the daily structure of activities we knew so well from our own TC in Denmark. We have also been able to recreate the special atmosphere that exists in a TC in our own prison treatment unit here in Denmark.

We currently have two treatment units at the prison – a residential unit treating 26 inmates, and an ambulant unit treating another 90 inmates. In order to provide drug treatment in Danish prisons, the treatment model in use has to be accredited by the Danish Prison and Probation Service. The accreditation process is extremely rigorous. We were required to produce extensive documentation about the TC treatment model and how it operated in our treatment unit at the prison. We had to present this documentation to a panel of leading Danish experts in the field of drug treatment. We did not succeed in our first attempt at accreditation. We were told that the panel of experts found our way of thinking and the TC treatment model foreign and strange in relation to their understanding of drug treatment. We often encounter this problem when we try to describe how a TC works. We were successful in being accredited in our second attempt, as we were better able to describe what we do at the TC in such a way that the panel could relate it to the theoretical framework for drug treatment, which they were more familiar with.

The focus of this chapter is not on the TC model and its elements, but rather on the various measures we have taken to ensure that the TC treatment model is able to function properly in a prison setting.

Opbygningsgården's drug treatment unit at Kragskovhede Open Prison

Before describing our drug treatment unit, it is necessary to describe a Danish 'open' prison, as this is not something which is well known or practiced to any great extent in other countries.

Virtually all inmates in the Danish prison system can serve part of their sentence in an open prison. However, it is usually inmates with relatively short sentences who are able to serve in an open prison. But inmates who have served a large part of their sentence in a closed prison (the more usual type of prison) can often serve the remainder of their sentence in an open prison.

An open prison has no high walls, but the inmates all know where the boundaries of the prison are. If an inmate goes outside the boundary without permission, he will probably end up back in a closed prison. It is therefore unusual for inmates to escape from an open prison, because they know the consequences of escaping. Such an action could also have a negative impact on an inmate's chances of being granted parole.

When a person is sentenced to prison and arrives at Kragskovhede Prison, he undergoes a screening process, conducted by one of the prison social workers. The inmate is then allocated a job at the prison – all inmates have to work between 8:00 a.m. and 3:30 p.m., Monday through Friday. A resource profile is also drawn up, using a variety of criteria, which outlines the measures required to support the inmate during his time at the prison, for example, help with literacy problems or anger management. The prison uses a Canadian screening tool called Level of Service/Risk, Need, Responsivity (LS/RNR) to conduct a risk assessment of the inmates, as they in addition to criminal behaviour, a criminal way of thinking and violent behaviour, often have drug-related problems they need to address as part of their resocialisation process.

Inmates can apply for drug treatment at the prison – either in the drug treatment unit (residential care) or as ambulant treatment, where they continue to live in another wing of the prison and attend the treatment unit on a daily basis. Danish law stipulates that everyone in Denmark has the right to drug treatment within 14 days of applying, even those serving time in prison.

Opbygningsgården is the sole provider of addiction treatment at Kragkovhede Prison, be it for the treatment of drug abuse, alcohol addiction, gambling and so on.

The residents and their daily activities in the residential drug treatment unit

Most of the inmates have a long history of crime and drug addiction. They have led lives with a great deal of stress and pressure from their surroundings and their families. Many of them have lived a double life, where they have had to lie and deceive people to 'survive' on a daily basis. Some of the inmates in our treatment programme have described the relief they felt when they were arrested and were finally able to get away from the very pressurised and stressful lives they had been leading, and that they were finally able to come clean and tell their closest family members about the reasons for their errant behaviour.

It therefore became clear to us, how important restitution and learning to relax are in the treatment programme. The inmates need to have time to relax and not be doing chores all day. Relaxing is a difficult exercise for many of the inmates, especially for those who have never been able to relax or alleviate the chaos they feel inside without taking illicit drugs.

We can clearly see when the inmates start to relax and gain a greater sense of inner calm, as the harsh lines on their faces soften, and the tension in their bodies dissipates. We can see this in the new inmates after only a short time in the treatment programme.

It is also easier for the inmates to look inwards and reflect on their behaviour, attitudes and beliefs, when they let their guard down and are not in such a state of high alert the whole time.

Ethnicity

Historically speaking – we are talking here about a year ago – we seemed to have difficulty in attracting inmates with other ethnic backgrounds than Danish to apply to enter our treatment programme, and the ethnicity of our unit's inmates did not therefore reflect the ethnicity of the prison population in general. As there have been many inmates with other ethnic backgrounds at the prison over the years, we were keen for such inmates to apply for treatment as well. We have not really taken any concrete action to investigate *why* it might be that inmates with other ethnic backgrounds do not apply to our treatment programme. But in our experience the best way to attract inmates to apply is to explain clearly to them what they can expect from the programme. We do now have some inmates from different ethnic backgrounds in the programme, so the unit better reflects the ethnicity of the prison population as a whole. These inmates have proved to be good role models, which in turn helps attract other inmates from different ethnic backgrounds to apply for treatment. We have not experienced tensions/problems between the various ethnic groups. Individual dietary requirements, such as inmates who do not eat pork, are also taken into account by the inmates, when planning the weekly meals.

Relaxation

Relaxation is one of the interventions we use in the programme, both in terms of relaxation such as mindfulness and yoga, which are a planned part of the weekly programme of activities, and more spontaneous relaxation where the inmates have time to relax and do nothing, which is not always easy for them!

The resocialisation of the inmates is a high political priority. Achieving successful resocialisation, so inmates are drug free and able to provide for themselves when they are released from prison, or are able to live on social benefits with a minimum amount of drug taking (harm reduction), requires more than action plans and setting goals, if the desired changes in the way the inmates think and behave are to become fully integrated into the way the inmates live their lives after prison.

It is important that the inmates learn to make time for themselves to reflect on how they feel about life, whilst serving their sentence and after prison, so that they do not feel that their time in the programme is simply a pointless treadmill they have to endure for a short time, because they have not understood what is meaningful, but are just trying to live up to other people's expectations in terms of making changes to their lives.

Mindfulness has many elements, involving both introspection and medi-tation, and the inmates learn to focus and gain an insight into how the mind, with its thoughts and feelings, works. They learn to separate thought from action and not identify themselves with their thoughts.

Teaching the inmates about philosophical reflection is also an element of our treatment programme. We introduce them to the ideas of various 'great' thinkers. Immanuel Kant's moral philosophy is one example we use, with regard to how you wish to act in the world and the environment you live in.

In our experience, the inmates are generally very interested in thinking more deeply about things and questioning their own views and attitudes, and they find to their surprise, that it can give them a new view of themselves and the world around them.

Yoga classes are a popular element of our programme, but it gave rise to some scepticism at first, because it is so different from the weight training and physical exercise which the inmates are more used to doing when they go to the gym. The inmates are, however, very quick to unite 'mind and body' and to understand the rationale behind it.

The challenges involved in providing drug treatment in a prison setting

It is a fact that there are many drugs in circulation in an open prison, and it is very easy for the inmates to get hold of drugs. If an inmate appears to be high, the staff will tell the inmate about their suspicions. We make it clear at the initial interview with any inmate wishing to enter our treatment programme, that the programme is a *collaboration* between the staff and the inmates, and that collaboration involves the staff expressing their thoughts and commenting on what they see as regards an inmate's behaviour. (A representative for the inmates in our treatment programme is always present at the interviews.)

The criminal element, for example, exchanging 'good' ideas and tips about criminal activities, is also a large part of prison life. The prison only has male inmates, and there are both so-called strong and weak prisoners. It can some-times be difficult for the staff to fully make sense of the various agendas the inmates might have.

Not all the inmates regard their criminality as a problem, apart from the problem that they have been caught and sentenced to prison for their criminal activities. Some of the inmates have grown up in an environment where drug taking and crime have been the order of the day. Many of them have grown up in very dysfunctional families.

We need to provide input and raise awareness amongst the inmates about many other issues than simply those related to drug taking.

We often use videos and give talks to the inmates as a way of helping them understand the nature of addiction in all its forms. For example, when we are unhappy as children, it affects our brains and our way of understanding and tackling the world we live in.

We played a YouTube video called 'Addiction' for the inmates, which they found very thought provoking, as it graphically demonstrated how addicts react to dysfunction. They could also relate to Gabor Mate's TED talk, as it filled them with a sense of relief. The rationale is that people react to something, which is not good for them. Drugs are 'pain killers', albeit just for a short time, but drug taking is an understandable and in some cases necessary escape when a person's life is not functioning properly.

Our approach and the philosophy behind it

Part of the philosophy of our treatment model is that when some problem, issue or inappropriate behaviour emerges, then it needs to be brought out into the open, discussed and constructive action taken. If an inmate refuses to be open about (repeated) relapses or other inappropriate behaviour, which is not conducive to collaboration between the staff and the inmates (the 'community'), then there could be consequences for him, in terms of whether he will be allowed to remain in the treatment programme or not. In a situation where an inmate's behaviour is a cause for concern, the well-being of the whole community will be taken into account when deciding whether to expel him from the treatment programme or not. The problems faced by one inmate are often taken up in general terms by the therapists with the whole group, as the treatment unit is relatively small and the inmates often know about each other's problems before the therapists hear about them.

It takes a lot of work on the part of the therapists to make the environment in the programme feel safe for the inmates and conducive to dealing with the serious problems they have, with regard to their drug taking and other social problems. The expertise of the therapists is fundamental to making this happen. They do this by breathing down their necks, confronting and challenging the inmates, but in a supportive and caring way.

Physical activity

Physical activity is very important. The inmates take part in physical activities several times a week. This includes ball games, going to the gym, jogging and so on. The treatment unit has its own garden, and the inmates have built a beach volley court and a boules green. Both are used extensively by the inmates and the staff, and this strengthens the sense of community amongst the inmates, promoting both physical and mental well-being amongst the inmates and the unit's staff.

The garden also has a small area where the inmates can grow vegetables, to everyone's benefit.

Food

We place a great deal of importance on providing healthy and varied food in the treatment unit. The inmates are responsible for preparing the meals and ensuring that there is salad and/or vegetables with every meal.

Once a week, two inmates and a prison warder drive to the nearest supermarket to do the weekly shopping. The inmates take turns preparing meals, and they have just introduced a 'chef of the week' award, which the inmates give to the inmate who has made a particularly tasty evening meal during the week. The inmates also eat lunch together.

Harm reduction

Opbygningsgården and Kragskovhede Prison take the issue of harm reduction very seriously. Unfortunately, not all inmates are able to stop taking drugs totally, not even when they are in residential drug treatment. We therefore provide support to inmates who find it difficult to quit drugs completely, and we work in collaboration with the health professionals at the prison. It might be that a particular type of medication can replace the joints an inmate usually smokes to help him go to sleep at night, and in the long term this might help give the inmate more hope for the future, that legal forms of medication can provide relief rather than having to resort to illegal drugs which require criminal activity to acquire.

Influence

The inmates often come to the staff with their own ideas and suggestions regarding activities in the treatment unit. An inmate once suggested the idea of having a 'Christmas comes early' activity, in the form of one chosen inmate receiving 'presents' from the other members of the community. The inmates meet in one of the group rooms, and each person has in advance written on a piece of paper (anonymously and without conferring with the others), what he regards as positive attributes about the chosen inmate. The inmates can also give well-meaning advice. The comments on the slips of paper are read aloud to the inmate who has been chosen to receive the 'presents'. It is a very constructive and affirmative process. Sometimes the inmate in question learns new things he did not already know about himself. The inmates often write similar things on their slips of paper.

We have found that the inmates on occasion have felt that the staff, that is, the therapists, social workers and prison warders, have led privileged lives and have never faced any problems of their own. This sometimes causes a 'them and us' mentality, which may or may not be justified. It has meant, though, that some therapists have decided to tell the inmates about their lives and backgrounds – not to belittle or denigrate the many problems which the inmates have to deal with, but rather as a way of giving them a different perspective and adding some light and shade to the picture the inmates have of the staff.

Most of the therapists are in their forties and fifties and they have suffered ups and downs in their lives, as all people do, and they have told the inmates about them, especially the downs. This has won them a certain respect from the inmates and has meant that the 'them and us' mentality has been downplayed for a while, but it will probably emerge again at some point, as inmates leave the programme and new ones enter it.

Our collaboration with other professions at the prison

Opbygningsgården's treatment unit currently has 26 inmates. We have two sections, with 16 inmates in one and ten in the other. The sections are located next each other, along one long corridor, with a staff office for the prison warders and the therapists in the middle, dividing the two sections.

We also has an ambulant section, providing drug treatment in the form of individual therapy and group therapy to an average of 90 inmates living in other sections of the prison.

We work closely with the prison warders in the day-to-day running of the two sections. They are an important resource, helping and supporting the therapists in their work. We are constantly trying to improve and extend our collaboration with the other professions working in the prison. From a historical perspective it has been a process of getting very different professions and cultures to meet and work together, developing their practice in the drug treatment programme, ensuring the control and the care aspects of running the programme work in harmony, with respect for each profession, in a credible, trusting and authentic collaboration.

It is our belief that the level of collaboration amongst the staff in the programme – both therapists and other professionals – is reflected in the inmates and how they collaborate. It is worth pointing out that in all the time that Opbygningsgården has been running the drug treatment unit at the prison, there have never been any incidences of violence or threats of serious violence in the unit.

We also have a social worker attached to the treatment programme. She helps the inmates with problems concerning housing, social benefits, debt and so on. It is very important that the action plan drawn up by the social worker (in collaboration with the inmate) complements the action plan our therapists draw up in collaboration with the inmate.

Unfortunately – or maybe fortunately – it is often the case that an inmate who has been released from prison, enters our programme for a second time, due to being sentenced to prison again. This is unfortunate, meaning that things did not go as planned for the inmate, but also fortunate, meaning that the inmate wishes to continue his drug treatment and build on what he learned during his previous time in the programme.

Inmates who have spent time in our treatment unit often wish to come back to it again. If an inmate's participation in Opbygningsgården's treatment unit is curtailed due to repeatedly breaking our ground rules or guidelines, or due to a lack of motivation, we take great pains to ensure that the inmate leaves the programme in a proper and sober fashion, so the inmate can apply to return to Opbygningsgården in the future, once he feels that he is more ready and motivated to deal with his drug addiction.

It often happens that when an inmate stops his treatment and leaves the residential programme, he continues receiving treatment in our ambulant section. This is usually because the inmate already knows the therapists in the ambulant section, (either because the inmate has had treatment in our ambulant section before entering the residential unit, or because he has met the ambulant section therapists, who also spend time in the residential unit, from time to time). This ensures continuity in the inmate's treatment, and the inmate is not made to feel excluded, despite having left the residential programme, but feels he is still being taken seriously in his desire to do something about his addiction problem.

It might appear to outsiders that inmates who have taken part in our residential treatment programme apply to come back again because they think it is the easiest way to serve out their prison time, rather than because they are serious about receiving drug treatment. But this is not generally the case. The community (which is involved right from the beginning, as an inmate representing the community takes part in the preliminary interview with all inmates applying to enter the programme) makes it clear to all potential inmates that it will make certain demands on the inmates, which in fact are harder to fulfil than the demands an inmate faces in an ordinary section of the prison, where the inmates are left more to their own devices and are not accountable to a community, as is the case in Opbygningsgården's treatment programme.

Our view on humanity

Our approach to drug treatment is based on a phenomenological view of human beings and is also reflected in the respect with which the inmates are met in everyday life in the programme. Openness and a total lack of prejudice from the therapists provide the ideal environment for the inmates to really relax and be who they are, and for helping them find out who they are, or who they want to be!

Our focus is on the *process* of change and on ensuring that all the inmates experience progression in relation to their own goals – either in a qualitative or a quantitative sense.

There are laws and regulations, which have to be adhered to, and we work very hard to ensure that we follow the action plans which have been drawn up for the inmates. Our ultimate aim in an ideal world is that all the inmates become drug free or reduce their drug intake. It is obviously the ultimate achievement if they can earn their own living and contribute positively to society. But if that is not possible, then receiving state benefits, having a greater appetite for life, where values such as reciprocity, honesty and caring for themselves are manifested in their lives and are helping them towards their goal of leading a happier and more peaceful life, are also great achievements.

We ask the inmates to complete a self-evaluation form before leaving the unit, and the things they write are often very moving and touching.

How we organise our treatment programmes

The treatment provided by our ambulant section takes the form of a series of individual conversations between the therapist and the inmate, and we also offer NADA (a type of acupuncture in the ear which has been shown to relieve withdrawal symptoms and improve treatment engagement and retention) and mindfulness – both of which are also offered in our residential unit.

The ambulant and the residential sections work closely together, and we use the ambulant section as a forum for preparing inmates for the move to the residential unit, and for treating inmates who have finished the residential programme but have not yet been released from prison.

We currently have six therapists working in the residential unit, and three therapists working in the ambulant section.

Continuous development and refinement of our treatment concept

We use the TC's elements but have had to adapt and refine them, so that they are applicable to the prison setting. Opbygningsgården is a TC, but we have obviously had to adapt our treatment model, as times, culture and society have changed, and to meet the ever-changing requirements and demands of the authorities who pay us to provide drug treatment.

During our six years running the prison programme we have stuck to the TC treatment model, but we have had to rename some of the TC elements to make them more contemporary, as many of the TC terms we used to use stemmed from the 1970s and 1980s and had become outmoded.

The therapists have become team players to a much greater extent in the treatment setting in the prison, as it is extremely important, especially for new inmates, that the therapists are very visible in the day-to-day running of the unit. This is also a result of the need for shorter and more intensive treatment programmes, due to shorter sentences.

The therapists have their job to do as therapists, but they are on a level footing with the inmates and are very happy to do things with the inmates, preparing meals and participating in other activities in the residential unit. The therapists are very visible 'on the floor' so that they can support and help the 'community as method' treatment method to function properly.

We have musical instruments in the residential unit, and we organise many other recreational activities, for example, painting and making bracelets.

We are convinced that creative activities help form and develop the brain, and being involved in a creative process also gives the inmates a sense of peace and calm.

Eclectic interventions

Our 50-page-long accreditation document describes our methods on a more theoretical level. We work eclectically. That is, we use different types of interventions, based on the competences of our various therapists, and not least according to the given situation. We do not, however, take action without careful consideration of the situation, and we do not, for example, use the 12-stage model. Our therapists need to know what they are doing, and why they are doing what they are doing.

Our professionalism and an awareness of which interventions to use and why in any given situation are extremely high on our agenda in the daily running of the treatment unit, and there is room for differences of opinion and discussion. Displaying a sense of humour, using appropriate language and showing respect play a large part in the working relationships we have with each other.

We describe our approach to treatment as being 'deliberately naive' – both in terms of our professional approach and our view on humanity – which means that we believe that what is said and done are true. It usually proves to be the case that this naivete frees us from having to be paranoid and take on the role of policeman. If an inmate looks as if he is high on drugs but claims that he is not, we can choose to believe the inmate's explanation but still confront the inmate by saying, 'even though you say that you have not taken any drugs, your behaviour means that you need to go to your cell now, and you also need to change your behaviour, as it is having a bad effect on the other people in the community, when you look and behave like you are high'. In some instances the inmate will admit to having had a relapse, but sometimes his behaviour is due to other factors (e.g. illness, emotional problems or tiredness), which come to light when the therapist talks to the inmate.

We have no doubt that the *community* is the decisive factor for creating an effective treatment programme in a prison environment. The therapists have individual sessions with the inmates, giving them the opportunity to open up and explore the personal problems they are facing. Opbygningsgården has a broad range of interventions, which provide the inmates with an effective treatment programme in safe and caring surroundings, with competent staff who support and work closely with the inmates during their time in the unit.

The therapists' backgrounds and our range of therapeutic interventions

Many of the therapists have backgrounds as nursery nurses, having worked with children and adults with special needs. Our staff also includes a social worker, a criminologist, a therapist (formerly a prison warder), and a health assistant.

Motivational interviewing (MI), gestalt therapy, cognitive therapy, a narrative approach, philosophical pedagogy, mindfulness and NADA are among the range of therapeutic interventions used on a daily basis in our treatment programme, both on a one-to-one basis and in groups.

The therapists have monthly group supervision sessions, and also participate in group supervision with the prison warders and the social workers once a month.

Staff can also receive individual supervision as required.

We hold staff meetings on a weekly basis.

There are also meetings with Opbygningsgården's closest collaborative partners at the prison once a month, in which representatives from the prison's senior management team, prison warders, social workers, nurses and other relevant professionals participate.

The staff can also study for further qualifications and go on training courses as appropriate, in order to support and further develop our treatment programme. We must never allow ourselves to become complacent and just be satisfied with the status quo.

Working with criminal drug addicts on a daily basis requires mental flexibility and a high level of understanding of the inmates' situation.

A retrospective look at our six years providing drug treatment in a prison

In short, Opbygningsgården has been providing drug treatment at Kragskovhede Prison for six years now, and there have been some rocky periods along the way.

Developing and adjusting our treatment programme at the prison would not have been possible without the invaluable support we have received from our parent organisation in Thisted. Their many years of experience have helped us avoid making too many mistakes along the way and have facilitated the process.

It has been hard work building up a good working relationship between the two organisations – the prison and Opbygningsgården – each with its specific role to play in the prison setting, with legislation and rules that have to be adhered to.

As a group, the therapists working in our treatment unit now have a solid working relationship, where reciprocity, and personal and professional respect for each other are very much in evidence on a daily basis – this can clearly be seen by how well the inmates thrive in our treatment unit.

Establishing effective collaboration with the prison warders has also taken time and effort to reach the stage it is at now, with the therapists and the prison warders working together in an authentic way, not least in relation to the inmates.

There is still some scepticism in the prison towards the treatment unit. However, thanks to the efforts of the prison warders in our unit and the therapists, there is less scepticism and more respect than was the case earlier, with the work of Opbygningsgården now being viewed as an integrated part of the prison, and its therapists being seen as valid co-workers in the prison setting.

Visions for the future

Opbygningsgården is very keen on disseminating its knowledge and experience of setting up a drug treatment unit to other prisons. We are planning a so-called halfway house which aims to support the inmates in the process of re-entering society when they are released from prison.

Unfortunately, many of the prison inmates face problems after their release from prison, as not all local authorities, families and so on have the skills and knowledge to support the inmates in their re-entry to society. These problems are often of a practical nature, for example, finding housing, obtaining state benefits, work, education and so on, and this is the case even though our social workers do everything possible to help the inmates prepare for their release from prison.

Epilogue

It is often a long and arduous journey for inmates to find their way out of crime and drug abuse.

It can feel like climbing a mountain, and as with any process of change, it is important to be present in both mind and body every step of the way, so you can remember the whole experience as being part of life's infinite changeability.

Bibliography

Chödron, P. (2007). *When Things Falls Apart.* Shambhala.

Kabat-Zinn, J. (2013). *Full Catastrophe Living.* Piatkus – Little, Brown Book Group.

Leon, G.N (2000). *The Therapeutic Community, Theory, Model as Method.* Springer.

Reinhardt, J.L. (2018). *Glimpses and Echoes from Nothing* (writing under the pseudonym M.T. Ness). Notion Press.

Part II

Research perspectives

Evidence for the effectiveness of democratic therapeutic communities

5

Steve Pearce

Introduction

Democratic therapeutic communities (DTCs) are considered distinct from drug-free/hierarchical therapeutic communities, although the two approaches share so many elements that findings from effectiveness research on one is likely to give a strong indication as to the likely effectiveness of the other (see De Leon, Chapter 9, this volume for a treatment of the effectiveness of hierarchical therapeutic communities). Although there have been a number of experimental studies examining the effectiveness of DTCs, several of them in secure settings, the number is low, in common with studies of prison interventions generally. There are several factors which make it difficult to carry out randomised trials in prisons, outlined below, but there may be additional difficulties in DTCs, including staff reluctance, the lack of good adherence measures and manuals, and technical problems carrying out a randomised study in what is normally a long-term high-cost intervention (Pearce & Autrique, 2010).

There is disagreement about how the effectiveness of an intervention in prison should be judged. Given that a prisoner's time in a DTC is normally a small proportion of their time spent in prison; the fact that there is often a lack of proper community support after release; the antitherapeutic prison culture outside prison DTCs, from which prisoners come and to which they normally return; and the multiple influences on attitude and behaviour, it is difficult for a fairly brief time in a therapeutic community to produce long-lasting effects on outcomes with such complex components as recidivism, or self-esteem. On the other hand, if we do not expect the impact of a therapeutic intervention such as DTC to be detectable in this way, it may be difficult to justify investing in it.

An alternative approach is the argument that it is worthwhile providing a hopeful and humane setting in which self-improvement and self-knowledge is promoted, independent of scientifically detectable long-term outcomes. According to this viewpoint, all prisons should have a rehabilitative, or

DOI: 10.4324/9780429317460-7

therapeutic, intention. A humane and rehabilitative environment should produce improvements in prisoner well-being while they are there, compared to during time in the general population of the prison system, showing in such findings as lowered adjudications, lower suicide and self-harm rates, and greater well-being.

In 1998, Barbara Rawlings undertook a review of the research literature on democratic prison therapeutic communities for the UK prison service (Rawlings, 1998). She identified the main problems with the studies to that date, which serves as a description of the difficulties in carrying out such studies more generally. The problems she identified were:

1. Lack of a credible control group. Without a comparator group, it is impossible to decide how much of any improvement recorded in the intervention would have occurred in a similar group without the intervention. Control groups vary according to how closely matched to the intervention group they are in terms of type of offence, length of sentence and age, all of which might affect the probability of recidivism, as well as psychological measures such as motivation to change.
2. Lack of granularity when measuring recidivism. An example given by Rawlings is the McGill University clinic (Cormier, 1975), which failed to find a significant impact on recidivism of the intervention when compared to a similar group in mainstream prison, but noted on further inquiry that the majority of reconvictions in the intervention group were technical parole violations. Reconviction is not the same as reoffending. For example, in a reconviction study after treatment at Grendon prison, Gunn (Gunn, Robertson, & Dell, 1978) found men reported a substantially larger number of reoffences than reconvictions. Thus measures of reconviction will be confounded by the subject's ability to avoid detection, and measures of reoffending based on subject report will be confounded by the subject's honesty.
3. Selection bias. This is a common problem in trials of prison interventions, and is problematic is several ways:
   a. Prisoners in TC programmes may be volunteers, which may make them likely to do better, independent of the intervention.
   b. Prisoners may be selected for other features that differentiate them in important ways from the general prison population, such as by length of sentence, drug use, psychiatric history or type of offence. This kind of selection bias can be addressed by using a control group chosen with the same criteria, but often is not.
   c. Several trials found a differential effect according to how long the prisoners had been in the programme. This finding, in which a subgroup of prisoners from the intervention group do better than

the control group, relies on selection based on the willingness or ability of a prisoner to tolerate an intervention over a prolonged period of time.

4. Poorly defined interventions. Rawlings reports on a large number of interventions which are not precisely described, with names like 'therapeutic milieu program' (Lambert & Madden, 1976) and 'retraining group' (Kennedy, 1970). Where the elements of these programmes are described, they often include some elements of DTC practice, and add other significant elements. Even when a programme is described as 'therapeutic community', it is often not possible from the reports to be certain what elements of DTC practice were included, or how rigorously the model was enforced. This problem is not helped by the lack of adherence measures, and until recently of an agreed manual for DTC treatment (Pearce & Haigh, 2017).

The last of the problems noted by Rawlings is particularly problematic in countries other than the UK and US, where the concept of a DTC is either not widely known or is associated with purely psychiatric patients.

It is more difficult to demonstrate effectiveness when prison programmes are longer term (as dropouts increase), engage comparatively small numbers of inmates (as constructing adequately powered studies is more difficult), or are difficult to standardise. DTCs fulfil all these criteria. Even when a programme is short term, easily implemented, treats large numbers and is easily standardised, effectiveness can be difficult to establish. The most prominent recent example is the Sex Offender Treatment Programme in the UK, a group-based cognitive behaviour therapy (CBT) programme for those with sexual convictions. In 2017, an evaluation of the programme was published, based on findings from 2,500 treated and 13,000 untreated sex offenders (Henry, 2017). The two groups were compared using a sophisticated matching algorithm, and followed up for an average of eight years. The study, which used retrospective matching and did not use an experimental design (it was not, for example, randomised), found an increase in sexual offending in the treated group compared to matched controls. Results such as this contribute to the view of some that reliable rehabilitation of those who have committed serious offences is not possible, and it is against this background that DTC research should be considered.

An additional consideration is the type of prisoners treated in prison therapeutic communities, both whether they are different to those in the general prison estate, and whether populations can be stratified according to likelihood of benefit. An example is psychopathy. About a quarter of prisoners score sufficiently highly on the Hare Psychopathy Checklist to reach threshold for psychopathy, both in general prison populations and in therapeutic communities, and this group may do worse than others in rehabilitation settings (Hobson, Shine, & Roberts, 2000). Studies to date have not addressed stratification of inmate characteristics in a useful way.

When investigating possible measures of success in a prison programme, the following types of outcome are commonly used.

1. Recidivism. It should be noted that reconviction offers only a proxy measure of reoffending, as a small proportion of crimes result in conviction (Theobald, Farrington, Loeber, Pardini, & Piquero, 2014).
2. Behavioural outcomes after release – for example, employment, stable relationships, stable housing.
3. Behavioural outcomes during the programme – for example adjudications, suicides and self-harm events, drug use.
4. Psychological outcomes, measured by questionnaire – examples include self-esteem, impulsivity and extraversion.
5. Programme experience or social climate – what it is like to experience a prison programme.

Randomised evidence in non-secure settings

Studies of non-offending populations

There are very few randomised studies of DTC treatment for non-offending populations. As Lees, Manning, and Rawlings (1999) noted in a review of therapeutic community research in 1999, 'therapeutic communities have not produced the amount or quality of research literature that we might have expected, given the length of time they have been in existence' (p.9). At that time, the only randomised study of non-offending populations in non-secure settings they were able to find was Piper et al. (1996), who compared an 18-week DTC treatment for personality disorder and affective personality problems with a delay treatment group. At eight-month follow-up, TC patients fared significantly better than matched controls in interpersonal functioning, symptomatology, life satisfaction and self-esteem. Since that time a further randomised controlled trial (RCT) of DTC treatment in non-secure settings has been published (Pearce et al., 2017). This study randomised psychiatric patients with personality disorder to receive DTC treatment or crisis planning. At two-year follow-up, DTC showed significant advantages in client satisfaction, self- and other-directed aggression and self-harm. Participants receiving DTC also demonstrated significant improvements in social function and mental health. Both of the RCTs to date in non-offending populations have targeted people with personality disorder, making them relevant to secure settings, but neither included offending outcomes.

There are a large number of non-randomised outcome studies of DTC treatment in non-offending populations, which have invariably found evidence of effectiveness of DTC approaches, mostly in personality disordered patients. For a review of these see Pearce and Haigh (2017).

Studies of offending populations

Some studies of DTC treatment for offending populations have been carried out in non-secure settings, and some have included offending as outcomes. Early studies included in the Lees et al. review (1999) suffer from a lack of information about experimental method, making the quality of the study difficult to judge; poor characterisation of the interventions used; and diagnostic categories that are imprecise or superseded. For example, Miles (1969) studied 'subnormal male psychopaths', who appear to have been mainly adolescents who had committed an offence, in a non-secure DTC operating on an inpatient psychiatric ward. Participants not allocated to TC treatment received 'traditional psychiatric disciplinary treatment'. Compared to the control condition, the TC treatment produced improvements in interpersonal relationships, empathic ability, the formation of reciprocal friendships and an increased capacity to recognise other's feelings towards themselves. A 1964 study (Craft, Stephenson, & Granger, 1964) looked at a hospital inpatient TC modelled on the Henderson Hospital, a residential non-secure DTC operating from the 1950s to the early 2000s in London. Fifty male 'adolescent delinquents' with low IQs were alternatively admitted to an inpatient TC or another ward with a 'disciplinary programme'. Absconding was higher among the control group, but residents from the TC ward committed almost twice as many crimes after discharge, and were more likely to require continued institutional care. The authors concluded that an authoritarian and disciplinary regime is more effective for this group.

Since 2000, studies of DTCs in non-secure settings have been of non-offending populations, perhaps as non-secure treatment of offenders has fallen out of fashion.

Randomised evidence in secure settings

Carrying out experimental studies in secure settings poses challenges. Prisoner movements are restricted, and accommodation is often overcrowded, both of which make it difficult to quickly allocate prisoners to interventions that can only be provided in dedicated units, such as a DTC. In DTCs that form a part of a mainstream prison (in the UK, all prison TCs except HMP Grendon), empty accommodation may be required for prisoners not on the programme, which is likely to adversely affect the milieu, and at times the number of prisoners both ready and willing to undertake an intervention may not be sufficient to make randomisation practicable while maintaining admission rates. Some of these difficulties have been described in a study commissioned by HM Prisons Service to examine the possibility of evaluating the DTCs at HMP Grendon, as a possible component of the Dangerous and Severe Personality Disorder initiative of the UK Government (Campbell, 2003). The study did not lead to the commissioning of a randomised study of the therapeutic intervention at Grendon, and the conclusions go some way to explaining the lack of randomised studies of prison DTCs. A systematic review in the same year found ten studies of DTC interventions in people with severe personality disorder since 1992, none of which were randomised (Warren et al., 2003).

Early studies were imprecise in describing the nature of the settings, making it difficult to draw conclusions that might be directly applicable in prisons. Reviewing pre-1990 literature, Lees et al. (1999) describe 14 studies of DTC approaches in secure settings, of which two were randomised and controlled. Neither of these occurred in a prison setting. The first of these (Cornish & Clarke, 1975) studied adolescent boys who were randomly allocated either to a secure DTC house or to a conventional house in an approved school (non-secure schools to which children were sent by a court when convicted by a court or deemed out of parental control). No significant differences in reconviction rates were observed. The second (Auerbach, 1977) was a study of a secure DTC operating as a 'street prison', the definition of which is unclear. The TC intervention seems to have followed hierarchical (drug-free) TC principles. The study found lower reconviction rates at up to four-year follow-up in the TC condition, and a lower incidence of new crimes.

There are no other randomised studies of DTC interventions in secure settings.

Non-randomised evidence in secure settings

Due to the difficulties carrying out randomised studies of milieu interventions in secure settings, most of the evidence for effectiveness of complex interventions, including DTC, comes from non-randomised studies.

Reconviction

A meta-analysis of published and unpublished studies of drug-abusing and non-drug-abusing prisoner populations conducted between 1968 and 1996, which examined over 1,500 studies (Lipton, Pearson, Cleland, & Yee, 2002), concluded that '[hierarchical] therapeutic communities and milieu therapy significantly reduce recidivism', referring by milieu therapy to DTCs and German social therapy. German social therapy is not characterised in such a way as to allow a clear identification with DTCs, and the remaining group (once hierarchical TCs and German social therapy approaches are removed) of 11 studies of 'holistic milieu therapy and other TC/milieu' produced a strong trend to effectiveness that fell short of statistical significance (1-tailed probability 0.053).

In her 1998 narrative review study, Rawlings (1998) concluded from her review of the literature that the effect of TCs on reconviction and reoffending was positive (Rawlings, 1998). Having said this, the studies Rawlings reviewed were of variable quality, and the outcomes also varied, although with a tendency for well-designed studies to produce evidence of benefit.

Since these reviews a number of further studies have been published. Marshall's 1997 study, a direct comparison (case-controlled study) of 700 prisoners admitted to HMP Grendon Prison DTC programme, with 142 prisoners selected for the prison for whom a place did not become available (Marshall, 1997), looked at four-year follow-up data on Home Office and Police databases. Additional comparisons were made with a general prison group of 1,400 prisoners, weighted to match their index offence to those committed by the Grendon cohort. Waiting list prisoners were found to be significantly more likely to have been reconvicted, to receive a new custodial sentence and to be reconvicted following a violent offence compared to the general prison group, indicating that HMP Grendon was selecting prisoners at higher risk of reconviction. The researchers identified a trend to lower reconvictions for prisoners admitted to HMP Grendon compared to those on the waiting list ($p < 0.1$) as well as trends to lower rates of reincarceration and reconviction for violence.

Taylor followed these cohorts for a further three years, making seven years in total, using identical methodology (Taylor, 2000). Once again, significantly more prisoners from the waiting list group were convicted than the general prison group, and prisoners admitted to HMP Grendon were convicted of fewer crimes and fewer violent crimes, once again failing to reach the 5% significance level. Both Marshall (1997) and Taylor (2000) identified a treatment length effect, in that longer treatment produced greater improvements in reconviction rates, although this finding is difficult to interpret due to the bias introduced by prisoner choice and the impact of early discharge due to poor behaviour.

A 1996 study (Thornton, Mann, Bowers, Sheriff, & White, 1996) examined the impact on reconviction rates of treatment in the dedicated wing for those with sexual convictions at HMP Grendon. Prisoners with at least two previous convictions for sexual offences showed a significantly lower reconviction rate than a similar waiting list control group, and attitudes to women and children improved more the longer they spent in one of the therapeutic communities.

McMurran performed a retrospective study of 81 patients who had either been assessed or received treatment in a medium secure unit (MSU) operating as a DTC (McMurran, Egan, & Ahmadi, 1998). They found a reduction in later offences in both groups, but found no effect of either having entered treatment or for length of treatment. The study is handicapped by small subgroup sizes.

Finally, in 2010 Miller and Brown examined reconviction rates for 94 prisoners who had attended Dovegate Prison DTC, also in the UK (Miller & Brown, 2010). This was a follow-up study using the subset of a group of 250 prisoners previously studied (Brown, Miller, O'Neill, Philpin, & Sees, 2008) who had been released, and were therefore able to commit further crimes. They found that, at 48%, reconviction rates were lower than for national samples, but higher than for the small group of 22 who had applied to join the TC but failed the assessment, therefore not receiving the treatment. They note that these results should be interpreted in the context of Dovegate selecting high-risk and more personality disordered offenders.

Questionnaire-based change

There are a number of studies of psychological and behavioural change in prisoners who have lived in a prison DTC.

PSYCHOLOGICAL CHANGES

Newton (1998) reported on 94 HMP Grendon men tested at reception and discharge. Hostility, locus of control measures and Eysenck Personality Questionnaire scores all showed improvement. Ten years later, the study was partially replicated (Shuker & Newton, 2008). One hundred seventy-two men were tested before and after treatment at HMP Grendon. Once again, hostility, Eysenck personality scales and self-esteem all improved significantly. On the measures applied, scores improved to a clinically significant extent in between 24% and 39% of the population studied.

Beneficial effects of treatment at HMP Grendon were also found by Birtchnell, Shuker, Newberry and Duggan (2009), who compared Grendon with a psychiatric MSU specialising in personality disordered offenders. Both produced improvements in maladaptive interpersonal tendencies as measured on the Person's Relating to Others Questionnaire over 18 months' treatment. These results are difficult to interpret due to heterogeneity of timings of tests between the two groups, and perhaps more importantly because the MSU regime incorporated DTC elements, and was explicitly staffed with people who had TC experience (Milton, Duggan, McCarthy, Costley-White, & Mason, 2007). HMP Grendon prisoners showed significant improvements after nine months, maintained at 18 months (Shuker & Newberry, 2010).

In 2014, a study of patients with personality disorder who had also committed an offence followed up 47 patients after treatment for up to three years (Wilson, Freestone, Taylor, Blazey, & Hardman, 2014). Most patients had been diagnosed with antisocial personality disorder, and all were judged to pose a significant risk to others. They were treated at Millfields MSU, a DTC modified to accommodate additional approaches to criminogenic needs and substance misuse. An intention-to-treat analysis demonstrated improvements in risk (measured using the Violence Risk Scale (VRS) and the Historical Clinical Risk (HCR-20) instruments) and psychological symptoms (using the Symptom Checklist-Revised, SCL-90R), following treatment. The SCL-90R covers such problems as symptoms of depression and anxiety, as well as paranoia (interpersonal sensitivity and persecutory ideas), perfectionism and hostility.

Locus of control has also been examined after DTC treatment in prisons, and found to become more internal in a study of 94 prisoners treated at HMP Grendon Prison (Newton, 1998). This study also recorded significant reductions in hostility following DTC treatment.

BEHAVIOURAL CHANGES

Neville, Miller, & Fritzon (2007) used a behavioural checklist approach to track prosocial, antisocial and offence paralleling behaviours from the therapy notes of 68 Dovegate inmates, showing statistically significant increase in pro-social behaviours, and decreases in antisocial behaviours.

The implementation of a prosocial environment that challenges the prison culture of intimidation and opposition between staff and inmates should produce detectable reductions in behavioural markers of distress and aggression, such as self-harm and violent behaviour. A 2010 study demonstrated lower rates of self-injurious behaviour at Grendon Prison than would be expected from prison service-wide rates, at 29 per thousand prisoners per year compared to 130–137 per thousand per year (Rivlin, 2010). This is an important result given the high rates of self-harm and suicide in prisons, and the lack of information on effective ways of reducing levels of self-injurious behaviour in offending populations.

In a related finding, Newton (2010) found dramatically lower adjudication rates at HMP Grendon compared to other male closed training (i.e. comparable) prisons. For all offences, the rate at HMP Grendon was 22 per 100 men per year, compared to a training prison rate of 109. For violent offences, the difference was even more marked, at 7 (training prisons) to 1 (Grendon).

Newton also compared adjudication rates for men in Grendon with their rates prior to transfer, in other words while in mainstream prisons. She found a rate for all adjudications of 167 prior to transfer (compared to 22 at Grendon), for staff assaults of 5 (compared to 0.5), prisoner assaults 6 (0.5), and drug related offences 24 (2). After transfer from Grendon back to the general prison population, adjudications rose again, but remained (statistically) significantly improved compared to before treatment at Grendon. This study updates and confirms an earlier review (Cullen, 1994), which found Grendon to have the lowest level of prison offending measured by Governor's reports of any prison in its category in the UK over 30 years.

Recent developments link moral development with criminogenic needs. Ahonen and Degner (2012) surveyed the field, concluding that milieu therapy and DTC approaches target moral development in a way that currently used CBT approaches are unable to match due to a too-narrow focus on criminogenic needs at the expense of personal and societal moral values. They noted peer relationships and staff–resident relationships are particularly important in moral development in a youth institution. At the time there were no useful studies looking specifically at moral development in DTCs, but more recently the development of moral thinking has been demonstrated after DTC treatment (Siegel, Curwell-Parry, Pearce, Saunders, & Crockett, 2020), in particular moral character inference, a function related to mentalisation. Given that DTC, and milieu treatment more generally, involve regular feedback loops following behaviour that affects other people in the group, and that the main mechanism of change is social (Pearce & Pickard, 2013), this is not unexpected.

This area of work links to the emerging understanding of the influence of prison moral and social climate on reoffending. Data from regular Measuring the Quality of Prison Life (MQPL) surveys are correlated with reoffending data, showing that higher scores on 'moral quality of life' and interior legitimacy produce lower reoffending rates following release (Auty & Liebling, 2020). Therapeutic prisons, notably HMP Grendon, score consistently highly in the three yearly MQPL surveys, as noted elsewhere by Liebling (2012):

> Sometimes the results are so outstanding (that is, outstandingly good (see, for example, survey results for Grendon 2009 and 2012), or outstandingly poor (see, for example, the recent survey results for Pentonville)) they deserve a separate study aimed at explaining their outlier status. But this type of inquiry is not resourced […] and would inevitably be time consuming to carry out.
>
> (Liebling, 2012, p.5)

Various published and unpublished reports indicate some of the beneficial impacts of DTC practice on prison culture (Evans, Roberts, Jacobs, &

Shuker, 2009; Shefer, 2010; Tonkin & Howells, 2009), leading to organisational efforts to export the beneficial aspects of DTC prisons to the wider prison estate (Bennett & Shuker, 2010). It has historically proved difficult to provide a consistently humane environment in prisons. DTCs have demonstrated they have been able to do so longitudinally (Genders & Player, 2010).

Conclusion

Due to the difficulty in carrying out methodologically rigorous experimental studies on prison populations, the longer-term nature of DTCs and their small number, there is a dearth of high-quality studies producing clear evidence of their effect in reducing recidivism. Psychological and behavioural changes have been convincingly demonstrated, evidenced by such measures as levels of self-harm and adjudications, but data is lacking as to the extent to which these benefits persist once inmates leave the therapeutic community.

There is nevertheless an argument for implementing therapeutic community values, in particular explicit feedback and the expectation of change for the better, and moral dealings between prisoners and staff, between prisoners and prisoners, and between staff, in order to make prisons more humane and decent places (Stevens, 2011), and thereby to reduce incidents of violence and self-harm. Prisoners in DTC prisons feel safer (Tonkin & Howells, 2009), report higher levels of decency and respect (National Offender Management Service, 2015), and are more likely to invest in their environment and take responsibility (Rhodes, 2010). Full DTC programmes are not the only way to implement communitarian, mutually respectful environments in prisons. Environments based on DTC principles but requiring less motivation to change from prisoners, and which are easier to implement, are currently being implemented in English prisons on a wide scale (Rawlings & Haigh, 2017). Known as psychologically informed planned environments (PIPES), they bring DTC values to a wider population. Whether they produce similar benefits in prisoner well-being and prison environment is not yet known.

References

Ahonen, L., & Degner, J. (2012). Moral development as a crucial treatment goal for young people in institutional care: A critical comparison between milieu therapy and cognitive behavioral therapy. *Therapeutic Communities: The International Journal of Therapeutic Communities, 33*, 4–15.

Auerbach, A.W. 1978. *The role of the therapeutic community 'street prison' in the rehabilitation of youthful offenders*. [Unpublished Ph.D. diss.]. George Washington University.

Auty, K.M., & Liebling, A. (2020). Exploring the relationship between prison social climate and reoffending. *Justice Quarterly, 37*, 358–81.

Bennett, P., & Shuker, R. (2010). Improving prisoner-staff relationships: Exporting Grendon's good practice. *The Howard Journal of Crime and Justice, 49*, 491–502.

Birtchnell, J., Shuker, R., Newberry, M., & Duggan, C. (2009). An assessment of change in negative relating in two male forensic therapy samples using the Person's Relating to Others Questionnaire (PROQ). *The Journal of Forensic Psychiatry & Psychology, 20*, 387–407.

Brown, J.M., Miller, S., O'Neill, D.A., Philpin, C., & Sees, C., Simmonds, R., Bobstien, A., Burdett, S., Cahalane, E., Frith, S., Neville, L., Northey, S., & Vallice, N. (2008). *HMP Dovegate therapeutic community: Longitudinal Evaluation*. Guilford: University of Surrey. Unpublished Report.

Campbell, S. (2003). *The feasibility of conducting an RCT at HMP Grendon*. Home Office, Research, Development and Statistics Directorate.

Cormier, B.M. (1975). *The watcher and the watched*. Tundra Books.

Cornish, D.B., & Clarke, R.V.G. (1975). *Residential treatment and its effects on delinquency*. HM Stationery Office.

Craft, M., Stephenson, G., & Granger, C. (1964). A controlled trial of authoritarian and self-governing regimes with adolescent psychopaths. *American Journal of Orthopsychiatry, 34*, 543–54.

Cullen, E. (1994). Grendon: The therapeutic prison that works. *Therapeutic Communities*, John Wiley and Sons.

Evans, R., Roberts, J., Jacobs, L., & Shuker, R. (2009). *Survey of bullying at HMP Grendon*. Unpublished manuscript.

Genders, E., & Player, E. (2010). Therapy in prison: Revisiting Grendon 20 years on. *The Howard Journal of Criminal Justice, 49*, 431–50.

Gunn, J., Robertson, G., & Dell, S. (1978). *Psychiatric aspects of imprisonment*. Academic Press.

Henry, O. (2017). Evaluation of the core sex offender treatment programme. *Probation Journal, 64*, 425–27. https://doi.org/10.1177/0264550517740997a

Hobson, J., Shine, J., & Roberts, R. (2000). How do psychopaths behave in a prison therapeutic community? *Psychology, Crime and Law, 6*, 139–54.

Kennedy, F.C. (1970). The US Air Force prisoner retraining program. *Federal Probation Journal, 34*, 39–44.

Lambert, L.R., & Madden, P.G. (1976). The adult female offender: The road from institution to community life. *Canadian Journal of Criminology and Corrections, 18*, 319–31.

Lees, J., Manning, N., & Rawlings, B. (1999). *Therapeutic community effectiveness: A systematic international review of therapeutic community treatment for people with personality disorders and mentally disordered offenders*. University of York, NHS Centre for Reviews and Dissemination.

Liebling, A. (2012). What is 'MQPL'? Solving puzzles about the prison. *Prison Service Journal, 202*, 3–5.

Lipton, D.S., Pearson, F.S., Cleland, C.M., & Yee, D. (2002). The effects of therapeutic communities and milieu therapy on recidivism. In J. McGuire (Ed.). *Offender rehabilitation and treatment: Effective programmes and policies to reduce re-offending* (pp.39–77). Wiley.

Marshall, P. (1997). *A reconviction study of HMP Grendon therapeutic community.* Home Office.

McMurran, M., Egan, V., & Ahmadi, S. (1998). A retrospective evaluation of a therapeutic community for mentally disordered offenders. *The Journal of Forensic Psychiatry, 9,* 103–13.

Miles, A. (1969). Changes in the attitudes to authority of patients with behaviour disorders in a therapeutic community. *The British Journal of Psychiatry, 115,* 1049–57.

Miller, S., & Brown, J. (2010). HMP Dovegate's therapeutic community: An analysis of reconviction data. *Therapeutic Communities Journal, 31,* 62–75.

Milton, J., Duggan, C., McCarthy, L., Costley-White, A., & Mason, L. (2007). Characteristics of offenders referred to a medium secure NHS personality disorder service: The first five years. *Criminal Behaviour and Mental Health, 17,* 57–67.

Ministry of Justice. (2009). *Results from an MQPL Survey at HMP Grendon.* Audit and Assurance: NOMS.

Ministry of Justice (2012). *Results from an MQPL Survey at HMP Grendon.* Audit and Assurance: NOMS.

Ministry of Justice (2011). *Results from an MQPL Survey at HMP Pentonville.* Audit and Assurance: NOMS.

National Offender Management Service. (2015). *Measuring the quality of prison life: Survey research carried out at HMP Grendon 13th to 16th October 2014.* Audit and Assurance: NOMS.

Neville, L., Miller, S., & Fritzon, K. (2007). Understanding change in a therapeutic community: An action systems approach. *The Journal of Forensic Psychiatry & Psychology, 18,* 181–203.

Newton, M. (1998). Changes in measures of personality, hostility and locus of control during residence in a prison therapeutic community. *Legal and Criminological Psychology, 3,* 209–23.

Newton, M. (2010). Changes in prison offending among residents of a prison based therapeutic community. In R. Shuker and E. Sullivan (Eds.). *Grendon and the emergence of forensic therapeutic communities: Developments in research and practice* (pp.281–91.) Wiley-Blackwell.

Pearce, S., & Autrique, M. (2010). On the need for randomised trials of therapeutic community approaches. *Therapeutic Communities, 31,* 338–55.

Pearce, S., & Haigh, R. (2017). *A handbook of democratic therapeutic community theory and practice.* JKP.

Pearce, S., & Pickard, H. (2013). How therapeutic communities work: Specific factors related to positive outcome. *The International Journal of Social Psychiatry, 59,* 636–45.

Pearce, S., Scott, L., Attwood, G., Saunders, K., Dean, M., De Ridder, R., ... Crawford, M. (2017). Democratic therapeutic community treatment for personality disorder: Randomised controlled trial. *The British Journal of Psychiatry, 210,* 149–56. https://doi.org/bjp.bp.116.184366

Piper, W.E., Rosie, J.S., Joyce, A.S., & Azim, H.F.A. (1996). *Time-limited day treatment for personality disorders. Integration of research and practice in a group program.* American Psychological Association.

Rawlings, B. (1998). Research on therapeutic communities in prison: A review of the literature. Unpublished.

Rawlings, B., & Haigh, R. (2017). Therapeutic communities and planned environments for serious offenders in English prisons. *BJPsych Advances, 23,* 338–46.

Rhodes, L.A. (2010). 'This can't be real': Continuity at HMP Grendon. In R. Shuker and E. Sullivan (Eds.). *Grendon and the emergence of forensic therapeutic communities: Developments in research and practice* (pp.203–16). Wiley Blackwell.

Rivlin, A. (2010). Suicide and self-injurious behaviours at HMP Grendon. In R. Shuker and E. Sullivan (Eds.). *Grendon and the emergence of forensic therapeutic communities: Developments in research and practice* (pp.265–80). Wiley Blackwell.

Shefer, G. (2010). The quality of life of prisoners and staff at HMP Grendon. In R. Shuker and E. Sullivan (Eds.). *Grendon and the emergence of forensic therapeutic communities: Developments in research and practice* (pp.247–64). Wiley Blackwell.

Shuker, R., & Newberry, M. (2010). Changes in interpersonal relating following therapeutic community treatment at HMP Grendon. In R. Shuker and E. Sullivan (Eds.). *Grendon and the emergence of forensic therapeutic communities: Developments in research and practice* (pp.293–304). Wiley Blackwell.

Shuker, R., & Newton, M. (2008). Treatment outcome following intervention in a prison-based therapeutic community: A study of the relationship between reduction in criminogenic risk and improved psychological well-being. *The British Journal of Forensic Practice, 10*, 33–44.

Siegel, J.Z., Curwell-Parry, O., Pearce, S., Saunders, K.E., & Crockett, M.J. (2020). A computational phenotype of disrupted moral inference in borderline personality disorder. *Biological Psychiatry: Cognitive Neuroscience and Neuroimaging, 5*, 10–16.

Stevens, A. (2011). A 'very decent nick': Ethical treatment in prison-based democratic therapeutic communities. *Journal of Forensic Psychology Practice, 11*, 124–50.

Taylor, R. (2000). *A seven-year reconviction study of HMP Grendon therapeutic community* Home Office Research, Development and Statistics Directorate London.

Theobald, D., Farrington, D.P., Loeber, R., Pardini, D.A., & Piquero, A.R. (2014). Scaling up from convictions to self-reported offending. *Criminal Behaviour and Mental Health, 24*, 265–76.

Thornton, D., Mann, R., Bowers, L., Sheriff, N., & White, T. (1996). Sex offenders in a therapeutic community. *Grendon: A Compilation of Grendon Research*. HM Prison Grendon.

Tonkin, M., & Howells, K. (2009). *Social climate in secure settings: A report for HMP Grendon*. Institute of Mental Health Report. Unpublished.

Warren, F., Preedy-Fayers, K., McGauley, G., Pickering, A., Norton, K., Geddes, J.R., & Dolan, B. (2003). *Review of treatments for severe personality disorder*. Home Office Online Report, *30*(3).

Wilson, K., Freestone, M., Taylor, C., Blazey, F., & Hardman, F. (2014). Effectiveness of modified therapeutic community treatment within a medium-secure service for personality-disordered offenders. *The Journal of Forensic Psychiatry & Psychology, 25*, 243–61.

Relationships work
Experiences of therapeutic community residents

6

Gareth Ross and Natalie Bond

Background

In 2018, Gartree Therapeutic Community (GTC) marked 25 years of both the life on and the life of the TC since it opened in 1993. GTC is a 25-bed TC for men in prison who have long-standing emotional and relationship difficulties that are functionally linked to their offending behaviour. Uniquely among prison TCs, the GTC only accommodates men serving indeterminate sentences.

Relationships are considered central to the work on the GTC. The latest Chief Inspectorate Report for HMP Gartree (HMCIP, 2017) acknowledged that the GTC continued to be 'very effective' (p. 6) where staff/prisoner relationships were observed to be 'particularly impressive, with high levels of good-quality engagement and awareness of prisoner needs' (p. 27).

This chapter presents two studies focused on the lived experiences of men on the GTC. In an organisation that is increasingly recognising the need to build rehabilitative cultures and become more trauma informed, the studies aimed to capture the power of relational working. The first part of the chapter summarises work already undertaken, exploring the experience of change on the GTC (which is presented elsewhere in more detail: Ross & Auty, 2018). The chapter continues by describing research completed by the current authors (Bond & Ross, 2018) and explores the experience of GTC members' participation in a psychodrama group, and is presented here for the first time. Interesting common themes between the studies are discussed.

Gartree Therapeutic Community (GTC) regime and therapeutic model

On the GTC twice weekly community meetings attended by all residents and available staff are held to discuss various factors associated with the running of and dynamics within the community and to provide opportunities to discuss problematic behaviour or breaches to community rules. In addition, residents attend open-ended psychotherapy groups, each lasting 90 minutes, three times a week. These are facilitated by a combination of specially selected and trained prison officers, psychotherapists, forensic psychologists and probation officers. Attendance in psychodrama and other creative therapies (when available) is optional. Residents also interact with the wider host organisation, typically in the afternoons when they attend employment and education.

As with other TCs, the GTC provides an environment to engage people with complex needs flexibly by integrating diverse therapeutic approaches (Shuker, 2010). The GTC operates in accordance with the principles set out by Rapoport (1960): *democratisation*, the emphasis on each community member participating in decision-making; *communalisation*, the building of relationships through shared involvement in domestic tasks, social activities and day-to-day living; *permissiveness*, a degree of tolerance for problematic behaviour so that it may be therapeutically explored; and *reality confrontation*, the process through which residents receive feedback on themselves via other community members.

TCs have famously been described as 'living-learning situations' (Cullen, 1994, p. 239), and everything that happens between members on the GTC is used as a learning opportunity. Life histories, including adverse life experiences and offending behaviours, are discussed in detail. Connections and parallels between past experiences, current day-to day behaviour and offending are identified and explored in order to facilitate change (Shine & Morris, 2000). Though facilitated by staff, the GTC model presents the community as the 'doctor' (Rapoport, 1960) holding the expertise and understanding of the residents required to facilitate change. See Stevens (2010) for a more detailed description of forensic therapeutic communities and Pearce and Haigh (2017) for a more general account of therapeutic community practice across settings.

Psychodrama on the GTC

Psychodrama has been a treatment method in prison-based TCs for over 30 years but has only been a core part of the therapeutic regime at HMP Gartree since 2014. It is a form of group psychotherapy that uses guided dramatic action and role playing to explore past, present and future scenarios. Scenes can be created and worked with including memories, conflicts, inner thought processes, fantasies, dreams or anticipated events (Jefferies, 2010). The person at the centre of the enactment is encouraged to develop insight into their patterns of relating.

The weekly psychodrama group on the GTC is delivered in Moreno's Classical Style (Moreno, 1985). This style encourages the use of here-and-now scenarios in the first instance which lead to a 'presenting scene' that is then carefully tracked back by the psychodramatist to establish the origins of the presenting issues – typically childhood adverse experience and/or trauma. Once the underlying trauma is established, the psychodramatist implements a variety of strategies to enable reparation and healing. The original presenting scene is then revisited to allow the individual to come back into the here and now and integrate that experience and allow for reflection. The main body of the work is bookended by creative warm-up exercises and space and time at the end for a debrief.

To allow for adjustment to the therapy unit and attachment to the community, men are required to have been in therapy for nine months or more before they engage in psychodrama on the GTC. There is an expectation that men will commit to a minimum of 12 months on the group. The group runs weekly for a two-hour session, includes a maximum of eight GTC residents and is supported by one other member of the wider GTC staff team. The psychodramatist is an experienced prison officer who has worked on the GTC for a number of years.

To date there has been no in-depth account of the experience of psychodrama in these settings, from the point of view of those engaging in it.

The need to understand how things work

Much of the literature about TCs has focused on evidencing their effectiveness (Newton, 1998; Shine, 2001; Shuker & Newton, 2008). In a non-forensic context several studies have indicated residential and non-residential TCs are an effective intervention for people with a personality disorder. Reported positive outcomes have included a reduction in acute psychiatric admissions (Davies & Campling, 2003) and improvements in mental health and social functioning (Barr et al., 2010). Greater improvements in patients who participated in TC treatment compared to treatment as usual has been found (Chiesa, Fonagy, & Holmes, 2006; Pearce et al., 2017). There is also a large body of research demonstrating that TCs can be successful in a prison setting (see Lees, Manning, & Rawlings, 2004 for a review).

However, studies focusing on outcomes have been criticised for telling us little about *how* people change (Duggan, 2004). Gibbons et al. (2009) suggest understanding the mechanisms by which people change is the most likely way of improving current treatment options. Arguably these mechanisms are not well understood (Higginson & Mansell, 2008; Duggan, 2004). Similarly, Ward and Maruna (2007) suggest that focusing on 'what helps' in reducing reoffending, alongside the traditional 'what works', might help give a better understanding of the processes people go through when making changes.

Smith (1996) has suggested that qualitative methods are appropriate when there is interest in understanding dynamic processes or slow-moving complex events. In recent years there has been much research into psychological change and recovery from various problems utilising qualitative methods that emphasise the patients' perspective and experience (Higginson & Mansell, 2008). There are few examples of a similar approach in forensic populations.

Research at HMP Grendon used prisoners' autobiographies to construct an understanding of the therapeutic process (Wilson & McCabe, 2002). They found that change takes time and requires social inclusion, a conducive environment and good relationships with staff. Miller, Sees and Brown, (2006) found that residents at HMP Dovegate identified change as a process involving self-referential properties, interpersonal facets and challenges. Ethnographic fieldwork at HMP Grendon and HMP Gartree by Stevens (2013) identified several change processes in prison TCs including identity reconstruction and narrative reframing. Dolan (2017) found that residents feeling safe, as well as having trusting and supportive relationships with peers and staff were an integral part of the process of change at HMP Grendon.

Exploring the client's perspective can provide new insights in identifying *what* changes and the processes of change in treatment for people with complex and long-standing problems. TC residents will have a broad perspective of the changes that they experience and the factors that promote change that are less likely than those of professionals to be shaped by training or theoretical allegiances.

The two studies reported here looked to add to this small field of research attempting to identify how people change on a TC. For the first study, the central research question was, 'how do residents experience change on a therapeutic community?' In the second, the central research questions was, 'how do residents in a prison therapeutic community experience psychodrama?'

Methods used

In both studies, small numbers of participants were interviewed individually and in depth about their experiences. Interviews were analysed using interpretative phenomenological analysis (IPA) following the guidelines suggested by Smith and Osborne (2003). IPA is an idiographic approach in which each case is analysed in detail before moving on to the next, slowly working towards more general themes. This method allows for a detailed examination and interpretation of lived experience.

Data collection and participants

In both studies, interview schedules were developed to set the frame of the interview and encourage participants to provide detailed accounts of their experience of making changes on the GTC and of their experience of psychodrama respectively. At these times the schedules were deviated from in order to focus on the lived experiences of the participants and ensure their narratives were fully investigated. Interviews lasted between one and one and a half hours, were audiotaped and later transcribed verbatim by the researchers.

For the first study, five former residents of the Gartree Therapeutic Community who 'completed treatment' were contacted with information about the research and asked if they wished to participate. To 'complete treatment' is to have a planned ending and to have completed at least 18 months in therapy (Paget, Thorne, & Das, 2015). Participants were aged between 34 and 58 and had spent between 34 and 41 months in therapy. All were serving life sentences for the offence of murder. None of the men in the first study had participated in psychodrama.

For the second study, four participants were recruited who each had completed at least 12 months of psychodrama whilst resident on the GTC. Participants were aged between 24 and 51. All were serving life sentences; three were convicted of murder, one of armed robbery.

Participants' names have been changed to ensure anonymity.

Study 1: the experience of change in a prison therapeutic community

Four main themes emerged and were labelled Motivation to Change (subthemes, Engagement, Determination); Environment (subthemes, Boundaries, Experience of care); Removal of Masks (subthemes, Embracing vulnerability, Emerging authenticity); and Relationships (subthemes: Re-enacting the past, Challenge from peers). Brief vignettes with extracts from transcripts are used to illustrate themes.

Theme 1: motivation to change

The process of **Engagement** seemed to be important, especially the idea that the desire to enter therapy was self-directed. Many were motivated by their index offence and the realisation that in some ways it represented not an isolated event but part of a pattern of behaviour. Participants were also

motivated by a desire to progress through the prison system and give themselves the best chance of a positive future. In addition, all participants referred
to therapy as being difficult and requiring **Determination**.

Theme 2: environment

Though some of the rules and processes are described as 'petty', the general
feeling was the rules and **Boundaries** held by the community helped people
feel safe enough to engage with the therapy and strive to make changes.
Relationships are encouraged between staff and residents: '*They're not just
a uniform are they*' (Edward), and participants expressed an **Experience of
Care.** Though acknowledged as only '*for now*' (Edward), Richard was one
of many participants to explicitly compare the environment to a family. The
sense of caring for others and experiencing care was further emphasised
when participants talked of their relationships with other community
members.

Theme 3: removal of masks

Participants described battling with their defences as the expectation to talk
openly and to connect with and express emotions in therapy clashed with
norms around prison behaviour where displays of emotions other than anger
are seen as a sign of weakness. Participants realised they must **Embrace
Vulnerability** to make positive changes and that the process of therapy makes
avoidance difficult to maintain. Many participants expressed that knowing
and seeing other men go through similar processes encouraged them to be
open. As their defences came down, the men found common ground despite
their differences. Participants reported taking risks with self-disclosure and
not experiencing negative consequences.

Being open and embracing vulnerability is part of the process of change,
in that it facilitates discussion, challenge and reflection; however, it can also
be seen as a change in itself. Often this was related back to previous problems.
Experiences of vulnerability and support facilitated an **Emerging Authenticity**
in participants. Free from their masks, the 'brick wall' and 'bravado', they were
able to avoid less and experience themselves differently. Participants emerged
from this process as more accepting of themselves and their offending.
Openness and tolerance experienced in the community were generalised by
participants, leading to improved relationships, different experiences and the
beginnings of a new identity.

Theme 4: relationships

Participants spoke about how their relationships with staff and community members would mirror difficult relationships in their life, in effect **Re-enacting the Past,** helping them reflect on repeating patterns that they were previously unaware of. Here-and-now behaviour emerging in therapeutic relationships was linked to previous problematic patterns of behaviour.

A second major subtheme was the idea that changes can be made through the process of **Challenge from Peers.** Participants reported that as they spent more time in therapy, their tolerance for challenge increased. Less guarded and in the context of a safe and supportive environment, participants found they were increasingly able to receive feedback from more sources.

Illustrative vignettes

James

James had a long history of violent, gang-related offending. His **Motivation** to do something different came though noticing the similarities in his most recent offence to previous offending and the fear that the pattern may repeat.

> I thought well I've got this life sentence, this is sort of similar … the crime was similar to the crime before … and I thought I've gotta do something about this … I thought if don't do it now then I'll not get out of jail, have any chance of getting out of jail, get myself hurt, get myself killed, hurt somebody else.

Upon entering therapy, James was taken aback by the personal nature of the work. He had things from his past he wanted to talk about, but seeing other men allow themselves to be open and unguarded was frightening.

> I wasn't expecting people, certainly what I would call the **calibre** of some of the people up there to be so open about personal issues, for example abuse issues, upbringing. All this stuff I knew I had to, **really**, speak about at some point because they were my core problems. And even though I went up there **for** that, all of a sudden I wasn't sure about that.

> I should have gained a bit of strength seeing these fellas, who I would call strong characters, talking about it but I was thinking 'they're in bits here'. You know I didn't really wanna be like that.

Ultimately James had to **Embrace Vulnerability** so that he could work. He spoke about how the clear **Boundaries** and the **Experience of Care** allowed him to feel safe.

I done 33 months up there and I never saw one fist connect to anyone. Me being one of them, one of the lively ones up there I did lose my temper a lot ... and some of the things you do say to each other up there in anger you'd never get away with on another wing because you'd be in a lot of trouble. You'd get physically badly hurt for less. So it is safe.

The help I got up there from them was unbelievable you wouldn't get anywhere else. You wouldn't get that on the outside never mind jail.

You do get some quite close relationships there I feel. Close bonds because you're trusting people with your deepest and darkest secrets ... There's fellas up there know things about me my parents don't know.

By paying close attention to the relationships formed in therapy James was able to notice how often they **Re-enacted the Past** relationships he had had. Through this he came to understand his violence not as isolated incidents but part of wider patterns of problematic relating.

These past problems I've had they're all linked but it took me a while to get that. And I found links while I was up there, some strong links and, what I found it hard to get to was the links I found with all these negative behaviours even played a part in my index offence, my murder.

Sean

Sean was serving a life sentence for the murder of his partner. His relationships with other family members had broken down and he lived a relatively isolated existence. Typically, he would defend himself from negative feelings by externalising the blame for his problems, presenting as aloof and dismissive of others. For Sean, his initial, internal **Motivation** was to restore relationships.

I was very aware it was a case of if not now then probably never ... if you don't sort your shit out you might not be a part of your children's future.

Sean found the process of opening up in therapy extremely exposing and he was anxious about the potential for his personal disclosures to be used against him. In time he learned to **Embrace Vulnerability** which allowed him to connect to a more **Authentic** account of his relationships problems and index offence.

*The first couple of times it's ... it feels really **really** exposed ... you give people a lot of ammunition, in theory ... But I was up there 3 years, I've been gone a year. Yeah, well, still again nothing terrible has happened.*

As hard as it was and as much as it shook me it's also been really liberating … If I'd have stuck to 'oh it was a fight that got out of hand' I don't know how I would have been able to address any of the stuff I addressed.

Key to Sean's experience was the revelation that echoes of previous relationships would affect how he perceived here-and-now interactions. In therapy his conflicts **Re-enacted the Past.** He gave the following example:

I have this whole thing where, either real or perceived, I've always been let down. My dad's always done this movie thing where he would be everything you want him to be for 2 weeks then he'd bugger off and be completely emotionally unavailable.

*Then Phil [therapy manager] did once, he promised to be there, something happened, he didn't let us know, he didn't turn up. I put him on the agenda and had a five minute rant. **That wasn't about him,** that was about me standing outside where no one picked me up and I'm standing in the rain wondering, 'what the hell's going on here'. It wasn't about Phil.*

Realising that he was transferring anger towards his absent father onto other figures in his life helped him reassess his own role in current conflicts. As did **Challenge from Peers**:

It took me quite a while I don't know how long it was in the end, over a year of twenty-one people telling me 'what!?!' 'that's not ok' – I don't know it took quite a while to think 'could it be me – could I be in the wrong here' eventually the idea they must all be crazy – it kind of wore off.

Nick

Nick had a lifelong pattern of problems in intimate relationships. He found the experience of care from staff allowed him to **Re-enact the Past** conflicts with his partners, working through them in a different way and ultimately emerging as a more **Authentic** version of himself.

It was a close bond with Jane [a female prison officer facilitator] but again to me there was always this experience of it was kind of one of regret in the sense that I can have this open relationship kind of where I'm speaking how I'm feeling and thinking and yet I couldn't do that to my wife.

I look back now [at time in therapy], I was being vulnerable there … I didn't do that with my wife. I was always pretending to be strong and that kind of nothing, there's no problems there's no issues and yet inside me there was [now] I'm being reflective, being thoughtful, being kind that's the person I want to be.

This is the change and I need to do this to interact and this is how I can have better relationships with both men and women in the future.

Study 2: the experience of psychodrama in a prison therapeutic community

Three main themes emerged and were labelled Secure Base (subthemes, Wider Context, Group Process and Care and Connection); Core Experience (subthemes, Facing Fear, being Taken Back, Emotional Connection and Seeing the Unseen); and Impact (subthemes Growth, Compassion, New Meanings and Improved Relationships.). Brief vignettes with extracts from transcripts are used to illustrate themes.

Theme 1: Secure Base

Borrowing a term from attachment theory, the first major theme was labelled **Secure Base**. Psychodrama was experienced as anxiety provoking, and all participants described the importance of feeling safe in order that they could explore themselves and their relationships with others.

There were three subthemes, **Wider Context, Group Process** and **Care and Connection**. Participants described how the psychodrama group being situated in the **Wider Context** of the GTC was important. The men knew each other, their therapeutic issues and life stories, and so a sense of intimacy was created more easily than it would have been if the group were strangers. The capacity for the community to act as a container for the difficult emotional experiences that emerged in psychodrama was also articulated.

Elements of **Group Process** also aided the feeling that the group was a safe space in which to be doing the work. The structure of sessions was a 'warm-up' at the start and a 'debrief' space at the end, temporally containing the work that occurs in between. The role of the group in deciding what work is to be done, whilst being led by the psychodramatist seemed to strike the right balance between autonomy and guidance.

It could also be seen that the experience of **Care and Connection** was an important element of the experience of psychodrama. This partly relates to the **Wider Context** theme, in that participants felt an existing care from their peers. However, this was enhanced in the psychodrama space through the heightened emotional states they experienced themselves and saw others in. Participants felt connected to the emotions they saw in their peers, and witnessing and connecting to others' vulnerability made them in turn feel safe to reveal their own.

Theme 2: the Core Experience

The second theme was labelled the **Core Experience**. This amounted to all of the processes that seemed to be what psychodrama work really was to the participants, most especially those features that distinguished it from other forms of group therapy in which they were also participating.

This theme comprised four subthemes that were labelled *Facing Fear*, being *Taken Back, Emotional Connection* and *Seeing the Unseen*. The importance of the **Secure Base** concept is highlighted by the experience that participants had of *Facing Fear* in psychodrama. Participants reported feeling a heightened level of anxiety ahead of the group because of the emotional nature of it. Feeling vulnerable in the space was a common experience that was regarded by participants as inevitable if the process was to be engaged with authentically.

Central to the experience of psychodrama was the experience of being *Taken Back*, to memories, relationships, experiences and so forth. This was experienced very differently from other forms of therapy in which events might be described like a story. The way the director of psychodrama focused participants in the present tense, the emphasis on first-person description, and the use of other group members or objects to represent things or people of importance, were all very evocative for participants. Frequently participants reported that this process heightened their *Emotional Connection* to the scenario. Once activated, participants described being held in their emotions so that they may be safely explored. Through exploring the scenes created in detail, participants described *Seeing the Unseen* and developing new insights into themselves and others.

Theme 3: Impact

The third theme was labelled *Impact* and represents the various ways the participants described the effect that they believed participating in psycho-drama had had on their lives. This theme comprised of four subthemes, *Growth*, *Compassion* (for self and others), *New Meanings* and *Improved Relationships*.

Participants reported meaningful psychological and emotional shifts in themselves and their relationship to the world. This *Growth* was not always easy to define but seemed to emerge from working through past traumatic experiences in the group. More tangible was the participants' experience of developing **Compassion**, for themselves as well as others. There was a sense of people forgiving themselves for the things they have done and finding forgiveness for others.

The subtheme **New Meanings** captures another of the results of the work in psychodrama. By re-experiencing past events, relationships and conflicts, participants gained new perspectives that changed their understanding of the event or relationship.

Perhaps most importantly, participants were very clear that the experience of psychodrama had led to **Improved Relationships** with significant others in their lives. Profound shifts were reported in relationships with immediate family members in particular. Here-and-now relationships were also experienced as improved through the insights gained in psychodrama.

Illustrative vignettes

Johnny

Johnny was a male in his early twenties with a history of impulsive, angry, aggressive behaviour in the outside community and in custody. His motivation in therapy generally would fluctuate but he found himself engaged by the psychodrama process. Elements of **Group Process** helped engage Johnny.

> Sometimes you don't feel the group today, don't really fancy this, then there's the warm up and you feel a bit more active and bit more responsive.

Johnny was drawn further into the process through **Connection** with the emotional experience of others.

> You see someone being vulnerable or connected to something … It it's just a very powerful thing to watch.

Working on his own material he expressed a strong sensation of being **Taken Back** and becoming the child he was.

> It's safe but you don't feel safe, especially if you're working on past things like childhood trauma, you can quickly feel like you're there, that you're back in that room, back in to that child again.

In psychodrama Johnny worked on the difficult relationship he had with his father. The use of role play created an **Emotional Connection** that was experienced profoundly.

It's, it's strange, it's really strange, coz you're feeling the same emotions that you would do if you, if I, was speaking to my mother or father.

Through the enactments in psychodrama Johnny was able to develop more **Compassion** for his father.

It shifted from anger … The guy's not just this figure that I've got, this biological father is actually a person, probably had his own issues in life … Makes you see the person instead of just the parent.

Learning that some of the triggers to his anger were rooted in past events gave **New Meanings** to here-and-now conflicts and gave an opportunity for **Improved Relationships**.

After going back through the memories, you realise that's why you're doing it … I need to learn how to control these feelings, thinking this is where these feelings come from, from this very moment, from this very memory.

I learnt how to deal with someone who's not responding to you, to understand that person as well, try to keep calm, try to get through what you want to say … I learnt how to bite my tongue and how to come through clearly instead of ranting or just exploding on someone, I could, I could talk and say this is how I feel.

Mike

Mike was a middle-aged man serving a life sentence for a series of violent robberies. He had learned from a young age not to show emotion and that the world was hostile and unworthy of his trust.

The following quote highlights the themes of **Facing Fear** and being **Taken Back**. Mike's anxiety is linked to the anticipation of *re-experiencing* and not just remembering the past. He vividly describes a typical scene from his childhood and its assault on his senses.

You're just filled with anxiety … setting it up is kind of daunting cus you know what you're putting into place, your putting that kitchen scene of where so much of the trouble, um, stemmed from in your whole life … it makes you recall the actual memories if you like, of the cigarette smoke and the smell of alcohol, and the tears of my dad crying and of his nose running and, um, Irish rebel music playing in the background.

Mike described another scene in which he wanted to explore a memory that had been troubling him. He frequently recalled the distress of one of the victims of robbery and could not understand it.

Why she was screaming like that, because, um, I was kind of thinking, have I done anything? Just stood here with a mask on, pointed a gun ... why's she screaming? I couldn't work it out.

Seeing the Unseen by re-enacting the scene with a staff member playing the part of a masked robber gave him a different perspective.

I think it was the scene of Sarah [staff member] *wearing a mask and er, er, a baseball cap and making out she was a robber. And that was actually me in the scene ... me stepping out the scene and looking out at her in that role, it looked quite frightening to be fair ... it just gives you food for thought.*

Steven

Steven was a man in his late twenties who used psychodrama to work on a past experience of abuse which had impacted on his self-identity and relationships with his family. Ultimately, this had set in motion a pattern of relating that cumulated in a violent offence. Like others, Steven reported finding psychodrama anxiety provoking and **Facing Fear** was necessary.

I used to feel nervous quite a lot and quite anxious ... I didn't like feeling vulnerable but I knew that it was important to see that and do my piece of work.

Steven also experienced the profound sense of being **Taken Back**, '*you actually think "oh my god I'm actually here again"*' and becoming **Emotionally Connected**, re-experiencing these feelings in the here and now.

Because everything's slowed down to the point where you have no other way out other than to sit with the feeling you feel right there.

You start feeling the emotions that you would have felt but you can go through all of the feelings, like sadness erm, shame as well ... I started to shrink into myself and I was so ashamed of my vulnerability and it was making me feel like the young boy that I was, in the scene at the time.

Working through the scene allowed Steven to see different perspectives and completely transformed his understanding of one of the central conflicts in his family relationships, giving him **New Meanings**.

It's a penny drop moment where I was sad and I was tearful at that point, because I'd realised that there is a lot of love and affection in my family towards me and I wasn't reading it, I was shutting it, I was batting it away and it made me feel really sad.

Ultimately, working through traumatic memories had some reparative effects that led to a sense of personal **Growth** and **Improved Relationships**. Enacting the scenes, being held in his emotions and finding some acceptance acted as an emotionally corrective experience.

> *I kind of felt like that shrinking feeling was starting to leave, erm, I got feelings of starting to grow as well and I was able to pick myself up and say I've done it, I've confronted one of the biggest, you know ... traumas of my life.*

> *Now I'm actually comfortable now in my own skin.*

> *It feels like I've found my place in my family again.*

Discussion

Though quite different in approach, there were several distinct similarities in the experience of participants on the GTC to those experiencing psychodrama. Clear boundaries provided a safe space for participants to express themselves emotionally and to explore difficult personal material. The experience of care fostered attachments, and these provided opportunities for corrective emotional experiences. Facing fears and accepting vulnerability was important. There was an emotional (i.e. not only cognitive) experience of re-enacting conflicts rooted in earlier life experiences in the here and now. Participants emerged from both processes feeling less burdened by their past, more compassionate and more authentically themselves. Improved relationships with significant others was a highly regarded outcome. Some of these connections between the studies are now elaborated on.

Shared themes

In both studies, features of the environment, including the experience of care and the provision of clear and consistent boundaries, were highly valued by participants. There features were represented in the themes **Secure Base**, **Experience of Care** and **Boundaries**. Our observation was that these characteristics seemed important prerequisites to therapeutic work without which participants would not have felt sufficiently safe to be open. Care was experienced from other residents as well as staff. Giving and receiving 'care' may be countercultural in a prison context (Crewe, 2005) and some staff may be uncomfortable with the idea and language (Crawley, 2004). However, caring appears to be an important aspect of therapeutic relationships between officers and prisoners (Tait, 2008). The findings here echo the importance of staff relationships found by Wilson and McCabe (2002). In the TC context it is an important enabler of attachment.

Along with feeling cared for, the clear structures and boundaries of the GTC and psychodrama were experienced as containing. Learning to live within the constraints of defined rules and boundaries and, over time, coming to adopt and enforce them is one of the key principles of social therapy (Genders & Player, 1995). A consequence of the clear rules is a sense of safety that permits the expression of feelings and personal disclosures. This containment allows individuals to display negative behaviour which can then be challenged (TC concept of permissiveness) or to reveal more vulnerable feelings which can be attended to.

Participants turning towards vulnerability, rather than away from it, was another feature in both studies illustrated in the **Embracing Vulnerability** and **Facing Fear** subthemes. In prison environments challenges to masculinity and status are frequent (Butler, 2008), and expression of emotions other than anger is ordinarily perceived as weakness (Jewkes, 2002; Hua-Fu, 2005). The TC context provides an environment where these 'compulsions to conform to hypermasculine ideal could be jettisoned' (Stevens, 2013, p. 127).

In both studies participants described re-enacting past conflicts and the learning from this represented in the subthemes **Re-enacting the Past**, **Taken Back** and **Seeing the Unseen**. The past could either be experienced through a deliberate exploration in psychodrama or via an unconscious re-enactment in general living brought to participants' awareness through therapeutic processes. Attachment theory suggests that children who experience insecure or abusive attachments with primary carers are more likely in adulthood to intuitively, unconsciously seek and reproduce similarly impoverished attachments and ways of relating (Bartholomew, 1990; Hazan & Shaver, 1994). Participants described how these dysfunctional relating styles can be experienced and made conscious. Problematic schemas triggered in here-and-now relationships can be explored, understood in a context of lifelong functioning and, through 'corrective emotional experiences' (Yalom, 1995), be made to feel less inevitable.

Another similarity across the studies was the development of a more authentic and compassionate self, seen in the subthemes **Emerging Authenticity**, **Compassion** and **Growth**.

This can be understood as participants in both studies becoming more accepting of themselves and the things they had done, which in turn they experienced as allowing them to be more accepting of others. Acceptance forms an important part of many psychotherapeutic approaches (e.g. Hayes, Strosahl, & Wilson, 1999; Linehan, 1993; Segal, Williams, & Teadale, 2002) and considered an important aspect of psychological change (Higginson & Mansell, 2008).

Participants described the self that emerged from the therapeutic process as more authentic. This is consistent with Stevens' (2012) argument that psychological change in TCs involves a process of identity reconstruction and narrative reframing as well as Maruna's (2001) findings that successful desisters had developed a new life narrative.

One notable *difference* between the studies is the emphasis the psychodrama participants placed on the power of imagery and action to evoke emotional responses. Sometimes these were distressing and participants had to overcome an instinct to avoid. Experiencing that they could tolerate this distress was important in and of itself, but it also acted as a gateway to reframing their experiences. A question that emerges is whether some of the creative methods used in psychodrama could be integrated into other aspects of TC work rather than only being held in a distinctive group.

Concluding thoughts and questions

It is clear in both studies that relationships are being used as the central vehicle for change. This is consistent with TC principles where ordinary everyday living is used to enable people to explore themselves and their relationships with others. As an intervention within the GTC, psychodrama appears to act as an accelerant to this process rather than replace or detract from it, justifying its modern description as a *core* creative psychotherapy rather than the less integrated sounding *complementary* psychotherapy as it has historically been referred.

Men use the processes on the GTC and in psychodrama to work on their own relational trauma as well as their offending behaviour. Both studies appear to support the notion of corrective emotional experiences being powerful agents for change. The importance of relationships between participants and staff lends support for other environments such as psychologically informed planned environments (PIPEs) that have been shown to facilitate strong attachments (Bond & Gemmell, 2014).

The research reveals the importance of the TC as a container – could psychodrama be safely practiced in other prison settings such as enabling environments? This would need careful consideration as there is the potential for psychodrama to be emotionally destabilising if practiced within an inappropriate context.

Being idiographic, focusing on the detailed experience of a few individuals' experiences, these studies do not reflect an attempt to construct a theory of change or of how a TC or psychodrama works. They do offer some insights, however, into how these processes are experienced which could contribute to theory development or refinement. Further work exploring how the residents experience of change is similar or different from theories of change on TCs (e.g. Haigh, 2013) would be useful. Finally, more general theories of change would be enhanced with some of the insights gained from these investigations. For example, the counter-therapeutic urge to avoid vulnerability at all costs, so striking in this forensic context, is likely to have relevance to a broader range of therapeutic processes and settings.

References

Barr, W., Kirkcaldy, A., Horne, A., Hodge, S., Hellin, K., & Göpfert, M. (2010). Quantitative findings from a mixed methods evaluation of once-weekly therapeutic community day services for people with personality disorder. *Journal of Mental Health, 19*(5), 412–421.

Bartholomew, K. (1990). Avoidance of intimacy: An attachment perspective. *Journal of Social and Personal relationships, 7*(2), 147–178.

Bond, N., & Gemmell, L. (2014). Experiences of prison officers on a lifer psychologically informed planned environment. *The International Journal of Therapeutic Communities, 35* (3), 84–94.

Bond, N., & Ross, G.E. (2018). The experience of psychodrama on a forensic therapeutic community: An interpretative phenomenological analysis. Manuscript in preparation.

Butler, M. (2008). What are you looking at? Prisoner confrontations and the search for respect. *British Journal of Criminology, 48*(6), 856–73.

Chiesa, M., Fonagy, P., & Holmes, J. (2006). Six-year follow-up of three treatment programs to personality disorder. *Journal of Personality Disorders, 20*(5), 493–509.

Crawley, E.M. (2004). *Doing prison work: The public and private lives of prison officers.* Willan.

Crewe, B. (2005). Codes and conventions: The terms and conditions of contemporary inmate values. In A. Liebling & S. Maruna (Eds.). *The effects of imprisonment* (pp. 177–208). Willan.

Cullen, J.E. (1994), Grendon: The therapeutic community that works. *Communities for Offenders, 14*(4), 301–11.

Davies, S., & Campling, P. (2003). Therapeutic community treatment of personality disorder: service use and mortality over 3 years' follow-up. *The British Journal of Psychiatry, 182*(44), 24–7.

Dolan, R. (2017). HMP Grendon therapeutic community: The residents' perspective of the process of change. *Therapeutic Communities: The International Journal of Therapeutic Communities, 38*(1), 23–31.

Duggan, C. (2004), Does personality change and, if so, what changes?, *Criminal Behaviour and Mental Health, 14*(1), 5–16.

Genders, E., & Player, E. (1995). *Grendon: A study of a therapeutic prison.* Clarendon.

Gibbons, M.B.C., Crits-Christoph, P., Barber, J.P., Wiltsey Stirman, S., Gallop, R., Goldstein, L.A., Temes, S., & Ring-Kurtz, S. (2009). Unique and common mechanisms of change across cognitive and dynamic psychotherapies. *Journal of Consulting and Clinical Psychology, 77*(5), 801–13.

Haigh, R. (2013). The quintessence of a therapeutic environment. *The International Journal of Therapeutic Communities, 34*(1), 6–15.

Hayes, S.C., Strosahl, K.D., & Wilson, K.G. (1999). *Acceptance and commitment therapy: An experiential approach to behaviour change.* Guilford Press.

Hazan, C., & Shaver, P.R. (1994). Attachment as an organizational framework for research on close relationships. *Psychological Inquiry, 5*(1), 1–22.

Higginson, S., & Mansell, W. (2008). What is the mechanism of psychological change? A qualitative analysis of six individuals who experienced personal change and recovery. *Psychology and Psychotherapy: Theory, Research and Practice, 81*(3), 309–28.

HM Chief Inspector of Prisons. (2017). *Report on an unannounced inspection of HMP Gartree.* HMCIP.

Hua-Fu, H. (2005). The patterns of masculinity in prison. *Critical Criminology, 13*(1), 1–16.

Jefferies, J. (2010). Psychodrama as part of core therapy at HMP Grendon. In R. Shuker & E. Sullivan (Eds.). *Grendon and the emergence of forensic democratic therapeutic communities: Developments in research and practice,* (pp. 137–52). Wiley-Blackwell.

Jewkes, Y. (2002). The use of media in constructing identities in the masculine environment of men's prisons. *European Journal of Communication, 17*(32), 205–25.

Lees, J., Manning, N., & Rawlings, B. (2004). A culture of enquiry: Research evidence and the therapeutic community. *Psychiatric Quarterly, 75*(3), 279–294.

Linehan, M. (1993). *Cognitive-behavioural treatment of borderline personality disorder.* Guilford Press.

Maruna, S. (2001). *Making good: How ex-convicts reform and rebuild their lives.* American Psychological Association.

Miller, S., Sees, C., & Brown, J. (2006). Key aspects of psychological change in residents of a prison therapeutic community: A focus group approach. *The Howard Journal of Criminal Justice, 45*(2), 116–28.

Moreno, J.L. (1985). *Psychodrama* (Vol. 1). Beacon House.

Newton, M. (1998). Changes in measures of personality, hostility and locus of control during residence in a prison therapeutic community. *Legal and Criminological Psychology, 3*(2), 209–23.

Paget, S., Thorne, J., & Das, A. (2015). *Service standards for therapeutic communities.* Royal College of Psychiatrists' Research Unit.

Pearce, S., & Haigh, R. (2017). *The theory and practice of democratic therapeutic community treatment.* Jessica Kingsley.

Pearce, S., Scott, L., Attwood, G., Saunders, K., Dean, M., De Ridder, R., Galea, D., Konstantinidou, H., & Crawford, M. (2017). Democratic therapeutic community treatment for personality disorder: randomised controlled trial. *The British Journal of Psychiatry, 210*(2), 149–56.

Rapoport, R. (1960). *Community as doctor: New perspectives on a therapeutic community.* Tavistock.

Ross, G.E., & Auty, J.A. (2018). The experience of change in a prison therapeutic community: An interpretative phenomenological analysis. *Therapeutic Communities: The International Journal of Therapeutic Communities, 39*(1), 59–70.

Segal, Z.V., Williams, J.M.G., & Teasdale, J.D. (2002). *Mindfulness-based cognitive therapy for depression: A new approach to relapse prevention.* Guilford.

Shine, J. (2001). Characteristics of inmates admitted to Grendon therapeutic prison and their relationship to length of stay. *International Journal of Offender Therapy and Comparative Criminology, 45*, 252–65.

Shine, J., & Morris, M. (2000). Addressing criminogenic needs in a prison therapeutic community. *Therapeutic Communities, 21*(3), 197–219.

Shuker, R. (2010). Personality disorder: Using therapeutic communities as an integrative approach to address risk. In R. Shuker & E. Sullivan (Eds.). *Grendon and the emergence of forensic democratic therapeutic communities: Developments in research and practice* (pp. 115–37). Wiley.

Shuker, R., & Newton, M. (2008). Treatment outcome following intervention in a prison-based therapeutic community: A study of the relationship between reduction in criminogenic risk and improved psychological well-being. *The British Journal of Forensic Practice, 10*(3), 33–44.

Smith, J.A. (1996). evolving issues for qualitative psychology. In J. Richardson (Ed.). *Handbook of qualitative research methods for psychology and the social sciences* (pp. 189–201). Wiley-Blackwell.

Smith, J.A., & Osborne, M. (2003). Interpretative phenomenological analysis. In J.A. Smith (Ed.). *Qualitative psychology: A practical guide to research methods* (pp. 25–50). SAGE.

Smith, J.A., Flowers, P., & Larkin, M. (2009). *Interpretative phenomenological analysis: Theory, method and research.* SAGE.

Stevens, A. (2010). Introducing forensic democratic therapeutic communities. In R. Shuker and E. Sullivan (Eds.). *Grendon and the emergence of forensic democratic therapeutic communities: Developments in research and practice* (pp. 7–25). Wiley-Blackwell.

Stevens, A. (2012). 'I am the person now I was always meant to be': Identity reconstruction and narrative reframing in therapeutic community prisons. *Criminology and Criminal Justice, 12*, 527–47.

Stevens, A. (2013). *Offender rehabilitation and therapeutic communities: Enabling change the TC way.* Routledge.

Tait, S. (2008). Care and the prison officer: Beyond 'turnkeys' and 'care bears'. *Prison Service Journal, 180*, 3–11.

Ward, T., & Maruna, S. (2007). *Rehabilitation.* Routledge.

Wilson, D., & McCabe, S. (2002). How HMP Grendon 'works' in the words of those undergoing therapy. *The Howard Journal of Criminal Justice, 41*(3), 279–91.

Yalom, I.D. (1995). *The theory and practice of group psychotherapy.* Basic Books.

Evaluating the efficacy of core creative psychotherapies within therapeutic communities at HMPPS Grendon

7

Jo Augustus and Jinnie Jefferies

Introduction

This chapter will briefly outline the context of HMP Grendon, before outlining the context and history of the development of core creative psychotherapies (CCPs) at the prison. This will include a description of how each CCP modality is practiced, their basis and aims of treatment. Related research exploring the effectiveness of creative psychotherapies within forensics will also be summarised. The chapter will provide an overview of recent qualitative research conducted and also discuss the methodologies used for conducting this research, before finally drawing upon the dominant themes.

In drawing upon the various themes gleaned from this analysis, the authors will present examples of techniques and sessions to expand on and support the findings of this joint evaluative research.

Grendon is a category B male prison accommodating 230 men in England and Wales. It is currently the only HM Prison that consists entirely of thera-peutic communities (TCs) and is divided into six different communities. Each community, with the exception of the TC Plus (a wing dedicated to working with prisoners with a lower intellectual ability), consists of up to 43 prisoners, who live, work and invest in therapy together through the model of psycho-dynamic group work. There is also a dedicated enhanced assessment unit, where prisoners will reside initially to determine their suitability for this treatment model.

The men who reside at Grendon have committed a multitude of serious offences, including murder, rape, arson, robbery and a vast array of other vio-lent offences. Many have long prison sentences to serve, and in that respect their treatment at Grendon will often only form a part of their journey through the prison system. A good proportion of the men who reside at Grendon have a diagnosis of severe personality disorder/traits. A severe personality dis-order is present when there are severe problems in interpersonal functioning

DOI: 10.4324/9780429317460-9

affecting all areas of their lives. There is evidence demonstrating the success of TCs treating personality disorders (De Boer-van Shalik & Derks 2010).

The foundations of the democratic therapeutic community (DTC) model for treatment were inspired by the work of Maxwell Jones (1953) and his work with post- war veterans after the Second World War, and also his pioneering work that took place in the Henderson Hospital treating patients with social and interpersonal problems. Bowlby's work (1944) on attachment theory has further influenced and shaped the psychodynamic group work model within DTCs. He emphasised how our early experiences of attachment to primary carers fundamentally shape how we experience the world beyond. Not surprisingly, a large number of prisoners in the UK have experienced disorganised or insecure early attachments, often as a result of childhood abuse/neglect.

There are some basic principles which characterise or shape democratic TCs: Democratisation, Permissiveness, Communalism and Reality Confrontation. These principles underpin the ethos of a TC upon which all the psychodynamic group work is essentially built.

The residents who come to engage in therapeutic work at Grendon have usually experienced varying degrees of trauma, a reality that further compounds their early disorganised or insecure attachment history. The trauma they have endured through their lives may also include the extreme offences they have committed and the devastating impact these crimes have had upon them and others. There are also a considerable number of residents who have been diagnosed with post-traumatic stress disorder (PTSD) at Grendon.

Addressing extensive offending behaviours, alongside buried trauma and experiences of abuse within group therapy, can be a very challenging task, and one that requires careful, considered and patient facilitation. The commitment the residents are capable of giving to one another in this considerable task can have a powerful impact. Conversely, it can also be inherently destructive, specifically if the resident is not fully committed to the process of real change.

The history of core creative psychotherapies at HMPPS Grendon

Core creative psychotherapies were introduced 39 years ago in the form of psychodrama and later, art therapy. Today there are three core creative modalities practiced at Grendon, including music therapy (although this modality did not form part of this research study presented). Today, the CCPs at Grendon are considered a central component of the integral group work that takes place on each TC. The CCP groups are once weekly for two hours, and the membership to each group is between six and eight.

The CCP groups have been developed at Grendon in order to provide the residents with an alternative and supportive way to access their emotions and to crucially uphold and support the core work they are engaged in within their small groups. It is important that the work in their CCP groups is regularly shared in all other group forums on the community, and regular opportunities are structured and put into practice in order that communication remains fluid and transparent. The residents themselves take ownership of this sharing and communication, both within their small groups and on the large group/community meetings where allotted time is given each week for this to happen. Those in art therapy are also encouraged to regularly take pieces of artwork into their small group to share and reflect upon. Integrating the work in this way enables others on the community who would not necessarily have contemplated a CCP group previously to consider how they may benefit from it themselves.

Psychodrama psychotherapy

Psychodrama is an action-based group psychotherapy created and developed by J.L. Moreno in the twentieth century.

It employs action methods to encourage the expression of suppressed emotions and introduces the possibility of change by correcting the maladaptive learning that has taken place.

It uses dramatic format, theatrical terms and role analysis for participants to explore in the context of the group how their modes of procuring and dealing with significant others is influenced by their internal world and how their dysfunctional 'internal working models' (beliefs of self and others) have been brought about by early childhood experiences. The client is encouraged to find new ways of perceiving and reacting to past and present life experiences and to understand the process as to how he/she has come to offend.

The technique of role reversal increases victim empathy or reflective functioning and explores the state of mind of the other. The physical setting of scenes and the use of group members to play significant characters in their lives brings the 'there and then' of the past into the 'here and now' of the session. This process provokes memories and strong feelings from the past and the present and allows the protagonist to examine the distorted belief systems that have influenced his/her behaviour and how unexpressed feelings of anger have been displaced onto the innocent victim. Internal working models and dysfunctional attachment strategies are understood and challenged. Goldman and Morrison (1984) described the structure of a session as follows:

- begins with the presenting problem;
- finds similarities in the recent past;

- discovers linkages with the deep past;
- helps the client under the process in his life;
- achieves a catharsis, if necessary;
- concretises the issues, choices and actions that keep the client in the present dysfunctional state;
- helps the client understand the options in life;
- aids in the integration of the cognitive and affective; and
- achieves closure and healing so that the client can carry out in life what has been learnt in the therapy.

Psychodrama psychotherapy forensic research

Jefferies (1987) carried out a qualitative research study at Grendon as part of a Master of Science project into whether psychodrama improved the self-concept of prisoners. The study found that psychodrama improved gains in self-concept but there were no significant differences between psychodrama and the control group. The view that negative self-image may lead to a propensity to offend is a long-standing one in criminology: Cohen (1955), Becker (1963), Hewitt (1970) and Kaplin (1975).

Subjects were 26 male prisoners of British birth with a mean age of 32 years. Subjects were invited to participate in the research project and were divided into two groups across two wings; two newly formed psychodrama groups which met for two hours a week in addition to their normal scheduled activities, and two controlled talking only groups that were already meeting thrice a week. The Tennessee Self Concept Scale (Fitts (1964) was administered, and all members in the study were pretested using this scale and post-tested after a period of three months. The test shows levels of self -concept. The result of the statistical analysis found that there was a significant difference between the pre- and post-test self-concept scores.

The idea that other people's perception towards self enables us to reflect on ourselves and have a self-view is supported by Cooley and others (1922). Charney's (1975) research findings in which he recorded and analysed an example of role reversal (a psychodrama technique) suggests that the use of role reversal, particularly when linked with R.D. Laing's theory (1966) of interpersonal perception assisted clients in developing accurate self-identities by helping them discover how they see themselves and how others see them. Both groups' self-concept scales improved, but it was predicted that the gains in the psychodrama group would be greater than the gains in the control group; however, the results were insignificant.

Other psychodrama research undertaken

Baim, Allam, Eames, Hunt, and Dunford (1999) undertook a research study on the use of psychodrama to enhance victim empathy in those who have committed sexual offences. The capacity to empathise with others, to perceive and share emotional response is related to prosocial behaviour. Hudson et al. (1993) showed low levels of empathy (especially towards the perpetrators' victims) in sexual offending. This research study examined the effectiveness of using psychodrama to enhance victim empathy in a group of nine members who had committed sex offences attending a Probation Service Treatment Programme. The psychodrama programme was evaluated using a number of psychometric tests pre- and post-treatment. The results indicated that psychodrama can be effective in enhancing empathy.

Maxine Daniels (2011) undertook research into the use of role play as a therapeutic tool in clinical practice, exploring how sexual offenders experience role reversing with their victims during sex offender treatment.

The study presents an investigation into the experiences of 11 sex offenders from three separate prisons, who had completed the victim empathy module. Interpretative phenomenological analysis (Smith 2009) was used to analyse the data. Seven superordinate themes were identified, and the findings built on the theory of the Assimilation of Problematic Experience Scale (APES) scale (Stiles et al. 1992). The results highlight the use of role play in helping offenders embody the role of victim and enabling them to unlock previously suppressed emotions. They were able to gain action insight into the consequences to victims and self, which allowed them to humanise the victim in order to understand the problematic experiences. Once they processed their internal parts and integrated parts of self, they were able to self-reflect and reformulate the experience in relation to the victim and in general perspective-taking.

Art psychotherapy

Art psychotherapy emphasises the process of art making safely within the context of a therapeutic relationship in pursuit of beneficial psychological, social and rehabilitative goals for its participants. The British Association of Art Therapists (BAAT) suggests that art psychotherapy is a form of therapy in which the making of visual images in the presence of a qualified art psychotherapist contributes towards externalisation of thoughts and feelings that may otherwise remain unexpressed. The images may provide a diagnostic tool as well as a therapeutic function, in that they provide the individual and therapist with a visible record of the session and give indicators for further treatment. Art psychotherapists may work with transference, that is, feelings from the past, which are projected onto the therapists. Such feelings are often contained within the artwork itself, and such enables resolution to take place indirectly if necessary.

Smeijsters and Cleven (2006) described the use of art therapy to evoke and release aggression, exploring this safely. They further speculate that individuals with a lack of insight achieve such through exploring cognitions, feelings and behaviours, resulting in a less distorted reasoning; the reflection of the image created enables the individual to be confronted with no escape and to deal with what they have made.

Art psychotherapy forensic research

Previous studies in prisons regarding art psychotherapy have included a qualitative study analysing prisoners aggression whilst incarcerated (Smeijsters et al. 2006). The prevalence of aggression is high within UK prisons. Figures reported 16,195 assaults in prisons in England and Wales in 2014 (Prison Service Journal 2015). The Smeijsters et al. (2006) study found that art psychotherapy resulted in increased awareness of the participants' own aggression and decreased impulsivity. Consequently, the individual gained the capacity to talk about conflicts and feelings instead of acting them out due to an increase in emotional literacy.

Schouten, Niet, Knipscheer, Kleber and Hutschemaekers (2014) published a systematic review aiming to identify and evaluate empirical evidence of the effectiveness of art therapy in the treatment of traumatized adults. As a result of the systematic review, six controlled, comparative studies on art therapy for trauma in adult patients were identified. A significant decrease in psychological trauma symptoms was found in the treatment groups, and one study reported a significant decrease in depression. The most statistically significant decrease in trauma symptom severity was found after art therapy intervention in combination with (other) psychotherapy treatment. The authors emphasize this modality's strength in enabling the processing of traumatic experiences and accessing/integrating traumatic memories.

Chong (2015) carried out a study investigating the distinctive role art psychotherapy plays in the intervention for clients with early relational trauma. Through the lens of interpersonal neurobiology, Chong focuses on the impact early relational trauma has on the brain and its development. She refers specifically to damage to a major regulatory system, resulting in an inability to experience empathy and also deficits in memory function and cognitive reasoning. She concludes that there are limitations of purely verbal- and cognitive-based therapies, emphasizing that there is a need for an extra channel of communication beyond verbal means to connect with survivors of early relational trauma, hence the significance of art psychotherapy. Chong (2015) emphasizes:

> Although language and cognitive functioning occupy a privileged position in modern society, interdisciplinary findings have shown that they are not the only method of communication and, in addition, pose several limitations and could potentially turn into a treatment-resistant device.

(p. 125)

Interestingly, Wylie (2007) conducted research at HMPPS Grendon through the production of art therapy imagery on the assessment unit, investigating whether the residents were eligible for treatment at the prison. He identified that their art expression gave a clear indication of their suitability and that such correlated to the residents duration at Grendon. This suggests that art therapy also has diagnostic abilities as well as therapeutic benefits.

Current research methodology and design

The most recent research which will be described throughout this chapter used a qualitative approach to collect data through semi-structured interviews and was analysed using thematic analysis (Herrett 2017), where the common and prevalent themes were identified to determine how effective the therapies were. This type of research was chosen to capture the experiences of the men in a detailed and rich way in order to provide specific aspects of the CCPs. The questions also addressed how the CCPs may help the residents stay offence free post-release. A sample of 12 residents at HMPPS Grendon volunteered for this research. The residents were living in four different therapeutic communities and had completed either art therapy or psychodrama. Each of the men had participated in the CCP for at least one year and the maximum participation time was three and a half years.

The specific research questions for the study were:

1. What is the therapeutic progress made by the men in CCPs and how do these help meet treatment targets and the individual needs and deficits of the men?
2. What does the CCP contribute to residents treatment that other therapies do not?
3. Do the CCPs help with progress in the purely verbal therapies?
4. What specific areas of the CCP helped group members?
5. How do the CCPs prepare the men for life outside prison?

Data analysis strategy

The interviews were analysed using a thematic approach of identifying, analysing and reporting patterns using the model outlined by Braun and Clarke (2006). A six-step coding process was used to generate the themes from the interviews; this ensured the data was sufficiently organised and considered.

Results and discussion

The thematic analysis performed on the data identified four overarching themes:

1. Gained insight
2. Accessing subconscious trauma
3. Space to be supported
4. Behavioural management

Theme one: gained insight

Self-awareness

It was evident from the study that creating an alternative medium to talking for participants to reflect on themselves was helpful. For example, in psychodrama, the residents were able to witness aspects of their life through a different perspective where they could see their own behaviour. This feature of the therapy appeared to cause the residents to evaluate their behaviours due to the aversive feelings they felt towards the *actions* they observed.

The concept of triggers is a stimulant that can contribute to maladaptive behaviours in the offending context. These can take the form of negative feelings, usually originating from childhood and adolescence. Triggers were a common theme, especially in psychodrama. The residents became more able to recognise what caused them to act in an antisocial way, possibly leading to their offence.

Understanding feelings

This subtheme referred to the residents' feeling they had connected to their emotions and were able to better understand and order their thoughts and feelings. The residents emphasized that if they understood their feelings by understanding *why* they were feeling that way, they were more able to control their reactions. Such understanding included their life before prison, allowing them to make sense of their past feelings. The residents also cited being able to identify transference towards the facilitator and use the CCP to work through such feelings.

Gained perspective

The data suggested that art therapy and psychodrama did help residents achieve the skills to examine situations from other peoples' perspective. Furthermore, the ability to take another person's perspective can lead to improvement on gaining victim empathy, eventually preventing recidivism. Within the study the residents discussed how they previously showed no respect for the others' feelings but that after completing a CCP they felt they had more consideration than before. Through psychodrama, for example, they were able to play the role of their victims directly, realising the fear they inflicted on them, further enabling victim empathy. These results also supported Bairn, Allam, Eames, Dunford and Hunt (1999) regarding their study on psychodrama and victim empathy.

Theme two: accessing subconscious trauma

Accessing deep memories

Within the study it was highlighted that the residents described how there were memories and parts of themselves that they had not previously been able to access through purely verbal therapies, or had been averse to, and that the CCPs enabled them to access these memories. Through discussions it was highlighted that due to the medium of creativity, either through dramatization or art, the men could be transported back to memories to be able to explore and discuss these areas more directly. This aspect was powerful due to the emotions that were brought out for the men, and subsequently helped them work through these issues. Furthermore, the residents stated that they could make sense of the situations they had experienced either during their offence or childhood which brought them some resolution.

Dealing with trauma

The residents described the different ways that the CCPs helped them deal with their own trauma. It was summarised that the CCPs enabled them to more freely express problems and relieve feelings of guilt and shame held onto for many years. Many of the men stated how the CCPs also empowered them to distinguish their abuser from others and that this then assisted them in controlling their reactions and how they treated individuals. This property of CCPs is important due to the link between trauma and offending (Macinnes et al. 2016).

Specifically, in art therapy Herretts' study (2017) highlighted the power of the image regarding how there was no escape from what had been created. This was different to small verbal groups as there was no way to divert. It also gave the men the opportunity to develop self-acceptance due to being able to sit with the image in front of them for a period of time.

Theme three: space to be supported

Safe to be vulnerable

A common theme outlined in this study highlighted the increased sense of security felt in the CCP group, especially compared with their small group. The deconstruction of the mask was cited and their increased ability to feel able to be vulnerable, liberated them from their 'macho' persona. In addition, shy residents who struggled to speak in group experienced an increased ability to voice their thoughts and feelings in the CCPs.

Self-expression

Herretts' study (2017) refers to the expressive nature of the CCPs, which appeared to enable the residents to talk about their problems more than they had ever done before. Moreover, through psychodrama, they were able to re-enact their offence and choose to act in a different way. Within art therapy, the comparison to reverting back to being a child was prominent and the benefits of being free to express their feelings and experiences were discussed. The ability to emotionally regress in this way was reported to have felt very enabling.

Furthermore, it was cited that in their small group residents only expressed verbally, but in art therapy, for example, they are able to enjoy themselves, having fun on occasion, which seemed to aid their progress. The medium of creating an image bypassed the verbal explanations of the men's feelings which they found difficult to say out loud. The expressive aspect of art therapy is further supported by Sarid and Huss (2010) who compared cognitive behavioural intervention to art therapy, finding that both allow imaginative expression, but the use of art materials allows manipulation and more sensory control, which increases self- expression.

Group dynamics

Herrett (2017) stresses that the importance of the CCP group was emphasized throughout the interviews. Many residents felt that the support and honesty of the therapist was an essential component to their progress. The research suggested that the CCP therapist asked thought-provoking questions and encouraged them to examine different aspects of their lives, more so than their facilitators in small groups.

In addition, the importance of the group members interactions was emphasised, the sharing of experiences and connections and how well they interacted together through the creative medium. However, there were some negative comments regarding the burden of listening to accounts of other people's crimes and their traumatic childhoods, as this had a negative effect on some of them.

Theme four: behavioural management

Control reactions/emotions

Within this theme the study highlights that a common issue for residents at Grendon is their lack of ability to control their reactions and emotions, often resulting in negative behaviours and contributors to their crime. This is a common treatment target for the men, and the study highlighted a perceived improvement in the control of their reaction and emotions due to the CCP.

Consequential thinking

The concept of consequential thinking refers to the ability to assess choices and anticipate how other people will react in different scenarios. Within the study, Herrett (2017) states,

> Upon completion of the CCP the residents appeared to demonstrate an increased understanding of how their actions affected their lives and others around them. The residents described how the CCP's helped them to examine each event of their life in such scrutiny that the ripple effect of their actions was made clearer to them than previously. This was achieved through re-enacting parts of the mens lives and practising possible future scenarios for example.
>
> (pp. 35–36)

It has been evidenced that teaching consequential thinking can reduce impulsivity, which is a high-risk factor for many residents at Grendon (Ross & Fabiano 1985). Herrett (2017) suggests that through the newfound consequential thinking, the men were able to view their lives in a different way, realising they were in control of what happens to them. Through acknowledgement of the work achieved in the CCP, they were able to see there was more to life than being in prison, reducing their need to reoffend.

Limitations of the study

The retrospective nature of the study may have changed the way the men recalled their experiences. However, it did allow the experiences of the CCPs to be reflected upon and allowed a long-term view to be captured. It was clear that there is uncertainty regarding whether or not it was solely the CCPs alone that were responsible for the benefits described. However, the interview questions were focused towards the added benefits of the CCP to the residents' progress at Grendon, which may have reduced the overlap between the CCPs and small groups.

Evidencing the research outcomes: two clinical vignettes

What follows are two brief clinical vignettes from psychodrama and art psychotherapy group work at Grendon that seek to evidence and support the research outcomes outlined above.

Vignette 1 Psychodrama

Psychodrama supports the identified themes highlighted in the research project:

1. Gained Insight
2. Accessing subconscious Trauma
3. Space to be supported
4. Behavioural Management

The following session illustrates how one individual through the use of psychodrama was able to gain a clearer understanding of the process that led up to his offence, and with the group providing a safe supportive environment, the individual was able to access and express his feelings about early childhood trauma and explore different ways of managing his behaviour. The words in inverted commas are the actual words spoken in the session by John.

John came to the session wanting to explore his offending behaviour. He was serving a lengthy sentence for rape. 'It is hard to forgive myself; it is just filthy what I have done. I did worse by committing rape than my Mum ever did to me. I hope I get to understand it.'

On the night of the offence, John had been discharged from hospital having cut his wrist. He left the hospital with his arm bandaged. He stated, 'I kept wishing I had lost my arm, that the doctor had not saved it. I know it sounds crazy, but I wanted to rip myself to pieces. The only person I wanted to hurt was my mother, God knows what was happening that night, because I don't.' After the offence he walked around for two weeks, sleeping in bushes, in parks, drinking heavily.

With a few props we had in the room, we constructed the symbols of the bush and asked John to do his roaming and settle under the bush. When he was ready, he was asked, having created the 'there and then' in the 'here and now' of the session, to speak his thoughts aloud, 'I keep looking for excuses, but I cannot find them. I say my mother is to blame but I do not know if she is, it's just me wanting to hurt a woman for some reason.' The psychodrama director picked up on John's statement, 'The only person I wanted to hurt was Mum.' John had already made the connection (*gained insight*) between his present actions and past feelings.

Psychodrama provides a forum for the prisoner to consider in detail how his present behaviour may be influenced by past early childhood experiences. John raped a woman rather than deal with his relationship with mother, his childhood trauma, and his feelings of inadequacy. To explore the link between past and present, John was asked to set up a scene with his mother. His mother is in the bathroom, where he found her bleeding, having cut herself. In real life he said nothing, shut the door, went downstairs and phoned 999, but now in the scene he is asked to confront her: 'I wanted you dead many times. Sometimes I think if I had let you die, I would have been a man now. I hate you (there is a long pause as John views his helpless mother played by a member of the group), why did you beat me?'

At this juncture it was important for John to reverse roles with his mother so that he could struggle with, and hopefully understand why his mother did what he accused her of. By using the technique of role reversal (sometimes with his victim), the prisoner learns to see events as others see them and comes to a clearer understanding of the interactions as they occurred and in so doing adjusts his own view. In the role of his mother speaking her words, he says, 'You remind me of your father and I just wanted to hurt you. You are always sticking up for your father and telling people I am bad. I hated you and your father. You are just like your father – selfish mean and cruel.' (*gained insight*)

Back in his own role and through the conversation that followed, John was able to express his feelings about the trauma he experienced as a child. John had never spoken about his anger towards his mother; instead, he had displaced this anger onto the woman he raped, but as the auxiliary playing the role of his mother repeated her accusations, John began to shout, 'I hate you, I should have let you die. You kept doing these things in front of the kids, you made me clear up your sick, you abused me.' At this point another group member came onto the stage to make a doubling statement expressing the suppressed feelings of John, 'In fact you are not much of a mother, and what hurts most of all is that you do not love me.' This doubling statement stopped John in his tracks and helped John to get to the bottom of his issue with his mother as he struggled with his tears, 'That's true, what hurts is you don't love me. I think every mother should love her son.' Turning to the director, 'She caused me a lot of damage' (*accessing subconscious trauma*).

John went on to tell his mother about the damage she had caused him and began to make the connection between his past experiences, his offending behaviour and his difficulty in making personal relationships, 'I always questioned people when they said they loved me, I always wanted to ask why. If they tried to hold me or put their arm round me, I would push them away. I thought they were going to do things to me that you did, be all lovey dovey and then kick me in the teeth.'

John was provided with a *supportive space* to gain insight into his crime and to access the subconscious trauma. As the session continued, by reversing roles with his mother, he contemplated her story: a mother who had been betrayed and rejected by her husband and who as a result had become depressed, over ate and lost control of her emotions. Having begun to understand better his mother's position, having expressed his own anger, the action moved on and John was given the opportunity to have for himself what he was deprived of all these years. 'All I wanted to do when she was drunk or in a bad mood was to go up and hold her, but I was scared.'

Psychodrama in its use of surplus reality offers the emotionally hungry prisoner the experience, perhaps for the first time, of finding out what it would have been like to have been loved, to receive tenderness rather than cruelty. In his final scene, his mother lay dying in hospital. John, in tears, heard what he thought and hoped his mother might have said, had he been there to make his peace. The auxiliary in the role of mother tells him that he is loved. It is hard for him to hear this, but he says that he looks forward to the day when he could accept and return the love he desires. He ends the scene by telling his mother that he loves and forgives her, before returning to speak to his victim, sobbing as he engages in the encounter, aware of his process and the consequences of his actions (*behaviour* management) (Jefferies 1971).

Vignette 2 Art psychotherapy

This clinical vignette will aim, through the course of one residents' participation within an art therapy group, to demonstrate how this particular modality enabled and enhanced his progress in therapy, specifically within the areas of Gained Insight, Accessing subconscious Trauma, Space to be supported and Behavioural Management as per identified themes highlighted within the research outcomes. I will demonstrate this through the aid of his artwork made in the group alongside the verbal dialogue of his progression through therapy.

Peter was convicted of murder when he was 19 years old. He was given a life sentence. He killed an innocent passer-by. Years of built-up feelings of shame, resentment and rage were expelled onto this victim in a matter of seconds, resulting in his death.

In order for Peter to fully acknowledge the source of his deeply repressed feelings of shame, resentment, hatred and rage, he needed to access through therapy his childhood, where the early relational trauma and abuse were first experienced. This was difficult, because Peter was very protective of his family and lacked insight regarding the extent of how these experiences had damaged and affected him, for example, his propensity for violence. During one session in art therapy he made an image of his front door at home, drawn from the perspective of a child (Figure 7.1). Through this image he began to *gain insight* within the group and allow himself to connect with the emotions he experienced in going in and confronting life behind the door. These were feelings he had not previously allowed himself to reconnect with, as the buried feelings of shame, guilt, hatred and rage experienced in his childhood had previously been protected/denied.

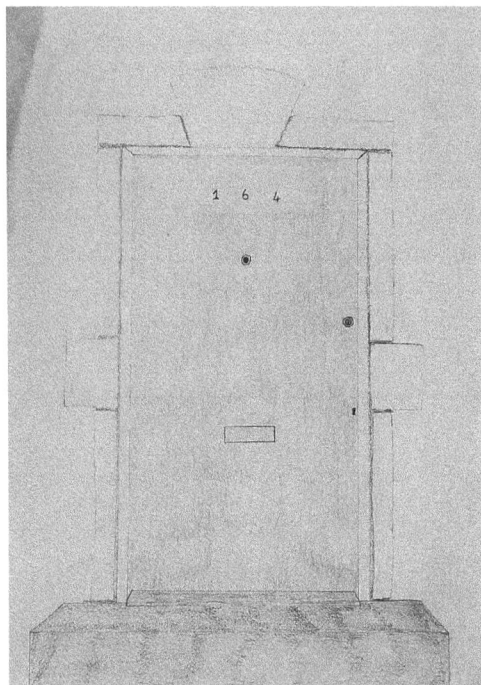

Figure 7.1 Image 1 – front door.

Subsequently, it took a few weeks before Peter decided to use a very large sheet of paper to express to the group what he had experienced *inside* the house he grew up in (Figure 7.2).

Peter was very emotional producing this image and began to share his experiences of witnessing severe domestic violence in the home, and his resulting feelings of hopelessness, anger, fear, rejection, distress and trauma (*Accessing subconscious trauma*). Accessing this subconscious trauma was extremely important for Peter, and eventually enabled him to reflect on his own extreme violence as a perpetrator, and some of its origins.

As Peters' index offence became more accessible within the therapy, he began to explore in more depth the source and impact of his own historical violence. He produced an image in which he confronted the moment he lost control of his rage and extracted his weapon (fencing) to attack his index victim with (Figure 7.3). Confronting the immense anger inside him during that moment enabled the whole group to consider any remaining residual anger (post-offence) that had previously been strenuously denied by him, attending to his *behavioural management*. Such also included his ability *now* to control his reactions/emotions, self-management and development of consequential

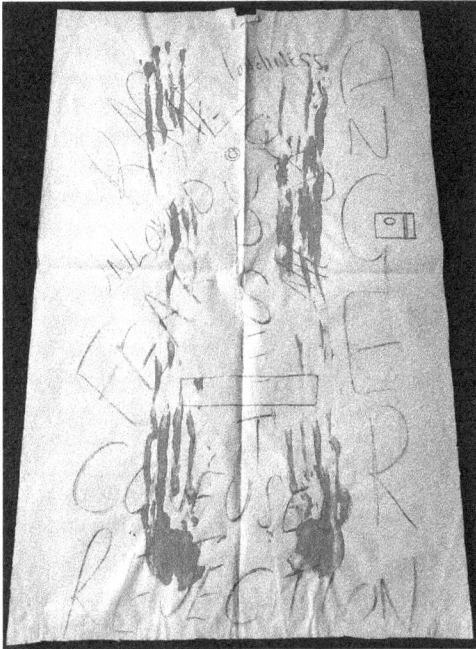

Figure 7.2 Image 2 – behind the door.

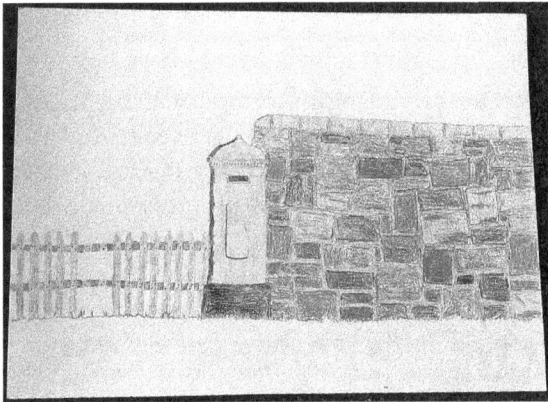

Figure 7.3 Image 3 – the offence.

thinking. This image also opened up further exploration regarding victim empathy.

As Peter progressed towards his recategorisation and potential release from prison, his ability to express himself and his vulnerabilities did increase

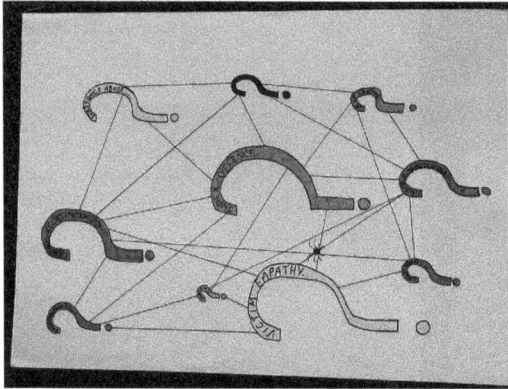

Figure 7.4 Image 4 – self-reflection.

significantly. He produced the image in Figure 7.4, which embodied the enormity of work he now recognised was needed in order for him to feel safe beyond prison from any subsequent acts of violence. He acknowledged that this image would not have been realized before he began art therapy, and that a *space to be supported*, in order to bear his vulnerability in this way, had enabled him to directly confront his own vulnerability and risk.

Conclusions

The research described demonstrates promising outcomes of these CCPs and was the first to conduct a qualitative study on the effectiveness of two CCPs at Grendon. Herrett (2017) concluded that the study indicates that CCPs clearly provide added value to the therapeutic progress made by residents at Grendon. These benefits are reflected through the themes of the data: Gained insight; Accessing subconscious trauma; Space to be supported; and Behavioural management, all of which can be contributing factors in reducing the individuals' risk of reoffending by increasing openness and control of their actions.

The clinical vignettes presented also demonstrate how both art psychotherapy and psychodrama psychotherapy serve to meaningfully enhance the overall TC work at Grendon – how they offer an alternative way to access emotions for residents and support the core work of forensic therapeutic communities. These also highlight the themes identified in the research and support its outcomes.

We continue to conduct six-monthly evaluations regarding how the residents experience their CCP groups. Each participant is invited to fill in a questionnaire. The results have consistently demonstrated how much the CCP groups are valued, and the ways in which they enhance the participants' core offending risk factor work within the whole framework of their group psychotherapy treatment. This feedback from the participants is invaluable and validates its relevance.

Regarding future research, a mixed-methods approach combining both qualitative and quantitative research will be of value, with the potential to provide empirical support for the themes identified. It would also be interesting to examine whether the type of crime committed by the individual has any effect on whether they choose to complete psychodrama or art therapy, and the benefits that they indicate, if any.

References

Baim, Allam, Eames, Hunt, S., & Dunford, S. (1999). The use of psychodrama to enhance victim empathy in sex offenders: An evaluation: *The Journal of Sexual Aggression, 4*, 4–14.

Becker, H. (1963). *Outsiders: Studies in the sociology of deviants.* Free Press.

Bowlby, J. (1944). Forty-four juvenile thieves: Their characters and home-life. *The International Journal of Psycho-analysis, 25*(19). https://doi.org/be442387fc5ald2ea8a802da11d5653

Braun, V., & Clarke, V. (2006). Using thematic analysis in psychology. *Qualitative Research in Psychology, 3*(2), 77–101. http://dx.doi.org/10.1191/1478088706qp063oa

Charney, M. (1975). Psychodrama & self identity. *Group Psychotherapy, 28*, 118–127.

Chong, C.Y.J. (2015). Why art psychotherapy? Through the lens of interpersonal neurobiology; The distinctive role of art psychotherapy intervention for clients with early relational trauma. *International Journal of Art Therapy, 20*, 118–126. https://doi.org/10.1080/17454832.2015.1079727

Cohen, A. (1955). *Delinquent boys: Culture of the gang.* Macmillan.

Cooley, C. (1922). *Human nature and the social order.* Scribner.

Daniels, M. (2011). *The use of role play as a therapeutic tool in clinical practice: What do sexual offenders experience when role reversing with their victims? Her Majesty's Prison Service Core Sex Offender Treatment Programme.* [Unpublished Doctoral thesis]. Metanoia in partnership with Middlesex University.

De Boer-van Shaik, J., & Derks, F. (2010). The Van der Hoeven Clinic: A flexible and innovative forensic psychiatric hospital based on therapeutic community principles. In R. Shuker & E. Sullivan (Eds.), *Grendon and the emergence of forensic therapeutic communities* (pp. 45–60). Wiley-Blackwell.

Fitts, W. (1964). *Tennessee Self Concept Scale.* Counselor Recordings and Tests.

Goldman, E., & Morrison, D. (1984). *Psychodrama experience and process.* Kendall & Hunt.

Herrett, N. (2017) *Evaluating the efficacy of core creative psychotherapies within Therapeutic Communities at HMP Grendon.* [Master's thesis]. Birmingham City University. Also published in *The Prison Service Journal* (2018), 238, 39–46.

Hewitt, J. (1970). Social stratifications of deviant behaviour. *Journal of Nervous & Mental Disorders, 159*, 172–181.

Hudson, S.M., Marshall W.L., Wales, D., McDonald, E., Bakker, L.W., & McClean, A. (1993). Emotional recognition skills of sex offenders. *Annals of Sex Research, 6,* 199–211.

Jefferies, J. (1971). What we are doing here is defusing bombs. In P. Holmes & M. Karp (Eds.), *Psychodrama: Inspiration & technique* (pp. 189–200). Routledge.

Jefferies, J. (1987). *The effect of psychodrama on the self concept of prisoners.* [Unpublished Master's thesis]. Surrey University.

Jones, M. (1953). *The therapeutic community: A new treatment method in psychiatry.* Basic Books.

Kaplan, H. (1975). *Self-attitudes and deviant behaviour.* Goodyear.

Macinnes, M., Macpherson, G., Austin, J., & Schwannauer, M. (2016). Examining the effect of childhood trauma on psychological distress, risk of violence and engagement, in forensic mental health. *Psychiatry Research, 246,* 314–320. https://doi.org/10.1016/j.psychres.2016.09.054

Prison Reform Trust. (2017). www.prisonreformtrust.org.uk/ProjectsResearch/Mentalhealth

Prison Service Journal. (2015). www.crimeandjustice.org.uk/sites/crimeandjustice.org.uk/files/PSJ%20221%20September%202015.pdf

Ross, R.R., & Fabiano, E.A. (1985). *Time to think: A cognitive model of delinquency prevention and offender rehabilitation.* Institution of Social Sciences & Arts.

Sarid, O., & Huss, E. (2010). Trauma and acute stress disorder: A comparison between cognitive behavioural intervention and art therapy. *The Arts in Psychotherapy, 37,* 8–12. https://doi.org/10.1016/j.aip.2009.11.004

Schouten, K.A., de Niet, G.J., Knipscheer, J.W., Kleber, R.J., & Hutschemaekers, G.J.M. (2015). The effectiveness of art therapy in the treatment of traumatized adults: A systematic review on art therapy and trauma. *Trauma Violence Abuse, 16*(2), 220–228. https://doi.org/10.1177/1524838014555032. Epub 2014 Nov 16.

Smeijsters, H., & Cleven, G. (2006). The treatment of aggression using arts therapies in forensic psychiatry: Results of a qualitative inquiry. *The Arts in Psychotherapy, 33,* 37–58. https://doi.org/10116/j.aip.2005.07.001

Smith, J., Flowers, P., & Larkin, M. (2009). *Interpretative phenomenological analysis: Theory, method and research.* SAGE.

Stiles, B. (2005). Assimilation of Problematic Experience Scale. *Psychology Quarterly, 18,* 85–93.

Wylie, B. (2007). Self and social function: Art therapy in a therapeutic community prison. *Journal of Brand Management, 14,* 324–334. https://doi.org/ 10.1057

Wylie, B. (2010). *Self and social function; Art therapy and readiness for treatment in a therapeutic community prison.* In R. Shuker, & E. Sullivan, (Eds). *Grendon and the emergence of forensic therapeutic communities: Developments in research and practice* (pp. 153–170). John Wiley & Sons.

Quality measurement 'from within' in Russian addiction rehabilitation centres

8

Background, design and results of a Norwegian–Russian cooperation project

Virginie Debaere, Kenneth Arctander Johansen and Ruslan Isaev

Background of the NORUS Project

The chapter presents the background, research design and findings of an innovative Norwegian–Russian cooperation project (NORUS) that aims at promoting service users' involved quality measurement and improvement in Russian substance addiction treatment services. This NORUS project started in 2018 from the Russian Strategy 2020 for the addiction field and the Norwegian policy of 'The patient's health service'. The idea for the project came to be when the Norwegian Ministry of Health issued a call to apply for a grant addressing Norwegian and Russian stakeholders to cooperate on health in the Nordic region, prioritising innovative projects contributing to users' involvement and the participation of vulnerable groups. The mixed-method design allows an in-depth view of service users' experiences in therapeutic community (TC)-like private rehabilitation centres in the Moscow region. Similarities and differences related to findings on the interrelatedness between residents' processes of change and treatment working principles in Western TCs are discussed. The particularity of quality improvement issues regarding addiction treatment in Russia are summarised and future steps for the continuation of the project are presented.

DOI: 10.4324/9780429317460-10

Russian challenge with regard to substance addiction (treatment)

Substance dependency issues are challenging for the Russian Federation. While official sources have published a steady number of 500,000 drug-dependent persons over many years (Information Agency RIA News, 2008), less official sources mention 1.5 to 2 million (Celinskiy, 2017; Information Agency RIA News, 2008), and recently even five million people with substance-misuse problems are mentioned, of whom 30% are dependent on illicit substances (Hamzaev, 2019). The high accessibility of new psychoactive substances might contribute to younger drug-using populations. High correlations are found between drug use and crime: 65% of all crimes are drug related, while nearly 80% of small thefts are thought to be committed by drug-dependent persons (Information Agency RIA News, 2008). The overall cost is estimated at 4.1 billion Russian roubles annually or 3.96% of Russia's gross domestic product (GDP) (Hamzaev, 2019) (i.e. 49,846 British pounds or 64,484 million American dollars or 57,726 million European euros (based on exchange rate on 2 November 2019)).

Russia's drug policy is part of its state policy on national security and socio-economic development. It was adopted in 2010 and outlined in *The Russian State Strategy for the Implementation of the National Anti-Drug Policy of the Russian Federation in the Period until 2020* (hereafter Strategy 2020) (Russian Federation, 2010). The strategy focuses mainly on substantially reducing the illicit drug trade and the impact it has on security, public health, society and the state, by focusing, amongst other measures, on the improvement of the system of law enforcement. Another goal is the reduction of the non-medical use of drugs through improving medical help and rehabilitation for people who use drugs (Russian Federation, 2009). However, according to the Russian government, the current drug treatment system overseen by the Ministry of Healthcare, is characterised by low efficiency and decreasing treatment services (Russian Federation, 2017). Therefore, a strategic goal is to improve access to treatment with the aim of reducing drug-related mortalities (Russian Federation, 2009).

Nonetheless, professionals in the rehabilitation field criticise the drug policy for not putting enough attention to demand reduction, development of rehabilitation and resocialisation programmes (Russian Ministry of Health, 2013). Furthermore, the *non-existence* of public quality standards for addiction rehab centres is what is experienced as most problematic.

As a matter of fact, the field of addiction treatment in Russia differs from that in most countries in Western Europe. Only a small segment is provided by the government. Nowadays, the system consists of four state rehabilitation centres and 20 rehabilitation departments (Federal Drug Control Service of

Russia, 2011). Officially, these centres focus on prevention and early detection (e.g. by the end of 2013, a drug-use detection test was implemented in the school system), but according to Ruslan Isaev (R. Isaev, personal communication, 20 October 2018), their professional activity remains rather opaque to the civil society. In fact, most addiction treatment services in Russia are organised by non-governmental commercial organisations. It is difficult to gain a clear overview of the Russian treatment sector. While there are also rehabilitation centres run by the Russian Orthodox Church (Chelischeva, 2015) and the labour communes (i.e. small communes based on the idea of work-as-therapy), the majority of today's addiction treatment is provided by private, commercial rehabilitation centres, of which there are about 1,500 in Russia (Rambler, 2018).

In dialogue with the researchers, Dr Isaev explained that it was only in 1996 that the first professional rehabilitation centres were established in Russia; they opened in Moscow and in St. Petersburg simultaneously (R. Isaev, personal communication, 20 October 2018). Near St. Petersburg, Louis F. Bantle opened The House of Hope on the Hill, the first and only Russian free rehabilitation centre for people with alcohol addiction, which is still operational today (House of Hope on the Hill). Next to another rehabilitation centre that started in 1996 in Moscow, The Recovery (which no longer exists today), attention was also focused on studying addiction treatment by opening a scientific centre in Moscow, which is the well-known Clinic of Marshak (Marshak's Clinic, 2007), still in existence.

From the beginning, psychologists have been employed alongside *experts by experience* in these rehabilitation centres. Important to note is that 'self-help' and 'peer support' have been widely used in Russia. This can be understood by the fact that many of these organisations have been influenced by the American drug-free TC model and/or the 12-step Minnesota rehabilitation model (Minnesota Model of Addiction Treatment). In 1997, the Russian Ministry of Health even prescribed the implementation of the 12-step philosophy to be part of the training programmes for professionals in addiction treatment (Isaev, 2015). After 1997, the 12-step programme together with the biopsychosocial approach to addiction became part of the mandatory programme of specialised higher education institutions. Today it is being taught in both the state universities and in the commercial (non-state) universities.

In recent years, the government has made some efforts to develop public quality standards for addiction rehabilitation centres, and to offer addicted persons financial support for treatment. In 2014, a state programme was launched in Moscow to subsidise addiction treatment for its citizens. Every adult experiencing drug addiction could apply for a governmental grant to pay his or her treatment programme in a private, qualified, addiction rehabilitation centre, while remaining anonymous. Hundreds of addicted persons and their relatives were helped successfully because of this financial aid from the state (which is, of course, a very low percentage of all persons in need) (Ivushkina & Raskin, 2015). It is also interesting to note that during the mentioned period, there were some legal developments. According to the legal changes, dependent people who were convicted could opt for addiction treatment in a qualified rehabilitation centre as an alternative to going to prison (Russian Federation, 2016). However, more work should have been done with the concerned stakeholders to translate it into a large-scale good practice. Then, unfortunately, the Federal Service Control of Drugs (FSCD) was disbanded in 2016. At present, it is not certain what government agency is responsible for services. Still, rehabilitation centres continue to emerge. These have been criticised for not being able to achieve remission and even for adding additional harm to the mental and somatic health of the service users (Russian Ministry of Health, 2013). Many of them do not have professional staff; basic requirements are not followed (e.g. fire safety, sanitary needs, etc); and violence has occurred, in some situations even with fatal outcomes (Starkova, 2019).

Norwegian experience of quality measurement and service users' involvement

In Norway, since 2004 dependency treatment became a state-managed specialised health service within the hospital sector (Nesvaag & Lie, 2010). Service provision consists of public hospital services and non-profit organisations that have contractual agreements with the health authorities at the cost of 3.6 billion Norwegian crowns in 2018 (i.e. 335.8 million European euros or 338.3 million U.S. dollars or 300 million British pounds (based on exchange rate on 18 November 2020)) (Norwegian Directorate of Health, 2018).

The principle of the Norwegian government's health policy is epitomised by the slogan 'The patient's health service'. The policy aim is that the service apparatus is of a certain capacity, that it is organised so that service users are able to choose freely the treatment they feel that they need (Norwegian Government, 2014), and that their voices are heard in the development of these services (Norwegian Government, 2018). In 2015, the health minister, Bent Høie, asked: 'If the service user could decide, what would the health system look like?' and stated that the answer has to be taken seriously (Sykepleien, 2015). The involvement of service users is part of Norwegian legislation; The Patient Rights Act (Norwegian Government, 2014) emphasises that service users shall be informed and be part of determining their treatment; and The Health Authorities Act and The Municipal Health and Care Services Act require service providers to establish systems for obtaining (service) users' experiences.

As a consequence, quality measurement 'from within' is central to Norwegian addiction treatment policy. Service users' involvement and feedback are crucial to quality measurement and improvement. Together with other quality measurements on clinical processes and results, service users' experiences are used to assess whether quality changes occur over time and patient experiences are seen as correlative with clinical efficacy and patient safety (Norwegian Directorate of Health, 2017).

Since 2013, the service users of all Norwegian residential addiction treatment services are asked annually to complete the Service Users' Survey, a questionnaire issued by the Norwegian Public Health Institute (Norwegian Directorate of Health, 2017). The accomplishment of that survey is counted as one of the eight quality indicators that measure overall quality of addiction treatment (Norwegian Directorate of Health, 2019). It documents the service users' satisfaction with the treatment. The surveys have been carried out amongst service users who were admitted to 24-hour cross-disciplinary specialised addiction treatment services, who were at least 16 years old (Norwegian Directorate of Health, 2017).

In the second quarter of 2020, Norwegian service users felt that they were generally sufficiently informed about the rules and routines of the treatment institutions upon admission and that they were welcomed in a satisfactory way. Normally, they did not have to wait long to start treatment. They had quite good experiences with the staff members. The service users perceived treatment to be useful and generally they had satisfactory access to the staff. To some degree they felt prepared for their life after discharge (Norwegian Public Health Institute, 2020).

Published annual reports based on the results are intended to reach political leadership, sector leadership, health professionals, service users and citizens (Norwegian Directorate of Health, 2017). They have been used to feed policy discussions and to improve strategies with regard to addiction treatment. For instance, civil society organisations and professional associations have raised political demands for a strengthened presence of certain professions in specialised health services (NTB, 2014), for improved integration of services and for more funding for re-entry programmes (Mathiesen, 2015).

The 'NORUS match'

Given the stated need of the Russian Federation, located in their white paper 'Strategy 2020', with regard to the development of quality treatment services for people suffering from substance addiction, a 'match' was found with the Norwegian quality measurement and improvement approach that is based on service users' experiences with treatment.

The first NORUS Project year

Stakeholders and working group

The two stakeholders that joined hands in the NORUS project are the Norwegian Interest Organization for Substance Misusers, or RIO (https://rio. no) and the Russian/international Independent Narcological Guild or ING (http://nng.com.ru/).

RIO is a Norwegian NGO advocating for the interests of people who suffer from substance misuse problems and consists solely of persons who have struggled with addiction problems. ING is an association of leading Russian and some European NGOs providing professional help to people suffering from drug and alcohol addiction. Its main goal is to offer qualitative/professional, effective and safe help to service users.

The first NORUS working group consisted of four members: Kenneth Arctander Johansen, communication manager at RIO and who has become general manager since 1 February 2020; Dr Ruslan Isaev, president of ING and director of a member organisation, the Clinic of Dr Isaev; Elvira Ikoeva, former employee of the Clinic of Dr Isaev and Russian-English translator; and Dr Virginie Debaere, clinician and researcher at Ghent University, where she has studied service users' processes of change in Belgian TCs.

The research project

To start investigating addiction treatment quality 'from within' in Russia, all service users from the four Moscow rehabilitation centres of the Clinic of Dr Isaev were asked to participate in completing questionnaires. The research design, implementation and results are explained below.

A multi-method research design

The starting point for the Russian survey was the Norwegian Service Users' Survey that comprises 42 multiple choice (MC) questions covering five themes: arrival at the rehab centre, treatment/therapy, treatment environment, staff members, and preparation for discharge (all but one question are answered on a five-point Likert scale). After translating the questionnaire into Russian, some content adaptations were made because of cultural differences (e.g. the Russian rehabilitation centres under study are private and they do not have the problem of waiting lists; substitution drugs are forbidden in Russia, so the Russian working group members stressed that it was inappropriate to refer to this product in the questionnaire); and 36 MC-questions were kept.

Three open questions were added to the questionnaire to gather more in-depth information. Before presenting the questionnaire to all residents, a pilot study was done with five random residents to test comprehension and applicability.

Two extra sources of information were added to the investigation: a visit to one of these four rehabilitation centres and a spontaneous focus group with its residents' group.

Results

General information All residing service users of the four Moscow rehab centres (n = 106) were invited to complete the questionnaire (after signing the informed consent). One person refused and three left the questionnaire blank, resulting in a very high response rate. The group of 102 participants consisted of 76% men and 24% women; their mean age was 29 years. Most of them have been using several substances, with alcohol being most popular and heroin/morphine least, as shown in Table 8.1.

Multiple choice questions The main result from the MC-questions is that most service users answered very positively to most questions – all mean scores are presented in Table 8.2. No significant differences were found between the rehab centres, between men and women or between ages.

A parallel response trend was noticed which is illustrated with the histograms of some questions in Figure 8.1. These skewed left histograms show that most respondents agreed to some, high or very high degrees with the MC-questions.

As seen in Table 8.2, the mean score is lower on five questions (Q9, Q13, Q24, Q33 and Q35). Q9 and Q33 asked for derogatory behaviour or mistreatment by staff; therefore, the respondents' disagreement is a good sign. The less positive result on Q35 indicates that the respondents who had been in rehab centres before (n = 26) had very divergent experiences with aftercare. Their disagreement with Q13 and Q24 indicates that they had not experienced

Table 8.1 The number of respondents who have been using these substances.

What substances have you been using mostly?	n?
Alcohol	71
Stimulants	44
Cannabis	37
Medication	25
Other	24
Heroin/Morphine	11

Table 8.2 The mean scores of all MC-questions.

	N	Min	Max	Mean	SD
Q3_info_at_arrival	102	1	5	**4,08**	1,087
Q4_welcomed_at_centre	102	1	5	**3,78**	0,897
Q5_understood_by_staff	102	1	5	**3,78**	0,828
Q6_staff_takes_time	102	1	5	**3,82**	0,709
Q7_staff_professional	102	1	5	**3,84**	0,869
Q8_feel_respected	102	1	5	**3,38**	0,881
Q9_neg_exp_by_staff	*102*	*1*	*5*	**2,25**	*0,941*
Q10c_help_from_group_therapy	96	1	5	**3,96**	0,845
Q10e_help_from_indiv_therapy	101	1	5	**4,19**	0,913
Q11_helped_by_treatm	102	2	5	**4,07**	0,926
Q12_informed_on_treatm	102	1	5	**3,67**	0,988
Q13_influence_on treatm	*102*	*1*	*5*	**2,8**	*1,275*
Q14_teatm_relevance	102	1	5	**3,52**	1,051
Q15_physical_help	102	1	5	**3,69**	1,09
Q16_emotional_help	102	1	5	**3,97**	0,928
Q17_staff_access	102	1	5	**4,05**	0,837
Q18_GP_access	102	1	5	**4**	0,965
Q19_feel_safe	102	1	5	**4,2**	0,975
Q20_social_contact_encouraged	102	1	5	**4,09**	0,986
Q21_soc_cont_opportunities	102	1	5	**4,59**	0.65
Q22_Participates_in_activities	102	1	5	**3,75**	0,927
Q23_meals_good	102	1	5	**3,92**	1,14
Q24_enough_privacy	*102*	*1*	*5*	**2,69**	*1,235*
Q25_staffhelp_discharge	84	1	5	**3,65**	1,081
Q26_staffhelp_life_after	74	1	5	**3,89**	0,837
Q27_satisfied_general	88	2	5	**3,92**	0,746
Q28_understand_probs	98	2	5	**4,32**	0,781
Q29_helped_to_cope	99	1	5	**4,07**	0,895
Q30_hope_better_life	99	2	5	**4,14**	0,881
Q31_family_involved	99	1	5	**3,88**	1,033
Q32_felt_forced	99	1	5	**3,33**	1,558
Q33_felt_mistreated	*99*	*1*	*5*	**1,56**	*0,823*
Q35_pleased_with_aftercare	*36*	*1*	*5*	**2,56**	*1,319*

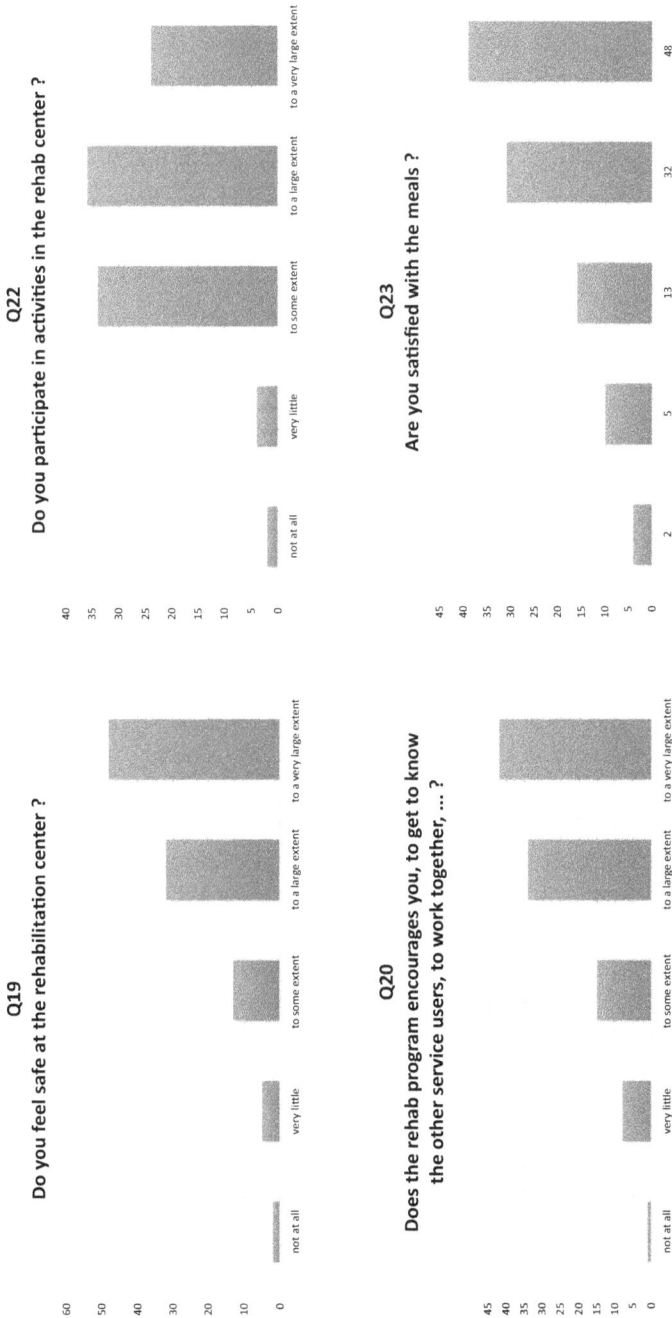

Figure 8.1 Four examples to illustrate the uniform response tendency to the MC-questions.

having much influence on their treatment and enough privacy. Interestingly, this last finding reflects a common comment by residents in TCs for addicted people (30), given that persons are expected to participate in a programme with a tight day schedule with exigent requirements and to start reconnecting with peers/staff members and talking about what they are feeling/experiencing, and not to keep from others their mental and emotional life (26).

Visit to a rehabilitation centre and focus group with residents The researchers visited one of the rehab centres, named 'Independence'. The residents' group consisted of 25 persons. The staff group consisted of one responsible clinician, four psychologists, ten counsellors, one cook, two nurses and one driver (and two cats).

Although this rehabilitation centre is not really considered a TC, it has assimilated several crucial features from the TC culture/approach. The residents follow a tight day schedule. All weekday mornings are charged with therapeutic group sessions. These daily 'small groups' start from a comment or task the psychologist has given to a resident on which the person can elaborate in the peer group and receive feedback from his/her peers and the psychologist. The daily 'dynamic group' in the evenings consists of all residents and deals with the group dynamics. It addresses, for instance, conflicts that have come to the fore because of the group life. In the afternoons, the residents take part in more relaxing/sports activities. Along with these formal group sessions, the residents bear several responsibilities in running the household, everyday responsibilities (e.g. turning on/off all lights), or weekly responsibilities (e.g. being the kitchen representative; organising the weekly cleaning of the house by residents; being the representative for small technical defects etc). The responsibilities are assigned to residents by taking into consideration their therapeutic process (e.g. has the person given enough/good feedback to others?). Also, very much like the state of affairs in Western drug-free TCs, residents receive privileges and/or consequences based on their engagement in the group programme and their therapeutic process/progress (e.g. a first meeting with a resident's family members is dependent on his/her engagement in the group program) (Debaere, Vanheule, & Inslegers, 2014).

Though the researchers had not planned to attend a group session, they were spontaneously invited to join a group that was taking place. After presenting themselves and the aim of their visit, they spontaneously asked a question to learn more about the residents' process of change/therapeutic journey: '*If so, in what way has the treatment programme been helpful to you (until now)?*' Very spontaneously, one resident after the other responded in a concise, clear way. The talking culture was obvious: these persons were used to talking about themselves, their difficulties and/in their interactions with others. Their responses revealed the in-depth psychotherapeutic work that they had been doing (e.g. they had been confronted with destructive

Table 8.3 The residents' answers to the question 'If so, in what way has the treatment programme been helpful to you (until now)?' in the 'pop-up' focus group.

resident 1	It has helped me to fall in love with life, to trust myself and to have good relations with my family members. With the help of staff, I have learned to open up more, which is hard, but every feedback they give is with love.
resident 2	I have learned that other persons are friends and I respect others' opinions.
resident 3	Now I can see the negative sides I have had.
resident 4	For the first time in my life, I can enjoy the city outside in the summertime; before, I couldn't.
resident 5	I have started to notice the consequences of my behaviour; I have become more stable; I have stopped blaming other people for who I am and what I did/do; I learn to interact with other persons (while I used to manipulate others).
resident 6	When I was addicted to alcohol, I had destructive patterns (e.g. cheating, doing robbery, …); here I learn to feel things I have never felt before, normal things, feelings.
resident 7	I had lost the sense to live, now this has changed. Before, the aims I had in life were not realistic; I have changed, now I have realistic aims/goals.
resident 8	Since being here, I learn to get along with my relatives; I have found a spiritual orientation (I learned this here).
resident 9	I have become more confident about me, about what I do, thanks to the interactions with other persons.
resident 10	Here I found out that I can be happy, also when I am sober … before I couldn't.
resident 11	I have been helped to face my fears … I used to be a 'psychotic sociopath'.

behaviour patterns in a way that had allowed them to accept and start making changes; they had been getting in contact with painful emotions that used to be anaesthetised by using substances; relations with relatives had been changing in a constructive way; people had started to love life again etc). Table 8.3 briefly presents the answers of all responding residents to the question in the pop-up focus group.

Responses to the open questions With the first open question, the respondents had been asked to describe their rehab experience in just one word. An overview of all given words is presented in Table 8.4.

A first finding is that most words have a positive connotation, designated in bold (e.g. useful, productive, good, maturation, helping, excellent, etc). In a next step, an attempt has been made to cluster words that fit together in meaning. As such, five word groups were created, which are presented in Table 8.5.

By looking at these words through the lens of successful processes of change in Western TCs (e.g. Debaere et al., 2016; Debaere, Verhaeghe, & Vanheule, 2017), the hypothesis can be forwarded that the group of respondents highlighted different aspects of a rewarding (= 'positive connotation'), yet

Table 8.4 Overview of all given words by the service users of the four rehabilitation centres to the question: 'How would you describe your experience at this rehabilitation centre in just one word?'

rehab 'Dual Diagnosis'	rehab 'Independence'	rehab 'Rise'	rehab "Development'
start	grateful	growth	useful
useful		maturity	useful
recovery	sobriety	vitally necessary	normal
learning	maturation	way	long
productive	hard	hard	excellent
salvation	hard	freaking annoying (to stop using)	unusual
good	new	bearable	good
useful		changes	useful
not easy	inventory	satisfactory	for the 1st time
reversion ('unfreeze')	useful	need	to recover
to get into a mess	boring	step	good
	discovery	massacre	hope
it's helping	educational	I am satisfied	excellent
God ('a miracle')	valuable	hope	productive
hope	control	shit	hope
hard	true life	good	productive
	necessary	need	sad
long (the time is passing slow)	normal	disconnection (from drugs)	normal
	beginning	qualitative	useful
analysing/recogniz. my mistakes	beginning	hope	positive
rehabilitation	life	growing up	a possibility (not to use)
serious	life	productively	
it's necessary	mindfulness	test	
give	metamorphosis	Euro (valuable)	
I don't know		reality	
excellent	knowledge		
maturity			
super			
satisfaction			
successful			
horror			
start			

Table 8.5 Meaningful word groups with some examples.

the word groups:	examples:
'timing' (possibility/beginning of something)	start, beginning, new, step, …
'utility / importance'	useful, productive, necessary, …
'content' (what is it about)	growth, recovery, maturation, sobriety, …
appreciation: 'positive connotation'	grateful, excellent, super, positive, …
appreciation: 'negative connotation'	hard, shit, boring, sad, …

difficult, frustrating (= 'negative connotation') process of change (= 'content/ what it is about') that is considered being worthwhile (= 'utility/importance'), and experienced it as an opportunity to take a new direction in life (= 'possibility/beginning of something').

The service users' responses to the second open question, 'Do you feel helped with your addiction problem by the service?' are in line with the foregoing: 76% responded 'yes', 23% 'maybe', and only 1% 'no'. They had also been asked to explain why they think so, and again, their capability of putting into words the processes and the experiences they had been going through and the changes that reflect psychotherapeutic work and the importance of the community was interesting, as illustrated with some quotes in Figure 8.2.

With the third and last open question, the respondents were asked whether they had experienced something that they consider important to quality improvement. Not all respondents wrote down something – many of

"I have begun to sleep, to eat, to **live normally as a Human** being and not as an Animal"

"I have confidence that I'll stay alive, that I am really ill and that a **community is hope**"

"I am not living in illusions anymore, I have a **realistic view of life**"

"They gave me back pure consciousness and **opened my eyes**"

"**Addiction itself isn't the only problem.** That is why skills of building relationships, recognizing your mistakes, asking for help, talking about yourself, helping others, are very important to me"

Figure 8.2 Some quotes from respondents who explained why they think the rehabilitation program is helping them.

those who didn't, were satisfied with how things were going on a daily basis. The 'shortcoming' that was mostly addressed by the respondents of all four rehabs, was that they wanted to have 'more free time' (for sleeping, walking, watching movies, etc). As mentioned before, such comments are also similar to those given by residents of Western TCs for drug-addicted persons. This kind of longing has been related to one of the two crucial dimensions in the relational atmosphere of drug-free TCs, the 'frustrating' dimension (which has also been described as 'tough' or 'strict' by other researchers, e.g. Infante, 2012; Perfas, 2004), that coexists with the 'holding' dimension (also described as 'humane' or 'caring') so that their suppressed emotional life awakens and the service users become able to mentalize affective tension (Debaere, Vanheule, & Inslegers, 2014). Therefore, the fact that the service users give expression to their longing for more relaxation is not an issue that seems to be alarming with regard to quality in these TC-like rehabilitation centres for drug-addicted persons, on the contrary.

Discussion and continuation of the NORUS project

With the NORUS project, the lived experience of 102 service users of four private addiction rehabilitation centres in Moscow region were studied. The researchers conclude that these centres seem to offer treatment of high quality, in which persons with substance-use problems are allowed to go through profound life-changing journeys by which a changed lifestyle becomes thinkable. The researchers were at first surprised by the results, since the residents' appreciation of all aspects of the treatment was much higher than anticipated, and even higher compared to the Norwegian results. However, the researchers do not consider it to be meaningful to compare the results from this limited service user survey with the Norwegian annual surveys. As mentioned before, in Norway, the service users of all residential addiction rehabilitation centres are invited to participate in the annual survey (e.g. in 2017, 110 institutions – also including non-profit organisations – were addressed and 1,173 questionnaires were completed), while in Russia only 102 persons from four centres of only one private organisation have participated. Moreover, social factors have to be considered, given that life circumstances for drug-addicted persons in Russia appear to be worse than in countries such as Norway. And from discussions with Russian experts, the researchers learned that these studied rehabilitation centres were of a very high quality according to Russian standards, and that service users and drug-dependent people most likely have very negative experiences with both treatment and overall stigmatisation and social exclusion from society, which was also suggested in previous studies (Lunze, Lunze, Raj, & Samet, 2015).

Although differences with 'Western' drug-free TCs have been noticed (e.g. not all aspects of daily life are to the same extent run by service users in a rotating hierarchical job structure), crucial and typical 'TC ingredients' are present in the studied services. For instance: problems and conflicts that arise in the daily life of the service users are used as the material that is worked with in the group therapy sessions; profound explorations of the residents' intra- and interpersonal relationships are at the heart of the daily practice in the services; the service users are expected to take responsibility for the choices they have made in the past and will make in the future. Perhaps more important is that the involvement of the perspective from people with dependency and service user experience is at the heart of these services: about 70% of all staff in the centres of the Clinic of Dr Isaev are 'experts by experience', that is, former substance-dependent people. In addition, family involvement, normally believed to correlate with improved treatment outcomes, is also included in the treatment approach.

As mentioned before, 'quality improvement' issues regarding addiction treatment in Russia are of another type compared to Norway or most other countries in Western Europe. First, the investigated treatment approach only exists in some private, commercial centres, so that it is only affordable for families who can pay for it. Second, there does not seem to be a clear, comprehensive list of available treatment in Russia for people with substance dependency problems. And third, there is not an overall policy plan to counter the problems as described in the paragraph 'Russian challenge with regard to substance addiction (treatment)'.

Since its first year, the NORUS project has been continuing. The questionnaire has been developed into an online survey to offer Russian service providers a tool to monitor their service users' experiences. This is done in order to promote a quality measurement 'from within' and to document results to policymakers as a way to respond to the policy suggestions in 'The Strategy 2020' of the Russian Federation. In addition to that, conversations have started between former service users of the centres of the Clinic of Dr Isaev and employees of RIO to explore the possibility of undertaking a policy analysis of the Russian treatment management situation based on discussions in the Civic Chamber of the Russian Federation that highlighted the need for a defined responsible agency. Finally, more visits are taking place in rehabilitation centres of other organisations and in other Russian regions to broaden the researchers' horizons further with regards to quality in Russian addiction treatment rehabilitation centres from the perspective of the service users' processes of change.

Acknowledgements

A special thank you goes to two persons without whom this (writing) project would not have been doable. Thank you Elvira Ikoeva and Alexey Knuazev for bridging our language gap in such a professional way, and for the many other ways in which you have been helpful and cooperative in our project. You have helped to make this project a real pleasure!

The information in this box is completed by a staff member

> *Drug rehabilitation centre number : .....*
> *Questionnaire copy number : .....*

Questionnaire

What is your experience with the treatment offered in the rehabilitation centre?

The purpose of this questionnaire is to gather information on clients' experiences in rehabilitation centres. This is done in order to improve the quality of the services offered in these centres. We are interested in your experiences in the facility you are staying.

The information is gathered anonymously.

There are two types of questions: closed questions and open questions.

- With the closed questions, you can choose an answer by putting a cross (X) in one of the boxes. Sometimes it is indicated that you can choose more than one answer;
- With the open questions, you are asked to write down the answer or your opinion.

Date: ..... / ..... / ....

What is your age?   ...... (years old)

Are you a woman or a man?

Man   Woman

Your background

1. What substances were you using the most before being admitted (this time)?

    You can choose more than one.

    alcohol   medicaments   cannabis   stimulants   heroin/morphine   other

    ☐   ☐   ☐   ☐   ☐   ☐

2. How long have you been staying in this centre?

    0–2 weeks   3–11 weeks   3–6 months   7–12 months   more than 12 months

    ☐   ☐   ☐   ☐   ☐   ☐

Reception and waiting times

3. Did you get any information about the rules and routines of the centre at your arrival?

    No   A little   Some   Much   Very much

    ☐   ☐   ☐   ☐   ☐

4. Were you met in a satisfactory manner when you arrived at the centre?

    No   A little   Some   Much   Very much

    ☐   ☐   ☐   ☐   ☐

Staff and practitioners

5. Do you feel like the staff understand your situation?

    No   A little   Some   Much   Very much

    ☐   ☐   ☐   ☐   ☐

6. Did/do you have the impression that the staff took/takes the time to talk and be in contact with you?

No A little Some Much Very much

☐ ☐ ☐ ☐ ☐

7. Did/do you feel confident about the professional competency of the staff?

No A little Some Much Very much

☐ ☐ ☐ ☐ ☐

8. Did/do you have the impression that you are respected?

Not at all A little Some Much Very much

☐ ☐ ☐ ☐ ☐

9. Did you experience any offensive or derogatory treatment by staff?

Never Yes, once Yes, a few times Yes, often Yes, very often

☐ ☐ ☐ ☐ ☐

Treatment

10. Indicate whether or not you have had the therapies listed below.

    And from the ones that you have had, indicate to what extent you have benefited from them.

    - Have you had **group therapy**?

      Yes No

      ☐ ☐

      If you answered 'Yes', specify what kind of group therapy (please give examples):
      ....

      If you answered 'Yes', to what extent have you benefited from this group therapy?

      Not A little Some Much Very much

      ☐ ☐ ☐ ☐ ☐

- Have you had **individual therapy**/conversations with one staff?

Yes   No

☐   ☐

If you answered 'yes', to what extent have you benefited from this individual therapy?

Not   A little   Some   Much   Very much

☐   ☐   ☐   ☐   ☐

11. To what extent has the treatment as a whole benefitted you?

Not at all   very little   to some extent   to a large extent   to a very large extent

☐   ☐   ☐   ☐   ☐

12. Do you feel that you have been informed enough about your treatment?

Not at all   very little   to some extent   to a large extent   to a very large extent

☐   ☐   ☐   ☐   ☐

13. Did you have any influence on your treatment?

Not at all   very little   to some extent   to a large extent   to a very large extent

☐   ☐   ☐   ☐   ☐

14. Did you feel like the treatment was relevant to your aims and goals?

Not at all   very little   to some extent   to a large extent   to a very large extent

☐   ☐   ☐   ☐   ☐

15. Did you receive help or treatment for physical illness or issues?

Not at all   very little   to some extent   to a large extent   to a very large extent

☐   ☐   ☐   ☐   ☐

16. Did you receive help or treatment for emotional issues?

Not at all   very little   to some extent   to a large extent   to a very large extent

☐   ☐   ☐   ☐   ☐

17. Did/do you have sufficient access to staff members?

Not at all   very little   to some extent   to a large extent   to a very large extent

□ □ □ □ □

18. Did/do you have sufficient access to a physician?

Not at all   very little   to some extent   to a large extent   to a very large extent

□ □ □ □ □

Environment and activities

19. Did/do you feel safe at the rehabilitation centre?

Not at all   very little   to some extent   to a large extent   to a very large extent

□ □ □ □ □

20. Does the rehabilitation programme help you, encourage you to get to know the other clients, to work together, …? (in other words: does the programme facilitate social contact between the clients?)

Not at all   very little   to some extent   to a large extent   to a very large extent

□ □ □ □ □

21. Do you have regular opportunities to meet clients and staff members?

Not at all   very little   to some extent   to a large extent   to a very large extent

□ □ □ □ □

22. Did/do you participate in activities at the rehabilitation centre?

Not at all   very little   to some extent   to a large extent   to a very large extent

□ □ □ □ □

23. Were/are you satisfied with the meals?

Not at all   very little   to some extent   to a large extent   to a very large extent

□ □ □ □ □

24. Did/do you have enough privacy?

Not at all   very little   to some extent   to a large extent   to a very large extent

☐   ☐   ☐   ☐   ☐

Preparations for discharge

The next questions on 'Preparations for discharge' (i.e. questions 25 and 26) should only be answered by service users who have been in the rehabilitation centre for at least three months!

25. Did/do you feel like the staff have helped prepare you for discharge?

Not at all   very little   to some extent   to a large extent   to a very large extent

☐   ☐   ☐   ☐   ☐

26. Do you feel like the staff have helped you towards achieving a meaningful life after discharge?

Not at all   very little   to some extent   to a large extent   to a very large extent

☐   ☐   ☐   ☐   ☐

Other

27. Are you satisfied with the total help and treatment you have received at this rehabilitation centre?

Not at all   very little   to some extent   to a large extent   to a very large extent

☐   ☐   ☐   ☐   ☐

28. Did/does the help and treatment received at the rehabilitation centre help you better understand your problems relating to substance abuse?

Not at all   very little   to some extent   to a large extent   to a very large extent

☐   ☐   ☐   ☐   ☐

29. Did/does the help and treatment received at the rehabilitation centre help you cope with your substance abuse?

Not at all   very little   to some extent   to a large extent   to a very large extent

☐   ☐   ☐   ☐   ☐

30. Did/does the help and treatment received at the rehabilitation centre provide you with hope for a better life after discharge?

Not at all   very little   to some extent   to a large extent   to a very large extent

☐   ☐   ☐   ☐   ☐

31. Did/do you feel like the staff involved your family in your rehabilitation programme, if possible and needed?

Not at all   very little   to some extent   to a large extent   to a very large extent

☐   ☐   ☐   ☐   ☐

32. To what degree did you feel pressured/forced to go to the rehabilitation centre?

Not at all   very little   to some extent   to a large extent   to a very large extent

☐   ☐   ☐   ☐   ☐

33. Do you believe that you were mistreated in the rehabilitation centre?

Not at all   very little   to some extent   to a large extent   to a very large extent

☐   ☐   ☐   ☐   ☐

Previous admissions

34. Have you previously gone to a rehabilitation centre for substance use problems?

No   Yes, once   Yes, twice   Yes, 3–5 times   Yes, more than 5 times

☐   ☐   ☐   ☐   ☐

35. If you have previously stayed at a rehabilitation centre, were you satisfied with the follow-ups and aftercare that you received after treatment? (Consider the last admission if you were admitted several times.)

Not at all   very little   to some extent   to a large extent   to a very large extent

☐   ☐   ☐   ☐   ☐

36. If previously admitted, was the last admission before this one at this treatment centre?

Yes   No

☐   ☐

Open questions

37. How would you describe your experience at this rehabilitation centre in one word: ……...

    Could you explain briefly what you mean by this word:

    ....
    ....
    ....
    ....

38. Do you have the impression that your stay at this centre is helping you with your addiction problem?

No   Yes   Maybe, I'm not sure

☐   ☐   ☐

    If you answered 'Yes', briefly explain why you think so:

    ....
    ....
    ....
    ....

If you answered 'No', briefly explain why you think so:

....

....

....

....

If you answered 'Maybe, I'm not sure', briefly explain why you think so:

....

....

....

....

39. Is there something you would like to add about your experience at this centre that you consider important with regard to quality improvement? Please answer below:

....

....

....

Thank you for cooperating in this survey!

References

Celinskiy, B. (2017, December 6). В России 5,5% населения – наркоманы. Официальная статистика – в 16 раз меньше [In Russia, 5.5% of the population are drug addicts. Official statistics – 16 times less]. Retrieved from www.newsru.com/russia/15jun2005/narkomany.html

Chelischeva, V. (2015, August 17). Количество православных реабилитационных центров с каждым годом увеличивается. [The number of Orthodox rehabilitation centres is increasing every year]. Retrieved from www.miloserdie.ru/article/pravoslavnye-centry-reabilitacii-dlya-narkomanov/

Debaere, V. (2014). *Beyond the 'black box' of the therapeutic community: A qualitative psychoanalytic study.* [Unpublished PhD dissertation, Ghent University].

Debaere, V., Vanheule, S., & Inslegers, R. (2014). Beyond the 'black box' of the therapeutic community for substance abusers: A participant observation study on the treatment process. *Addiction Research & Theory, 22*(3), 251–262. https://doi.org/10.3109/16066359.2013.834892

Debaere, V., Vanheule, S., Van Roy, K., Meganck, R., Inslegers, R., & Mol, M. (2016). Changing encounters with the Other: A focus group study on the process of change in a Therapeutic Community. *Psychoanalytic Psychology, 33*, 406–419.

Debaere, V., Verhaeghe, P., & Vanheule, S. (2017). Identity change in a drug-free therapeutic community: A Lacanian interpretation of former residents' perspectives on treatment process and outcome. *Therapeutic Communities, 38*, 147–155.

Federal Drug Control Service of Russia (2011). В РФ должен быть внедрен единый госстандарт реабилитации наркозависимых – ФСКН [A single state standard for the rehabilitation of drug addicts should be introduced in the Russian Federation – Federal Drug Control Service] (2011, October 21). Retrieved from https://ria.ru/20111021/466594306.html

Hamzaev, S. (2019). 'Трезвая Россия' подсчитала экономические потери страны от наркомании ['Sober Russia' calculated the country's economic losses from drug addiction] (June 21). Retrieved from https://ria.ru/20190621/1555767628.html?fbclid=IwAR1mIZiACH9FMXQODc3JWIwt_pn1pcldMuV5UpVW1yoVhPANQzWBqOK6Jgk

House of Hope on the Hill – The charitable rehabilitation centre on alcoholism treatment. Retrieved from http://houseofhope.ru/en/about-house.html

Infante, M.R. (2012). Preserving the integrity of the therapeutic community: Maintaining a manual of operations to prevent aberrations in TC practice. Paper presented at the 25th World Conference of Therapeutic Communities, Bali.

Information agency RIA News (2008). Проблема наркомании в России: статистические данные [The problem of drug addiction in Russia: Statistics] (June 7). Retrieved from https://ria.ru/20070626/67829656.html

Isaev, R. (2015). Лечение наркомании. Практическое руководство к выздоровлению [Addiction treatment. A practical guide to recovery] Moscow: Eksmo.

Ivushkina, A., & Raskin, A. (2015) Наркоманы смогут лечиться в частных клиниках за госсчет с 2016 года [Addicts will be able to be treated in private clinics for a state account from 2016] (October 17). Retrieved from https://iz.ru/news/592556

Lunze, K., Lunze, F.I., Raj, A., & Samet, J.H. (2015). Stigma and human rights abuses against people who inject drugs in Russia – a qualitative investigation to inform policy and public health strategies. *PLOS ONE, 10*(8), e0136030. https://doi.org/10.1371/journal.pone.013603

Marshak's Clinic (2007). История «Клиники Маршака» – Клиника Маршака (1996–2007) [History of the 'Marshak Clinic' – Marshak Clinic (1996–2007)]. Retrieved from www.marshak.ru/clinic/history/

Mathiesen, A. (2015, December 10). Rusomsorgen er en helsepolitisk forsømmelse [Substance care is a health policy neglected]. Retrieved from www.dagbladet.no/kultur/rusomsorgen-er-en-helsepolitisk-forsommelse/60163852

Minnesota Model of Addiction Treatment. www.rehabcenter.net/the-minnesota-model/

Nesvaag, S., & Lie, T. (2010). The Norwegian substance treatment reform. *Nordic Studies on Alcohol and Drugs, 27,* 655–666.

Norwegian Directorate of Health (2017, November 30). Pasienterfaringer fra tverrfaglig spesialisert rusbehandling [Patient experiences from multidisciplinary specialised drug treatment]. Retrieved from www.fhi.no/publ/2020/brukererfaringer-med-dognopphold-i-tverrfaglig-spesialisert-rusbehandling-kvartalsrapporter/

Norwegian Directorate of Health (2018). Kostnadsnivå og produktivitet i psykisk helsevern og TSB 2014–2018 SAMDATA spesialisthelsetjeneste Rapport [Cost level and productivity in mental health services and dependency treatment 2014–2018 SAMDATA specialist health services Report]. Retrieved from www.helsedirektoratet.no/rapporter/is-2852-kostnadsniva-og-produktivitet-i-psykisk-helsevern-og-tsb-2014-2018

Norwegian Directorate of Health (2019, April 10). Rusbehandling [Substance abuse treatment]. Retrieved from www.helsedirektoratet.no/statistikk/statistikk/kvalitetsindikatorer/rusbehandling

Norwegian Government (2014). Pasientens helsetjeneste [Patient's health service] (January 7). Retrieved from www.regjeringen.no/no/aktuelt/pasientens-helsetjeneste/id748854

Norwegian Government (2018, December 5). Sjeldent viktig i pasientens helsetjeneste [Especially important in the Patient's Health Service]. Retrieved from www.regjeringen.no/no/aktuelt/sjeldent-viktig-i-pasientens-helsetjeneste/id2621420/)

Norwegian Public Health Institute (2020). Pasienters erfaringer med døgnopphold i tverrfaglig spesialisert rusbehandling (TSB) 2. kvartal 2020 Nasjonale resultater [Patient experiences with inpatient specialist dependency treatment (TSB) 2. quarter 2020 National results]. Retrieved from www.fhi.no/publ/2020/pasienters-erfaringer-med-TSB-2-kvartal-2020/

NTB. (2014, July 11). Rusmidler – Mangelfull oppfølging av ruspasienter [Drugs – inadequate follow-up of drug addicted patients]. Retrieved from www.nettavisen.no/nyheter/mangelfull-oppfolging-av-ruspasienter/3732271.html

Perfas, F. (2004). *Therapeutic communities: Social systems perspective.* Lincoln, NE: iUniverse.

Rambler (2018, September 4). Как работают центры принудительного лечения наркоманов в России Об этом сообщает Рамблер. [How do the centres for compulsory treatment of drug addicted persons work?]. Retrieved from https://news.rambler.ru/other/40722848-kak-rabotayut-tsentry-prinuditelnogo-lecheniya-narkomanov-v-rossii/

Russian Federation (2009). Russian State Antidrug Policy Strategy. Retrieved from www.eegyn.com/pdf/Russian%20State%20Antidrug%20Policy%20Strategy.pdf

Russian Federation (2010, June 9). Указ Президента РФ от 9 июня 2010 г. N 690 'Об утверждении Стратегии государственной антинаркотической политики Российской Федерации до 2020 года' (с изменениями и дополнениями) [Decree of the president of the Russian Federation of June 9, 2010 N 690 'On approval of the strategy of the state anti-drug policy of the Russian Federation until 2020' (as amended)]. Retrieved from http://base.garant.ru/12176340/-friends

Russian Federation (2016). Статья 82.1. Отсрочка отбывания наказания больным наркоманией [Deferral of serving a sentence by a drug addict]. Retrieved from http://stykrf.ru/82-1

Russian Federation (2017). Уточненный отчет о ходе реализации и оценке эффективности государственной программы Российской Федерации «Развитие здравоохранения» за 2016 год [An updated report on the implementation and evaluation of the effectiveness of the state programme of the Russian Federation 'Healthcare Development' for 2016]. Retrieved from https://static-1.rosminzdrav.ru/system/attachments/attaches/000/037/752/original/%D0%A3%D1%82%D0%BE%D1%87%D0%BD%D0%B5%D0%BD%D0%BD%D1%8B%D0%B9_%D0%BE%D1%82%D1%87%D0%B5%D1%82_%D0%B7%D0%B0_2016_%D0%B3%D0%BE%D0%B4.pdf?1520932932

Russian Ministry of Health (2013). Ответ на письмо Президента ННГ из Минздрава России [Reply to a letter from the president of the NIS from the Ministry of Health of Russia] (March 15). Retrieved from http://nng.com.ru/files/otvet-na-pismo-prezidenta-nng-iz-minzdrava-rossii/

Starkova, A. (2019). Новый поворот: кто поплатится за смерть Марьянова [A new twist: who will pay for Maryanov's death] (December 2). Retrieved from www.gazeta.ru/culture/2019/02/12/a_12179611.shtml

Sykepleien (2015, January 7). Helseministerens sykehustale – Pasientenes helsetjeneste [Health minister's speech to regional health authorities – The Patient's Health Service]. Retrieved from https://sykepleien.no/2015/01/pasientenes-helsetjeneste

Therapeutic communities for substance abusers in correctional settings

9

The American experience

George De Leon

Therapeutic communities in corrections

The need for substance abuse treatment in correctional populations has been well documented over some four decades since therapeutic community (TC) programs first appeared in American prisons and jails. Research played a central role in the development of the prison TC model by providing information that influenced policy makers to support prison substance-abuse treatment for the purposes of improving public safety and public health. Notably, the effectiveness of community-based TC programs provided the empirical groundwork for implementing TCs in correctional settings. (See comprehensive reviews of TC effectiveness in De Leon, 2010; Vanderplassen, Colbert, Autrique, Rapp, Pearce, Broekaert, & Vandevelde, 2013). Specifically, in the early days a considerable number of admissions to community-based TCs had criminal justice histories. Outcomes for these showed significant reductions in recidivism (e.g., arrests, convictions, and incarcerations) as well as reductions in relapse to substance abuse (e.g., De Leon, 1984, 1988)

Beginning in the 1970s, with the development of the Cornerstone and Stay'n Out programs, and continuing thereafter, the community TC model was modified and adapted to correctional environments where it became the primary approach for treating substance abuse among inmates (Wexler, Falkin, & Lipton, 1990; Wexler & Prendergast, 2010)

The rapid expansion of prison TCs in the early years was documented in a national survey conducted by the Association of State Correctional Administrators (ASCA) (Rockholz, 2002). The survey identified over 250 TC programs in 40 states. The peak period of new start-ups occurred in 1997–2000. All programs specified substance abuse as the primary participant characteristic. A subset of programs focused on special criminal justice populations, for example, youthful offenders, sex offenders, those with co-occurring psychiatric disorders, and those with targeted problems, for example, driving-under-the-influence offenders,[1] violent–aggressive inmates, and parole violators.

DOI: 10.4324/9780429317460-11

The survey also underscored wide variability in the application of the TC approach. This issue illustrated the challenge of adapting the TC for special populations and special settings. While modifications of prison TCs are common, their effects on treatment outcomes remain unknown (Melnick, Hawke, & Wexler, 2004; Taxman & Bouffard, 2002; Welsh & Zajac, 2004). The following sections provide an overview of essential elements of the traditional TC and the special issues in adapting these elements to correctional settings.

The therapeutic community: essential elements

The TC perspective or theory shapes its program model and its unique approach, community as method. The perspective consists of four interrelated views of the substance use disorder, the individual, recovery process, and healthy living. Drug abuse is viewed as a disorder of the whole person, affecting some or all areas of functioning. Cognitive and behavioral problems are often present, as are mood disturbances. Thinking may be unrealistic or disorganized; values may be confused, nonexistent, or antisocial. Frequently, the patient exhibits deficits in verbal, reading, writing, or marketable skills. Moral or even spiritual issues, whether expressed in existential or psychological terms, are apparent. Thus, the TC perspective considers the problem to be the individual, not the drug, and addiction is a symptom, not the essence of the disorder.[2]

View of the person

In TCs, individuals are distinguished along dimensions of psychological dysfunction and social deficits rather than according to drug use patterns. Regardless of differences in social background, drug preference, or psychological problems, most individuals admitted to TCs share clinical characteristics (Table 9.1). Whether they are antecedent or consequent to serious involvement with drugs, these characteristics are commonly observed to correlate with chemical dependency. More important, in TCs, a positive change in these characteristics is considered to be essential for stable recovery.

View of recovery

In the TC perspective, recovery extends beyond drug freedom, involving a change in lifestyle and in personal identity. The primary psychological goal is to change the negative patterns of behavior, thinking, and feeling that

Table 9.1 Typical behavioral, cognitive, and emotional characteristics of substance abusers in traditional therapeutic communities.

- Low tolerance for all forms of discomfort and delay of gratification
- Problems with authority
- Inability to manage feelings (particularly hostility/anger, guilt, and anxiety)
- Poor impulse control
- Poor judgment and reality testing concerning consequences of actions
- Unrealistic self-appraisal regarding discrepancies between personal resources and aspirations
- Prominence of lying, manipulation, and deception as coping behaviors
- Personal and social irresponsibility (e.g., inconsistency or failure in meeting obligations)
- Marked deficits in learning and in marketable and communication skills

predispose the individual to drug use; the main social goal is to develop the skills, attitudes, and values of a responsible drug-free lifestyle.

In many TC residents, vocational and educational problems are marked; middle-class, mainstream values are either missing or not sought. Usually these residents emerge from a socially disadvantaged sector. Their recovery in the TC is better termed "habilitation," the development of a socially productive, conventional lifestyle for the first time. Among individuals from more advantaged backgrounds, the term "rehabilitation" is more suitable, which emphasizes a return to a lifestyle previously lived, known, and perhaps rejected.

View of right living

TCs adhere to certain precepts and values that constitute a view of healthy personal and social living that guide and reinforce recovery. For example, community sanctions address antisocial behaviors and attitudes; the negative values of the street, jails, or negative peers; and irresponsible or exploitative sexual conduct. Positive values are emphasized as being essential to social learning and personal growth. These values include truth and honesty (in word and deed), a work ethic, self-reliance, earned rewards and achievement, personal accountability, responsible concern (being one's brother's or sister's keeper), social manners, and community involvement. The precepts of right living are constantly reinforced in various formal and informal ways (e.g., signs, seminars, in groups and community meetings).

The TC approach: community as method

The TC approach can be summarized in the phrase "community as method" (De Leon, 2000). Theoretical writings offer a definition of "community as method" as follows: the purposive use of the community to teach individuals to use the community to change themselves. The fundamental assumption underlying the TC approach is that individuals obtain maximum therapeutic and educational impact when they engage in and learn to use all of the activities, elements of the community as the tools for self-change. Thus, community as method means that the community itself provides a context of relationships and activities for social learning. Its membership establishes the expectations or standards of participation in community activities; it continually assesses how individuals are meeting these expectations and responds to them with strategies that promote continued participation.

TC program model

The key components of the program model are its social organization (structure), peer and staff roles, groups and individual counseling, community enhancement meetings, community management elements, and program stages. Each component reflects an understanding of the TC perspective and each is used to transmit community teachings, promote affiliation, and support self-change.

Social organization

The TC social organization is stratified with relatively few staff of the TC at the top complemented by resident peers at junior, intermediate, and senior levels. This peer level-to-community structure strengthens the patient's identification with a perceived ordered network of individuals. More important, it arranges relationships of mutual responsibility at various levels in the program. The daily operation of the community itself is the task of the residents, who work together under staff supervision. The broad range of resident job assignments illustrates the extent of the self-help process. Residents perform all house services (e.g., cooking, cleaning, kitchen service, minor repair), serve as apprentices, run all departments, and conduct house meetings, certain seminars, and peer encounter groups.

The TC is managed by the staff, who monitor and evaluate client status, supervise resident groups, assign and supervise resident jobs, and oversee house operations. The staff members conduct therapeutic groups (other than peer encounter groups), provide individual counseling, and organize social and recreational projects. They make decisions about resident status, for example, discipline, promotion, transfers, discharges, furloughs, and treatment planning.

Peers as role models

Peers, serving as role models, and staff members, serving as role models and rational authorities, are the primary mediators of the recovery process. TC members who demonstrate the expected behaviors and reflect the values and teachings of the community are viewed as role models. TCs require multiple resident and staff role models in order to maintain the integrity of the community and ensure the spread of social learning effects.

Staff members as rational authorities

Staff members foster the self-help learning process through performance of their managerial and clinical functions described above but also as role models and rational authorities. TC residents often have had difficulties with authorities who have not been trusted or who have been perceived as guides and teachers. Therefore, residents need a positive experience with an authority figure who is viewed as credible, supportive, corrective, and protective so that they may gain authority over themselves (personal autonomy). As rational authorities, staff members provide the reasons for their decisions and explain the meaning of consequences particularly in terms of recovery and personal growth.

Therapeutic educational activities (groups and individual counseling)

Various forms of group process and individual counseling provide residents with opportunities to express feelings and resolve personal and social issues. They increase communication and interpersonal skills, bring about examination and confrontation of behavior and attitudes, and offer instruction in alternative modes of behavior. The main forms of group activity in the TC are peer-led encounter groups, staff-led therapy, and tutorial groups. Other groups that convene regularly or are held as needed supplement the main groups. These vary in focus, format, and composition and include gender, ethnic, age-specific, or health theme groups. Additionally, cognitive-behavioral tutorials using manualized curricula are employed for targeted areas such as relapse prevention, criminal thinking, trauma and post-traumatic stress disorder, and so on.

One-to-one counseling balances the needs of the individual with those of the community. Peer exchange is ongoing and is the most consistent form of informal counseling in TCs. Staff counseling sessions may be regularly scheduled or conducted as needed. The focus of staff counseling is to address issues that may impede progress and to facilitate the resident's adjustment to and constructive use of the peer community. Counseling is also employed for the purpose of developing an individualized treatment plan.

Community enhancement activities (meetings)

Community enhancement activities are the facility-wide meetings that convene daily. These include the morning meeting, the seminar, the house (evening) meeting, and a general meeting. Some of these are held almost daily while others are called when needed. These gatherings are necessary for building the spirit of community in which members are expected to participate actively. Though different in format, all meetings have the common objective of facilitating the individual's assimilation into the community. The purpose of the morning meeting is to instill a positive attitude in the community at the beginning of the day, motivate residents, create camaraderie, and strengthen unity. Seminars are community-wide teaching sessions led by peers or staff presenting topics that directly or indirectly relate to the TC perspective on recovery and right living. House meetings are coordinated by senior residents to transact community business. General meetings take place only when needed and are usually called so that negative behavior, attitudes, or incidents in the facility can be addressed. While these activities are often facilitated by senior residents, staff are available to oversee them.

Community enhancement also occurs in a variety of nonscheduled, informal activities as well. These include activities related to rituals and traditions, celebrations (e.g., birthdays, graduations, phase changes, job changes), ceremonies (e.g., those relating to general and cultural holidays), and memorial observances for deceased residents, family members of residents, and staff members.

Community and clinical management elements

Community and clinical management elements maintain the physical and psychological safety of the environment and ensure that resident life is orderly and productive. Thus, they strengthen community as a context for social learning.

The main elements that are staff managed, although with some input from the senior resident social hierarchy, are privileges, disciplinary sanctions, surveillance, and urine testing. However, peer confrontation in the form of verbal correctives (pull ups), affirmations (push ups), and feedback (e.g., reactions, advice, information) are ongoing community management activities.

Program stages and phases

Recovery in the TC is a developmental process that can be understood as a passage through program stages of learning. The learning that occurs at each stage facilitates change at the next, and each change reflects movement toward the goal of recovery. Three major program stages characterize change in long-term residential TCs – orientation-induction, primary treatment, and reentry – and may include additional substages or phases. The original time frame for these stages was grounded in a planned duration of treatment ranging up to 24 months. Current stage and phase durations are shorter, commensurate with decreased overall planned durations. Regardless of temporal changes, completion of each stage is a celebrated event marking acknowledged programmatic and clinical progress.

Completion marks the end of active program involvement. Graduation itself, however, is an annual event conducted in the facility for individuals who have completed all program stages and have successfully spent some time outside the treatment facility. Thus, the TC experience facilitates a process of change that must continue throughout life; and what is gained in treatment are tools to guide the individual on a path of continued change. Completion, or graduation, therefore, is not an end but a beginning.

Aftercare

Until recently, long-term TCs addressed key clinical and social adjustment issues of aftercare during the reentry stages of the two-year program. However, funding pressures have resulted in shorter planned durations of residential treatment and the stages and phases therein. This has underscored the necessity for aftercare resources to address both primary treatment as well as reentry issues. Thus, contemporary TCs offer post-residential treatment and social services within their systems, such as intensive day treatment and step-down outpatient ambulatory treatment, or through linkages with outside agencies.

Prison-based TCs: modifications and special issues

The advance of the prison-based TC in the peak period was based upon evaluation studies of an original cadre of prison TC programs that retained key elements of the traditional TC (see Table 9.2). The eligibility criteria for referral to the prison TC, typical inmate profiles, and planned duration of treatment were similar and are briefly summarized.

Referral criteria: The inmates referred to prison-based TCs are those who have a documented history of substance use or abuse (i.e., per a review of inmate files) and who do not meet the exclusionary criteria (such as documented in-prison gang) affiliations, assaultive behaviors, and Immigration and Naturalization Service holds. Additional exclusions may be those with sexual offenses and those who are actively violent. (As discussed below, however, modified prison TC programs have been implemented for co-occurring substance abuse and psychiatric disorder.)

Eligible inmates are those within two to three years of release or parole. Most of the prison TC programs surveyed in the evaluation research were similar in planned duration, 9–12 months, but additional programming beyond the prison TC has varied. Also, policies varied as to mandating participation in prison TCs and/or aftercare.

Typical profiles: Inmates entering prison-based TC treatment settings reveal deviant social and psychological profiles. Characteristically, they have histories of severe drug use (frequency, duration of use); criminal deviancy (arrests and incarcerations); psychological problems (depression, anxiety, poor self-esteem, antisocial personality, and other diagnoses); and social problems (poor employment and educational histories, lacking or deficient social skills) (e.g., Sacks, Sacks, McKendrick et al., 2004). Overall, it is a profile that is considered high risk, requiring an intensive treatment modality such as the TC.

Adapting the TC to correctional settings has required modifications that address specific characteristics of the criminal justice client (e.g., criminal thinking and lifestyle; low intrinsic motivation for change). However, adaptation has also involved issues and problems that have affected the optimal implementation of the TC approach itself. A more detailed review of these issues is contained in an early report by Kressel, Zompa, and De Leon (2002). Several are highlighted here in terms of three general areas: institutional, correctional policy, and clinical issues.

Institutional issues (prison limitations)

Program setting: Community-based TCs attempt to maintain "physical and psychological" boundaries between the program and the setting in which they

Table 9.2 Essential elements retained in the original prison TCs.

- Planned duration of in-prison residential treatment at least 9–12 months
- Planned duration of post-treatment aftercare in a community-based TC program 6–9 months recommended
- Program structure: 3 main phases, orientation main treatment, reentry
- Resident hierarchy to manage the community under staff supervision
- Staffing pattern that includes recovered addicts and former convicts in clinical management roles
- The TC program model: Critical program components include community enhancement meetings, encounter groups, and other forms of tutorial and clinical group processes
- A system of privileges and disciplinary sanctions
- Community and clinical management; peers utilizing verbal correctives (pull ups) and affirmations (push ups)

Note: The original programs that were evaluated included Stay'n Out, New York; Key Crest, Delaware; Amity-Vista, California; and Kyle New Vision, Texas.

are located. It is particularly important in prison settings to minimize potential negative influences from contact with the general prison population. The approach has been to designate wings or pods of the prison facility for the TC housing and programming. However, contact between the TC participants and general population inmates, for example, the recreational yards and dining areas, remains an issue.(As reported below a dedicated prison TC, Sheridan in Illinois, minimizes this mixed population issue.)

Physical space, acoustics and other impediments: The physical elements of prison institutions, specifically, space and acoustics, can limit or impede optimal functioning of the TC program. However, it is not uncommon for prison TC programs to conduct all program activities in a single large space with poor acoustics.

Unlike other treatment and/or educational prison programs, the TC approach (community as method) utilizes a daily schedule of activities that includes three community-wide meetings as well as various clinical and tutorial groups. Adequate space is needed to efficiently conduct these activities. Communal meetings require a large space and an appropriate *acoustical* environment (microphones and speaker system if needed) to assure that words (essential messages of therapeutic change) can be heard. Separate rooms for clinical and tutorial groups should be available to minimize distraction and to preserve confidentiality. Though mundane, these space issues can impede a difficult population from engaging in a demanding treatment process.

Staff integration: The interface between prison security requirements and essential TC activities is a challenging issue in correctional settings.

For example, the logistics of movement and the scheduling of activities in a prison is difficult. Lockdowns and population counts, though necessary, are often intrusions on treatment activities, as are prohibition of radios, CD players (for morning meeting music), the use of pencils, notebooks, flip charts, and so on.

Constructive resolution of these logistical and related issues depends upon an effective level of integration between correctional staff (administration and custody) and treatment personnel. Indeed, the importance of staff integration is evident in the 24-hour management of the TC program itself. For example, a key modification in prison programs is that the planned treatment activities, for example, community meetings, groups, seminars, are usually contracted to 20–30 hours a week. Beyond these formal activities the *informal* peer interactions must sustain their perceptions of a positive community and reinforce the TC teachings on right living to minimize negative prison influences. This requires a cooperative relationship between custody and treatment staff in the management of the program particularly in the hours when TC treatment staff leave the facility.

Participants perceive the treatment program as credible when custody and treatment staff are on the "same page" with respect to management. For example, physical and psychological safety is assured when custody supports enforcement of program cardinal rules prohibiting gang activity, drugs, gambling, and intimidation. In particular, treatment staff must be capable of discharging residents for violating cardinal rules and in some cases for persistent noncompliance. However, effective custody–treatment staff integration is difficult to achieve in prison TCs, reflecting various issues, for example, the lack of cross-training, the selection of appropriate custody staff, and embedded institutional norms.

Correctional policies

Staffing pattern: Historically, the primary professional staff for traditional TCs were recovering individuals who themselves may have completed a TC, some with criminal justice histories. However, in many prison systems policy precludes employment of ex-offenders, thus limiting recruitment of TC-trained personnel.

Referral and assessment process: Research and clinical experience in both community and prison-based TCs indicate that the TC approach is most appropriate and effective for those with bona fide substance abuse and related lifestyle problems and in particular those who are internally motivated to change. In many prisons, however, the assessment process is inadequate to optimize referral of inmates who are most appropriate for the TC program. The referral process itself is often influenced by administrative demands for utilization. For example, TC treatment staff may participate in classification meetings to identify appropriate inmates, but they often accept questionable clients under explicit or implicit pressures to "fill the beds." A disproportionate number of inappropriate clients invariably impacts negatively on program management and ultimately treatment effectiveness.

The assessment process is most efficiently conducted by the TC treatment staff using clinical interview. The main focus of assessment is to evaluate inmate motivation and suitability for the prison TC. Inmate decisions to enter a prison-based TC may be based on recovery as well as non-recovery reasons. The former refer to problem recognition and desire to change, the typical indicators of internal motivation. However, inmates may also enter a TC as a condition for parole or to avoid chaotic, monotonous, or unsafe conditions in the general prison population. These *non-recovery reasons* may explain why some inmates do not fully engage with treatment or community activities. For example, an inmate who enters a TC only to meet parole board expectations may have little incentive to invest in his treatment and, though completing the program, remains at high risk for relapse or recidivism.

TC programs can tolerate a diversity of clients with respect to motivation provided that all inmates *participate* in program activities and do not impede the progress of others. Moreover, research on community-based TCs shows positive post-treatment outcomes in a number of legal referrals who enter TC treatment primarily for non-recovery reasons (e.g., De Leon, 1988), a finding that supports common clinical observations that the TC treatment itself can change participant reasons for remaining and completing treatment. Nevertheless, a disproportionate number of "unmotivated" inmates strain overall program management (e.g., less participation, negative attitudes, low morale, more disciplinary actions).

Clinical program issues

A notable modification in prison TCs is evident in two essential elements of community as method. These involve peer face-to-face confrontation, namely, *pull ups/push ups* and *encounter groups*. Few programs practice these elements in accordance with TC theory. For example, rather than as face-to-face exchanges, pull ups are typically delivered in writing, which limits their effect in maintaining peer-managed accountability.

Properly trained and practiced, verbal correctives (pull ups) and verbal affirmations (push ups) are essential interventions in the mutual self-help process. This well-established clinical conclusion gains support from research demonstrating positive correlations between verbal correctives and affirmations delivered and received during program tenure and reduced post-release re-incarceration rates (e.g., Warren et al., 2007).

The encounter group (often misnamed as the confrontational group) is a critical component of the original TC approach. In prison settings, however, these groups have been eliminated or extensively modified, limiting their clinical efficacy. The primary aim of encounters is to raise participant awareness of how their behaviors and attitudes affect others in the community (De Leon, 2000, chapter 18). However, the utility and impact of encounter groups extend beyond behavioral management. Properly implemented, the encounter process involves *training appropriate affective expression* in those presenting and those receiving the confrontation, and indirectly in those observing the group. Participants learn to identify, and express their genuine feelings in appropriate words. This is a crucial training for many who lack such verbal skills or have histories of inappropriate or destructive expression of emotionality. In this regard, the social intercourse in community life gives rise to "real" feelings among participants that provide the material for training constructive communication practices in the TC. These practices initiate changes toward the broader therapeutic goals of emotional maturity.

The modification of peer confrontation in pull ups and in encounters is commonly attributed to correctional concerns about safety and security: Indeed, inmates themselves are often hesitant to deliver peer confrontations, viewing these as defying prison or street culture norms (e.g., snitching and retaliation). Other than a few anecdotal reports, however, there is little empirical evidence to validate these security concerns. In contrast, studies report that the prison units housing TC programs appear to be comparatively safer than standard (non-TC) units, showing significantly fewer incidents of violence, higher morale among custody officers assigned to the TC, as well as lower administrative costs reflecting fewer disciplinary problems (cited in Hiller & Saum, 2018).

Collectively, the above modifications and issues of adaptations can affect participants' perceived credibility of the TC as *a culture of change*. Grounded in its perspective on recovery and right living, the TC must compete with prison culture that reflects a custodial perspective on security and safety as well as the negative socialization effects of prison life. TC theory asserts that individuals change when they participate fully in the TC, when they "buy in" to the program, its philosophy and method. Indeed, establishing a culture of change is a *prerequisite* for the effectiveness of the TC. This proposition is commonly supported by clinical experience and in developing research. Participants who score high on affiliation in community-based TC programs show greater clinical progress (Kressel, De Leon, Palij, & Rubin, 2000). Conversely, in a recently completed prison-based study participants report that mistrust, skepticism, and doubts about the program's credibility affected their engagement (e.g., Kreager et al., 2018).

Effectiveness of prison-based TC treatment

The above issues notwithstanding, some 40 years of research documents the effectiveness of prison based TCs. Hiller and Saum (2018) provide a comprehensive overview of the evidence base for in-prison TCs. This includes reviews and meta-analyses of the empirical literature (Mitchell, Wilson, & MacKenzie, 2007; Belenko, Hiller, & Hamilton, 2013; Galassi, Mpofu, & Anthansou, 2015; Vanderplasschen, Colpaert, Autrique et al., 2013), as well as evaluations of single programs (e.g., Griffth, Hiller, Knight, & Simpson, 1999; Inciardi, Martin, & Butzin, 2004).

The literature on the effectiveness of prison-based TCs can be organized in terms of early and later studies. Early studies evaluated the original, first generation of prison-based TC programs that launched and adapted the TC approach in correctional settings (e.g., Stay'n Out (New York); Amity-Vista (California); Key Crest (Delaware); New Vision (Texas)) and evaluated modified prison-based TCs for co-occurring disorders. Although a critical review of this research is beyond the scope of this chapter, key findings and conclusions are summarized.

In the early research, emphasis is on criminal justice outcomes such as re-arrest and re-incarceration since recidivism is of key interest for the correctional system, but results included substance use, employment, and psychological outcomes. Reductions in recidivism at one to three years post-release are consistently higher for TC participants compared to non-treatment and other treatment groups, although the comparative impact of the TC on reducing drug use is less than on crime.

Aftercare's contribution to maintaining reduced recidivism has been reported by studies conducted in Delaware (Inciardi, Martin, & Butzin, 2004); Texas (Knight, Simpson, & Hiller, 1999); and California (Wexler, De Leon, Thomas et al., 1999). The aftercare findings were also obtained in studies of federal inmates (Pelissier, Gaes, Camp et al., 1998).

The general conclusions drawn from the early evaluation studies is that in-prison TCs are most effective when continuity of care is maintained during re-entry through community-based aftercare and when used with inmates with the most severe clinical profiles (Hiller & Saum, 2018). In addition, the TC impact appears to be larger on recidivism than on drug use, particularly in the first years following re-entry to society.

The earlier period of research also witnessed the application of the modified TC for special populations and special settings (see De Leon, 1997), including women in prison TCs (e.g., Hall, Prendergast, Wellisch et al., 2004) and for those with co-occurring psychiatric disorders in community and prison-based programs (Sacks, Sacks, McKendrick, Banks, & Stommel, 2004). Most of the elements of the TC were retained in these applications, but key modifications were guided by the unique needs of the client (e.g., less structure, lower intensity of group interactions, focus on skills development, as well as medication needs).

A comprehensive summary of the research on the modified prison-based TC for co-occurring disorders is contained in Sacks (2010). Single program evaluations yielded positive outcomes contrasted to comparison groups in terms of drug and crime reductions and psychological improvements as well as reduced re-hospitalization.

In prison-based studies of the modified therapeutic community (MTC), offenders who received MTC in prison and aftercare had significantly lower reincarceration rates at one-year post-prison release (5%) than offenders in a mental health control condition (33%) or those who received prison MTC treatment only (16%), which confirmed the added value of TC-oriented aftercare. (Sacks, Sacks, Kendrick, Banks Banks, & Stommel, 2004).

In a later Colorado prison study, upon release, male inmates with co-occurring disorders were randomly assigned to either to the Experimental (E) reentry modified therapeutic community (RMTC) condition or to the Control (C) parole supervision and case management (PSCM) condition. An intent-to-treat analysis 12 months post-prison release showed that the (E) RMTC participants were significantly less likely to be re-incarcerated (19% vs. 38%), with the greatest reduction in recidivism found for participants who received MTC treatment in both settings. These findings support the RMTC as a stand-alone intervention and provide initial evidence for integrated MTC programs in prison and in aftercare for offenders with co-occurring disorder (Sacks, 2010).

A second wave of evaluation studies utilized improved methodologies such as single program and multisite designs, measures of program quality, and analyses of client risk–outcome interactions (e.g., Jensen & Kane, 2010, 2012; Duwe, 2010); Olson & Lurigio, 2014; Welsh, Zajac, & Bucklen, 2014). Overall, findings supported the conclusion that prison TCs are comparatively more effective in reducing recidivism when clients completed both the prison TC treatment and participated in post-prison aftercare. However, other studies reported diminishing positive effects for the TC over time, variability in program outcomes, and low participation rates in aftercare. Two studies in particular underscored the issues of aftercare and treatment fidelity in interpreting TC effectiveness.

In a well-designed randomized trial, prison TC outcomes did not differ significantly from prison based non-TC treatment comparisons (Welsh,

Zajac, & Bucklen, 2014). Although all inmates participating in the study were mandated to receive six months of post-prison outpatient aftercare, investigators were unable to assess the utilization, or quality of aftercare services provided.

A large-scale study of the California Substance Abuse Treatment Facility (SATF at Corcoran Prison) showed no differences in improved outcomes TC and non-TC matched comparisons (at Avenol Prison) at five years post-release (Zhang, Roberts, & McCollister, 2011). At the two-year follow-up of this sample, the researchers conducted focus groups with program participants, treatment staff, and facility staff that revealed a number of problems and issues with implementation of the TC program at the SATF. These include: treatment staff being poorly trained; high treatment staff turnover rates; conflicts and lack of coordination between treatment and custody staff; a program curriculum that was repetitive and dull; overcrowded sessions that countered a TC culture; and the fact that some participants were not interested in participating but were mandated to do so. In addition, participation rates in residential and non-residential aftercare were quite low (Anglin, Prendergast, Farabee, & Cartier, 2002).

The future of TCs in correctional settings: going forward

The research and clinical experience over several decades supports the conclusion that prison-based TC programs are effective in reducing recidivism and substance abuse. However, this conclusion is tempered by two major issues, aftercare and the fidelity of TC treatment. This last section addresses these issues to illustrate how the TC in correctional settings can meet its promise and potential going forward.

Recovery-oriented aftercare

The most consistent findings in evaluation studies document the importance of aftercare in the effectiveness of the prison TC. Clients transitioning from prison-based TCs *require* a *continuum of care* to sustain positive post-release outcomes.

An ideal aftercare system is one that provides seamless continuity of care. It is a system capable of coordinating a diversity of treatment, correctional (surveillance), and social services to meet the changing needs of clients as they transition from prison-based treatment to re-entry into the larger community. Rather than a system, however, the past and current status of aftercare can be described as a loose aggregate of providers with diverse approaches and philosophies (De Leon, 2007). The research on community aftercare programs for those released from custody is limited, and there is no standardized conceptualization of what constitutes aftercare. Neither the core intervention components nor the core implementation components associated with the aftercare phase of the continuum of care are well understood (Welsh, Zajak, & Bucklen, 2014).

A recovery-oriented integrated system (ROIS) conceptualized in other writings (De Leon, 2007) consists of treatment interventions, social services, and surveillance activities *guided by a common perspective on the disorder, re-entry, and recovery*. The term "re-entry" designates a client's *social status* with respect to their return to the macro society. Typically, this status is assessed in terms of the familiar issues and needs associated with return to society, such as housing, education, employment, and family reintegration. Recovery refers to a client's *clinical status* with respect to changes in cognitive, emotional, and social-lifestyle characteristics associated with their substance abuse disorder.

In a ROIS, the convergence of the terms re-entry and recovery is evident. Individuals reveal their treatment needs (clinical status) in how they cope with their re-entry issues. Conversely, the timing and constructive utilization of re-entry social services will depend upon progress in their clinical status. (A familiar example is readiness for employment; re-entry clients may be ready to *get* a job, but clinically, not be prepared to *keep* a job.) This distinction between re-entry and recovery captures the basic rationale of a ROIS – to facilitate a *recovery-oriented re-entry* for those returning to the larger society.

In a recovery-oriented continuum, the cornerstone programs are the prison TC followed by the post-prison TC re-entry residence. For those completing prison-based TCs, managing their clinical issues and re-entry needs is most efficiently coordinated in a post-prison TC-oriented program that provides *continuity* of perspective (recovery -oriented), of approach (community as method), and of support (peer relationships).

That the effectiveness of the prison TC is considerably enhanced when treatment continues in TC-oriented aftercare settings is affirmed in the research literature (e.g., Wexler, De Leon, Thomas et al., 1999; Sacks, Sacks, McKendricks et al., 2004; Martin, Butzin, Saum, & Inciardi, 1999). Specifically, best outcomes are obtained among those clients who complete a 12-month prison TC and 6–12 months of a TC-oriented residential re-entry program. Indeed, this prison TC finding *reconstitutes* the well-established time in treatment effects obtained in studies of community-based TCs. Namely, duration of treatment is directly related to post-treatment success (De Leon, 1984).

Motivation and mandated aftercare

Although stable recovery is time correlated, sustaining individuals in the recovery process itself remains a challenge. Specifically, strategies are needed to increase client motivation to utilize any system of post-release aftercare. The importance of internal motivation in seeking and remaining in treatment has been emphasized in all subgroups of criminal justice substance abusers (Farabee,Prendergast, & Anglin, 1998), including coerced clients, that is, drug court referrals (Taxman & Messina, 2002).

Of particular relevance is the research showing that the majority of substance abuse offenders completing prison-based TC treatment do not voluntarily participate in aftercare treatment (Zhang, Roberts, & McCollister, 2011). Notably, one study has shown that among admissions to the Amity prison-based TC, those with higher internal motivation were more likely to volunteer for Vista, the post-prison TC-oriented aftercare program. (Melnick, De Leon, Thomas et al., 2001). However, this group represented less than a third of the prison completers.

Related to motivation is a common clinical observation that illuminates the issue of low participation in aftercare. Participants in prison TCs often view the completion of the prison program as the end of their treatment. As they approach completion of the prison TC, their focus shifts from primary *problems* (the cognitive, emotional, and behavioral characteristics of their disorder) to re-entry *needs* associated with moving into society (e.g., housing, vocation, education--training, family reintegration, finances). Giving priority to their re-entry needs and the understandable desire for release from incarceration, they are disinclined to elect any aftercare program, particularly the demands of another post-prison residential TC.

These clinical observations and motivational findings provide a rationale for a *mandated strategy* that requires completion of both prison and post-prison TCs. Support for a mandated aftercare can be drawn from the experiences of the original community-based TCs. The most stable long-term positive outcomes were obtained among the graduates -who completed 12 months of primary residential treatment plus 6 six months in residence in transitional re-entry (live in and work out) followed by six months of independent living (live out and work out), including participation in weekly groups and staff contact. (e.g., De Leon,, 1984). Over a third of these graduates initially entered residential treatment under some form of mandated status.

In the original cadre of prison TCs, aftercare was voluntary. Graduates of Amity in California had the option to enter Vista, a post-release community-based TC. Similarly, in the New York prison-based TC Stay'n Out graduates were encouraged to continue in aftercare treatment in the community. In the multistage Delaware program (Key -Crest), those completing the 12-month institutional TC (Key program) had the option of completing their sentence requirement in the 26-week TC (Crest) housed in a correctional work release facility. However, a third stage of aftercare following Crest was voluntary. The Key Crest five-year follow-up findings showed best results for completing the two stages + voluntary participation in TC-oriented outpatient aftercare groups.

A 2009 evaluation of the Sheridan Prison-based TC program in Illinois included mandated participation in various aftercare services. Over 56% of the prison TC graduates completed some modality of aftercare. However, the strongest predictor of aftercare completion was whether one was referred to residential aftercare, which included residential treatment, half-way houses, and recovery homes. (Olson, Rozhon, & Powers, 2009).

Overall, more research is needed to clarify predictors of completion of aftercare. However, a reasonable hypothesis for voluntary admissions is that mandating participation will increase completion rates of both the in-prison and post-prison TC-oriented aftercare program, which will significantly improve longer-term outcomes.

The issue of fidelity of the prison-based TC

Adapting the TC approach for correctional settings has impacted the fidelity of treatment in prison-based TCs. Examples of limitations that undermine the culture of the prison TC were provided in the earlier discussion on special issues. That treatment or program fidelity has been a long-standing issue was identified in the national survey of corrections-based TCs conducted by Rockholz (2002). A key conclusion by Rockholz was that many programs "only vaguely resemble what is understood by TC experts to constitute a real TC." This conclusion led to the development of national standards for prison TCs (ONDCP, 1999), an accreditation process implemented by the America Correctional Association (ACA) and to published recommendations to improve the fidelity of prison-based TCs (Kressel, Zompa, & De Leon, 2002). Nevertheless, maintaining TC fidelity is an ongoing challenge that requires appropriate training and fidelity assessment capability. This final section briefly outlines a general perspective and specific strategies toward meeting this challenge.

Perspective

Fidelity, meaning "faithful" to the TC approach, may be understood in terms of two dimensions. *Model fidelity*, refers to the extent to which programs a) are guided by the TC perspective on recovery and "right living' for treating the whole person; b) adhere to its mutual self-help approach (i.e., community as method); and c) retain essential components of the program model (e.g., community meetings, a resident work structure, a phase system, peer encounter and other groups, etc.). The second dimension, *practice fidelity,* refers to standards of clinical and program management, that is, the extent to which the activities and essential components of the program are appropriately and effectively implemented. TC effectiveness and fidelity of treatment are closely related (Dye, Ducharme, Johnson, Knudsen, & Roman, 2009).

Strategies

The key strategies needed to assure *high-fidelity* TCs are appropriate training models and ongoing fidelity assessment. Training to fidelity requires a teaching curriculum based on a uniform definition of community as method, and appropriate training models.

a. *A uniform definition*: The TC can be distinguished from other approaches and other communities in its use of community as the primary method of treatment. Community as method is defined as *the purposive use of community to teach individuals to <u>use</u> the community to change themselves.*

b. *Teaching curricula:* Teaching materials and manuals based upon a uniform definition of the TC must focus on the relationship between theory and practice: This can be summarized in three questions: *what, how, and why we do what we do* in TCs? All members of the community, participants, and staff (treatment and ideally, custodial) must understand that every element and activity has a therapeutic and/or educational purpose (e.g., morning meeting, house meeting, privilege, sanctions, encounter group).

c. *Appropriate training models:* Five decades of experience indicate that training for work in TCs requires combinations of didactic teaching of theory and practice as well experiential learning as participants in TCs. Thus, TC training is most efficaciously implemented in high-fidelity prison TC programs that serve as *centers of excellence.* Cadres of staff would rotate through these proposed centers as interns for several months, learning and experiencing how and why community as method works. Analogous training models are found in conventional graduate and postdoctoral medical settings based on the well-grounded assumption that staff should learn their specialty in the "best teaching hospitals."[3]

Fidelity Assessment

A key insight from decades of clinical and research experience is that fidelity is in a "constant state of erosion." Sustaining a high-fidelity TC program requires not only training but regular observation of fluctuations in program quality. Thus, fidelity assessment is necessarily an ongoing activity best conducted by expert teams of TC workers who periodically review not only *whether* program elements are present (*model fidelity*) but how well they are being implemented (*practice fidelity*).

Protocols for assessing both model and practice fidelity remain to be developed for prison-based TC programs and TC oriented aftercare programs. Relevant generic TC training curricula are available (e.g., CSAT Therapeutic Community Curriculum, 2006) but are not specific to Prison-based TCs. The corrections version of the Survey of Essential Elements Questionnaire (See De Leon & Melnick, 1999), a useful tool for assessing model fidelity, is contained in a published report (ONDCP, 1999).

Finally, the utility of expert assessment teams has been demonstrated by the American Correctional Association (ACA). However, their focus has been credentialing rather than training to improve the quality of TC programming and practice toward better outcomes.

Summary and conclusion

The current status of Prison TCs may be viewed from an evolutionary perspective. The success of community based TCs for substance abusers, many with criminal justice histories, laid the groundwork for launching prison-based TC programs. Evaluations of the first generation of these prison-based programs yielded impressive outcomes and potentiated a rapid expansion of prison based TCs. A later wave of evaluations with improved research methodology generally replicated the positive outcomes of the prison based TCs. However, firm conclusions concerning effectiveness are clouded by several factors e.g., diminishing effects in long term outcomes, reductions in planned duration of treatment, low aftercare participation and wide variability in program quality.

Advancing the TC approach in corrections will require creative efforts to maintain high-fidelity programs and implement systems of aftercare that sustain individuals in the recovery process. In this regard decades of research and clinical experience offer three key insights (1) TC based programs are more successful in correctional institutions in which staff, policies and practices are integrated to maximize the TC as a culture of change and minimize the negative influences of prison and street culture. (2) Prison based TC (9–12 months) programs are the initial components of a recovery-oriented continuum of care that includes a post-prison transitional TC (6–12 months) followed by after-care services. Completion of both residential components should be mandated to optimize long term outcomes.

(3) The fidelity and effectiveness of TC programs are closely related. Establishing high-fidelity prison TC programs requires intensive didactic and experiential training for both treatment and correctional staff optimally implemented in TC programs that are designated centers of excellence. Finally, maintaining high-fidelity programs is an ongoing process conducted by highly trained fidelity assessment teams.

Notes

1 In the North American literature on prison TC treatment, the terms offender, inmate, and resident are conventionally used.
2 A comprehensive description of the therapeutic community theory, model, and method is contained in De Leon, 2000.
3 Ironically, the early prototype of such centers appeared in the first generation of community-based TCs. Well-known programs (e.g., Phoenix House, Daytop Village, Amity) were the sources for developing residents into experienced staff whose expertise evolved from their participation in high-fidelity programs. Many of these staff helped launch new community and prison-based programs. Informed by research, formal *didactic* curricula emerged later that articulated theory concepts and rationales such as presented in section 1. Today, *experiential and didactic* understanding are essential for managing and maintaining high-fidelity TCs.

References

Anglin, M.D., Prendergast, M.L., Farabee, D., & Cartier, J. (2002). *Final report on the substance abuse program at the California Substance Abuse Treatment Facility (SATF-SAP) and state prison at Corcoran: A Report to the California Legislature*. Sacramento, CA: California Department of Corrections, Office of Substance Abuse Programs.
Belenko, S., Hiller, M., & Hamilton, L. (2013). Treating substance use disorders in the criminal justice system. *Current Psychiatry Reports, 15*(11). https://doi.org/10.1007/s11920-013-0414-z
CSAT Therapeutic Community Curriculum. (2006). U.S. Dept. of Health and Human Services, Substance Abuse and Mental Health Services Administration, Center for Substance Abuse Treatment. Rockville, MD: DHHS publication, no. (SMA) 06–4121.
De Leon, G. (1984). The therapeutic community: Study of effectiveness. *National Institute on Drug Abuse Treatment Research Monograph Series* (DHHS Publication No. ADM 84–1286). Rockville, MD: National Institute on Drug Abuse.
De Leon, G. (1988). Legal pressure in therapeutic communities. In C.G. Leukefeld & F.M. Tims (Eds.). *Compulsory treatment of drug abuse: Research and clinical practice, NIDA Research Monograph 86* (DHHS Publication No. (Adm. 88–1578, pp. 160–77). Rockville, MD: National Institute on Drug Abuse.

De Leon, G. (2000). *The therapeutic community: Theory, model, and method*. New York, NY: Springer Publishing.

De Leon, G. (2007). Toward a recovery oriented integrated system (ROIS). *Offender Substance Abuse Report*, Nov./Dec., *V11*(4).

De Leon, G. (2010). Is the therapeutic community an evidence-based treatment? What the evidence says. *Therapeutic Communities, 31*, 104–28.

De Leon, G., & Melnick, G. (1993). *Therapeutic community Scale of Essential Elements Questionnaire (SEEQ)*. New York, NY: Center for Therapeutic Community Research at National and Development and Research.

De Leon, G. (Ed.) (1997). *Community as method: Therapeutic communities for special populations and special settings*. Westport, CT: Greenwood.

Dye, N.H., Ducharme, L.J., Johnson, A.J., H.K. Knudsen, & Roman, P.N. (2009). Modified therapeutic communities and adherence to traditional elements. *Journal of Psychoactive Drugs, 41*(3), 275–83.

Farabee, D., Prendergast, M., & Anglin, D. (1988). The effectiveness of coerced treatment for drug-abusing offenders. *Federal Probation, 62*(1), 3–10.

Farabee, D., Prendergast, M., Cartier, J.E., Wexler, H., Knight, K., & Anglin, M.D. (1999). Barriers to implementing effective correctional drug treatment programs. *The Prison Journal, 79*, 150–62.

Galassi, A., Mpofu, E., & Athanasou, J. (2015). Therapeutic community treatment of an inmate population with substance use disorders: Post-release trends in re-arrest, re-incarceration, and drug misuse relapse. *International Journal of Environmental Research and Public Health, 12*, 7059–72.

Griffith, J.D., Hiller, M.L., Knight, K., & Simpson, D.D. (1999). A cost-effectiveness analysis of in-prison therapeutic community treatment and risk classification. *The Prison Journal, 79*, 352–68.

Hiller, M.L., & Saum, C.A. (2018). Substance abuse treatment in prison: The therapeutic community. In W.T. Church & D. Springer (Eds.). *Serving the stigmatized: Working within the incarcerated environment*. New York, NY: Oxford University Press.

Hiller, M.L., Knight, K., & Simpson, D.D. (1999). Prison-based substance abuse treatment, residential aftercare, and recidivism. *Addiction, 94*, 833–42.

Inciardi, J.A., Martin, S.S., & Butzin, C.A. (2004). Five-year outcomes of therapeutic community treatment of drug-involved offenders after release from prison. *Crime & Delinquency, 50*, 88–107.

Jensen, E.L., & Kane, S.L. (2010). The effect of therapeutic community on time to first re-arrest: A survival analysis. *Journal of Offender Rehabilitation, 49*, 200–9.

Jensen, E.L., & Kane, S.L. (2012). The effects of therapeutic community on recidivism up to four years after release from prison: A multisite study. *Criminal Justice and Behavior, 39*, 1075–87.

Knight, K., Simpson, D.D., & Hiller, M.L. (1999). Three-year reincarceration outcomes for in-prison therapeutic community treatment in Texas. *The Prison Journal, 79*(3), 337–51.

Kreager, D.A., Zajac, G., Davidson, K., Haynie, D.L., Schaefer, D.R., Young, J.T.N., & De Leon, G. (2018). *The Therapeutic Community Prison Inmate Networks Study (TC-PINS): Evaluating peer-based processes in a prison substance abuse treatment unit*. Report to the Pennsylvania Department of Corrections.

Kressel, D., De Leon, G., Palij, M., & Rubin, G. (2000). Measuring client clinical progress in therapeutic community (TC) treatment: The Client Assessment Inventory (CAI), Client Assessment Summary (CAS) and Staff Assessment Summary (SAS). *Journal of Substance Abuse Treatment,19*, 267–72.

Kressel, D., Zompa, D., & De Leon, G. (2002, July/August). A statewide integrated quality assurance model for correctional-based therapeutic community programs. *Offender Substance Abuse Report, II*(4), 49–64.

Martin, S.S., Butzin, C.A., Saum, C.A., & Inciardi, J.A. (1999). Three-year outcomes of therapeutic community treatment for drug-involved offenders in Delaware: From prison to work release to aftercare. *The Prison Journal, 79*, 294–320.

Melnick, G., De Leon, G., Thomas, G., Kressel, D., & Wexler, H.K. (2001). Treatment process in prison therapeutic communities: Motivation, participation, and outcome. *American Journal of Drug and Alcohol Abuse, 27*, 633–50.

Mitchel, O., Wilson, D.B., & MacKenzie, D.L. (2007). Does incarceration-based drug treatment reduce recidivism? A meta-analytic synthesis of the research. *Journal of Experimental Criminology, 3*, 353–75.

Olson, D.E., & Lurigio, A.J. (2014). The long-term effects of prison-based drug treatment and aftercare services on recidivism. *Journal of Offender Rehabilitation, 53*, 600–19.

Olson, D.E., Rozhon, J., & Powers, M. (2009). Enhancing prisoner reentry through access to prison-based and post-incarceration aftercare treatment: Experiences from the Illinois Sheridan Correctional Center therapeutic community. *Journal of Experimental Criminology, 5*, 299–321.

ONDCP. (1999). *Therapeutic communities in correctional settings*. The Prison Based TC Standards Development Project (G. De Leon). White House Office of National Drug Control Policy.

Pelissier, B., Gaes, G.G., Camp, S., Wallace, S., O'Neil, J.A., & Saylor, M.A. (1998). Federal prison residential drug treatment reduces substance use and arrests after release. *American Journal of Drug and Alcohol Abuse, 27*(2), 315–37.

Rockholz, P. (2002). National update on Therapeutic Community Programs for substance abusers in state prisons. *Offender Substance Abuse Report, 2*(4).

Sacks, S. (2010). Research on the effectiveness of the modified therapeutic community for persons with co-occurring substance use and mental disorders. *Therapeutic Communities, 31*, 104–28.

Sacks, S., Sacks, J.Y., McKendrick, K., Banks, S., & Stommel, J. (2004). Modified TC for MICA offenders: Crime outcomes. *Behavioral Sciences and the Law, 22*, 477–501.

Taxman, F., & Bouffard, J.A. (2002). Assessing therapeutic integrity in modified therapeutic communities for drug-involved offenders. *The Prison Journal, 82*, 189–212.

Taxman, F.S., & Messina, N.P. (2002). Civil commitment: A coerced treatment model. In C.G. Leukefeld, F.M. Tims & D. Farabee (Eds.). *Treatment of drug offenders: Policies and issues*. New York: Springer.

Vanderplasschen, W., Colbert, K., Autrique, M., Rapp, R.C., Peace, S., Broekaert, E., & Vandevelde, S. (2013). Therapeutic communities for addictions: A review of their effectiveness from a recovery-oriented perspective. *The Scientific World Journal, 2013*, 427817. https://doi.org/10.1155/2013/427817

Warren, K., Harvey, C., De Leon, G., & Gregoire, T. (2007). I am my brother's keeper: Affirmations and corrective reminders as predictors of reincarceration following graduation from a corrections-based therapeutic community. *Offender Substance Abuse Report, V11*(3).

Welsh, W.N., & Zajac, G. (2004). A census of prison-based drug treatment programs: implications for programming, policy and evaluation. *Crime and Delinquency, 50,* 108–33.

Welsh, W.N., Zajac, G., & Bucklen, K.B. (2014). For whom does prison-based drug treatment work? Results from a randomized experiment. *Journal of Experimental Criminology, 10,* 151–77.

Wexler, H.K., & Prendergast, M.L. (2010). Therapeutic communities in United States' prisons: Effectiveness and challenges. *Therapeutic Communities, 31,* 157–75.

Wexler, H.K., De Leon, G., Thomas, G., Kressel, D., & Peters, J. (1999). The Amity Prison TC evaluation: Reincarceration outcomes. *Criminal Justice and Behavior, 26,* 147–67.

Wexler, H.K., Falkin, G.P., & Lipton, D.S. (1990). Outcome evaluation of a prison therapeutic community for substance abuse treatment. *Criminal Justice and Behavior, 17,* 71–92.

Zhang, S., Roberts, R., & McCollister, K. (2011). Therapeutic community in a California prison: Treatment outcomes after 5 years. *Crime & Delinquency, 50*(1), 88–107.

Part III

Narrative perspectives and developments

10

The 'gentle revolution' of new therapeutic communities for offenders with mental disorders in Italy

Closure of the forensic psychiatric hospital (FPH) and opening of the therapeutic residential facility for execution of security measures (RESM)

Simone Bruschetta

The development of Italian legislation

Ten years ago, on the Italian sociopolitical horizon, the need to complete the process of legislative reform that led to the closure of the psychiatric hospitals was delineated, which commenced with the 'Basaglia' law in 1978 (Basaglia, 1982), starting a process of transformation of legislation on security measures for those citizens with mental disorders, which led to the closure of the *ospedali psichiatrici giudiziari* (OPG). OPGs are old 'forensic psychiatric hospitals' (FPHs) reserved exclusively for the detention of psychiatric patients, previously called 'criminal asylums for insane offenders', created during the fascist regime, which have always remained separate from the NHS and under direct authority of the Ministry of the Interior. The years 2008–2017 were referred by Italian civil society as the decade of the 'gentle revolution', to use a definition coined by the 'single commissioner' for overstepping the OPGs, Franco Corleone (Corleone, 2016).

The political and social process of this 'gentle revolution' finally ended with the establishment of *residenze per l'esecuzione delle misure di sicurezza* (REMSs) for people with mental health disorders who have committed an offence, in which prisoners would officially become patients of the local

DOI: 10.4324/9780429317460-13

community mental health department like all other Italian citizens, as institutionally assisted by the NHS. REMSs are therapeutic 'residences for the execution of security measures' (RESMs) for users with severe mental illness. Moreover, if compared to the 1,500 inmates present in the old FPHs in the years around 2010, the limited and significantly lower number of beds that are today available in RESMs shows that residential treatment as a therapeutic solution has been employed, both politically and legally, under temporary and not definitive terms, and therefore with periods of stay that the necessity of a continuous turnover inevitably makes brief. The NHS thus assumed the risk of new skills that could transform its social function of guaranteeing the right to care for citizens, in two ways: regressively, through regulatory social control skills, or conversely, progressively, through political development skills.

Let's sum up the main stages of this 'gentle revolution'.

This process was officially initiated during the second government of Romano Prodi together with the health minister, Livia Turco. They issued the Decree of the President of the Council of Ministers (d.p.c.m.) on 1 April 2008, which transferred to the NHS both the functions and the forensic health system units, giving full equality to healthcare for free citizens and for those with restrictions due to offending behaviours and, consequently, the clear distinction between penitentiary functions and health functions in the management of old FPHs.

In 2008, the European Council Committee for the Prevention of Torture (CPT) also became interested in the old Italian FPHs, undertaking a series of visits, the first of which was carried out in Aversa between 16 and 26 September, which produced a report containing numerous complaints about the scandalous living conditions of the people held there.

In the same year, with the 30 July 2008 deliberation of the Senate, a Parliamentary Commission of Inquiry was established aiming to evaluate the effectiveness and efficiency of the NHS, which, three years later, in the session of 20 July 2011, approved a 'Report on the Living Conditions and Care within old FPHs', which stated the need to 'put a stop to the phenomenon of systematic extensions of detention orders, based on a broad interpretation of the concept of social danger: often the extension is the result not of the subjective condition of persistent danger, but because of the lack of an adequate supply of external residential and rehabilitation facilities'.

Legislation for overcoming the old FPH has definitely compromised the fundamental structure of the original regulation of personal security measures, without changing the Italian Penal Code, which has lasted for more than 85 years. Thanks to the fact that the exclusion of criteria relating to the examination of social danger for prisoners with mental illness (referred to in art.2 co. 4 cp as established in co.4 of art. 3-ter dln211 / 2011) is now allowed by the two prerequisites for the application of personal security measures, even if only in cases of 'non-imputability due to reduced liability' and in those of 'semi-imputability due to partial mental disability'. This was a historic first blow to what is known as the 'Rocco Penal Code', which still survives unchanged since the fascist regime.

In the same vein legislation decreed that all 'provisional or definitive custodial security measures, including admission to the RESM, cannot last beyond the established time limit set out by the sentence given for the crime committed'. And this is a second blow, perhaps even heavier than the first, to the above-mentioned fascist era.

Today, admission to the RESM is intended for all those individuals in a position of social danger such that they are expected to be detained, and those experiencing mental health difficulties. The RESM can therefore be definitively understood as residences established by the NHS to primarily guarantee mental health care for people subjected to the execution of personal security measures, and only secondarily their custody. For this reason, these are managed directly by the community mental health department, in collaboration with the judicial authorities only for those functions concerning the administration of measures that restrict personal freedom.

The RESM is therefore a residential health facility belonging to the local community mental health department which as such must meet the accreditation requirements provided by the Decree of the President of the Republic of 14th January 1997 and the Decree of the Minister of Health of 1 October 2012, thus falling within the regulation and administration of health services by the regions and the autonomous provinces. In the 2012, the Unified State Conference, Regions and Autonomous Provinces, expressly reiterated that each individual interned in the RESMs must be 'guaranteed all the rights that are already intended for those admitted to old FPHs, but in a broader perspective'. This agreement also explicitly invites each region to define operating procedures that avoid the risk of new forms of institutionalisation, guaranteeing the exercise of the main civil rights starting with that of the entitlement to treatment, but also pointing out that security and surveillance services must remain in the perimeter and be activated on the basis of specific agreements with the prefectures, and the information contained in the patient's file.

At this point, it is clear that, with its establishment, the RESM is facing today the same power conflicts that took place in the sociopolitical processes that characterised the so-called Basaglia reform (Basaglia, 1982), in which legal and health demands confront each other. The RESM could therefore be better represented not only as a physical place for the execution of detention security measures, but also as a place, mental and social at the same time, where the aforementioned conflict can be, dangerously but democratically, revealed or denied.

RESM as a forensic therapeutic community

Against all denial, opacity and manipulation of the conflict of power in the RESM and therefore in the society that conceived it, the culture of enquiry (Lees and Manning, 2004) of the tradition of the democratic therapeutic community (DTC) (Jones et al., 1952), represents today a methodological principle which the organisation of residential treatment in compliance with the 2012 definition of the Unified State Conference, Regions and Autonomous Provinces, should be inspired by. Exploring what occurs within the RESM community boundaries requires not quiet any event without a recognized and shared meaning, and commits all its members to exercising critical thinking about the reality, starting from that what happens during the cohabitation and daily collaboration that takes place within, and ending with social institutions that influence these (first of all, the health and juridical ones).

Thus, the RESM can be thought of as a therapeutic environment organised to support and implement a transformational process of relational functioning and of exploration of the patients' mental suffering. In other words, RESM is like a stable, coherent and structured organisation that works therapeutically with mental health difficulties, and performs the function of a specialised *community psychotherapeutic setting*, because it is explicitly aimed at the treatment of serious mentalness, through the definition of its operational and symbolic boundaries.

The RESM can thus become for each of the people who comprise it (practitioners, service users, officials, administrators, family members, etc), each with its own social function, the operative and symbolic place to experience and explore conflicts of power, and learn more democratic ways for their composition. All this happens by analysing the events and responsibilities of the here and now, integrating multiple points of view on the facts and their motivations, reworking the past before being included in the RESM and opening a thought of hope for the future, after leaving the RESM. Main (1989) has indicated the culture of enquiry as the fundamental requirement of every therapeutic community (TC), a concept that has become an indispensable parameter of evaluation of the therapeutic processes foreseen by the theoretical-scientific model of the DTC of the English tradition. Furthermore, Haigh (2013) suggests to consider it as a parameter that defines the level of development of the ideological theme of 'communalism' and the quality of the therapeutic principle of 'communication' within all human environments that perform therapeutic and developmental functions for their members.

'Communalism' as described by Rapoport (1960) indicates a mode of community functioning based on a set of strictly interpersonal and intimate relationships, encouraged within the boundaries of the same residential environment by the sharing of facilities, by the informality and by the expectation of all its members to participate to the community life. According to this ideological theme, today called methodological, the construction of the meaning of individual and collective events occurring within the RESM community boundaries commits everyone to a continuous transition from an inquisitive thought to a reflective one, and vice versa. The work on significant events, from time to time, depending on whether legal institutes or health institutes prevail in the culture of the RESM in that moment, can assume two different characteristics: an arid and inquisitorial enquiry of the past (with procedural formalities and meticulous examinations), or an opening to the future with open questions and free comments, able to convey a subjective sense of freedom and possibilities of change.

In the RESM there are two social cultures that meet/clash with the judicial one of control and the healthy one of care. For example, the judicial application of social danger for prisoners, a very frequent, I would say basic, object of work within the RESM, represents very well the conflictual space between culture of control and culture of care. This is the same conflict that underlies the establishment of the RESM: the conflict between investigative and reflective thinking. Another example are the institutions of clinical diagnosis and of therapeutic treatment. The former can be understood as a nosographic classification or as a process of knowledge, the latter as psychiatric rehabilitation or as a recovery process. In the RESM, these two social cultures create an environment of constant transition between care and control.

The authoritarian culture in the analysis of social danger

The legal institution of social danger is one of the two prerequisites necessary for the application of the personal security measures set out in the Italian Penal Code (Rocco Penal Code), and it is refers to a large number of work practices active in the RESM. The regular and periodical examination of social danger (a judicial review) is expressly set out as a fundamental practice of the job of the supervisory magistrate, who decides the suspension or the extension, and indicates the type of measure (custodial or non-custodial) that would be more effective in ensuring the exercise of the rights of the prisoners. In the case of patients admitted to the RESM, as well as all citizens who have committed a crime under the community mental health service managed by the NHS, this periodic review also serves to indicate the type of personal security measure most suitable to guarantee the entitlement to treatment, and therefore, in this case, the health institution may not be involved, thus activating that transitional space described above, between the institute of care and that of control, which is so dangerous for both institutions involved, as heuristic for the evolution of the living and working conditions of people who are part of it.

The normative definition of the criteria for the examination of social danger is decisive for the fate of the prisoners' personal freedom because of the application of custodial security measures, such as for those people hospitalised at the RESM. Italian Penal Code (art. 203) defines a person as 'socially dangerous' […] when it is more likely that he could potentially commit new acts foreseen by the law as crimes'. However, among the criminal capacity indexes it also refers to 'conditions of personal living standards, family and social life'. In a judicial review of social danger, these conditions are clearly deduced from the guidelines of the two separate institutions of the state system (judicial and healthy) that meet in the RESM.

1. The *local Offices of External Penal Enforcement*, which performs, at the request of the supervisory magistrate, the investigation useful to supply the necessary data for the application, the modification, the extension and the withdrawal of the security measures.
2. The *local community mental health department* – the *NHS* – which identifies the conditions and needs of those involved and in agreement with the prison officers identifies external resources useful for taking responsibility for both the health service and for the subsequent social reintegration.

The local community mental health department of which the RESM is a part, therefore, 'dangerously' assumes the responsibility for a different and certainly supplementary function to that for which it was instituted, which is in fact that of a health service which guarantees the right to treatment. Furthermore, if during the examination there is no 'data' on the 'criminal capacity' useful for the modification or revocation of the custodial security measure, and at the same time there are no 'useful external resources' for taking charge of the prisoner (as e.g., family contexts or alternative health and residential services), then for the patient admitted to the RESM, these conditions meet the requirement of affirming the persistence of social danger and, therefore, extending the same detention security measure. 'Dangerously' for the social function of the mental health department, this extension of detention security measures will also take place in all those cases in which the patient should be discharged under any other profile except for the lack of 'conditions of individual living standards, family and social life'. In this case, the RESM becomes only a place of detention and not of cure, destroying the social function of the mental health department managed by the NHS.

It is clear that if the criterion for the examination of social danger involves an acquisition in the Italian law according to which the social danger 'is not a biological or psychological factor exclusively linked to the personal characteristics of the individual, but it must be ascertained through the interaction of these elements with the complex of environmental factors', it should not therefore 'be understood in a situational sense, because the subject is not a monad, and must be placed in the social and family context of reference' (Pellissero, 2014). It is then that the health institution is radically integrated within the positivist matrix of determinism, not only biological but also social, which risk assesses its evaluating function of a type of social danger that we could call 'preventive'. In other words, this is evaluated on the potential risk of a person returning to commit crimes within individual, family and social life, which is unknown.

Here, a *Kafkaesque* vicious circle is activated:

>> Non-dischargeable patient due to the absence of alternative living conditions to RESM >> Impossibility to assess the risk to commit a crime in a social environment alternative to RESM >> Confirmation of the condition of social danger >> Impossibility to construct environments and ways of life alternative to RESM >>

Fortunately, the perverse effects of this circle are attenuated by the recent legislation that established that all the 'provisional or definitive custodial security measures, including the admission in the RESM, cannot last beyond the established time for the imprisonment sentence intended for the crime committed'. This, however, does not preclude the possibility of serious damage inflicted on the social function of the NHS, by distorting the value of its own institution that came into place through the law.[1]

In this regard, Michel Foucault's masterly lesson on the nature of the power within health institutions, necessary for the foundation of a modern state of law, which takes upon itself and transforms the functions of the sovereign and punitive power of the monarch into a civil and democratic power which, as an alternative to 'macro-physics of sovereignty', is based on 'micro-physics of discipline'[2] (Foucault, 1973–1974). With the arrival of modernity, power passed into the hands of those who exercise it through the evaluation of the distance from the norm or normality represented by a normal situation, that is, in the present case, a situation in which all the indispensable conditions and resources are assumed to be present so that it would not be is possible to recommit the crime. The more the situation, which constitutes the norm on which to evaluate the distance, is ideal and hypothetical, the more decisive is the value of the medical and psychological sciences, precisely because they are assigned the social role of evaluating the individual's hypothetical intentions in a not current environment. Here, it is evident that in the case of health, the conflict between two complementary social functions, competitors and antagonists, is played out in full: the disciplinary-normative and the protective-rescuer cases.

The examination of the 'preventive' social danger becomes a new function of 'risk assessment' for the medical and psychological sciences that submit themselves to a new form of law, the 'norm', whose power is exercised in a technocratic way, establishing organisations of life, of care and of work that become increasingly less human, such as all those practices that fall within the scope of so-called criminological science. In this way, once again the transformation identified by Foucault with the birth of the prison is realised, so that the delinquent is no longer defined by the criminal act committed outside the law, but by his deviation from the norm. Hence, the deprivation of freedom comes to play the social function of a political, economic and health discipline, exercised by an essentially technical power, precisely defined as 'penitentiary', which is also the responsibility of criminological science. In this regard, Foucault reminds us that, in the same way criminology is an illegitimate child of the scientific disciplines of medicine and psychology, the *penitentiary* is a state power, the illegitimate child of judicial power. This is a very dangerous vicious circle, always active, within that transitional space between the sanitary and legal instances activated by the RESM, which we recognise in the logic of the asylum that has never been totally overcome in Italian society, and that only an authentic democratic culture and an equally authentic culture of care (both in medicine and in psychology, both clinical sciences) could interrupt.

In this case, the RESM assumes, as an institution, the ambiguous and ambivalent function of the political and social process of which it is an illegitimate child, the exercise of a 'distorted' power not only for the treatment of mental suffering but also for the social control of the deviant, the author of crime with a mental disorder. This is the price that this 'special' residence for equally 'special' service users of the community mental health department, must pay on a daily basis, to represent today the symbolic fulfilment of that political and social process that officially decreed full equality of the health care system for free citizens and for those with restricted freedom.

But this 'gentle' revolution deserves to be translated, in full respect of its democratic ethos, into new practices of care of the social dimension, so that the most heuristic position, but also the most therapeutic to be employed, remains that of accepting the risk until the very end, with confidence in the future and change. The establishment of the RESMs as well as a potential danger for the NHS's public culture, it also represents the potential for all public administration services in Italy and therefore for the transformation of the most authoritative and less democratic legal aspects of society.

This has also a fundamental position in regards to the institution of social danger with which the RESM, together with its service users, operators and stakeholders, finds itself dealing with today. Furthermore, the institute of the community mental health department of which the RESM is a part, finds itself with the chance to radically transform the socio-institutional context that frames the analysis of the social danger of its patients. The RESM will be able to meet the challenge of constructing real alternatives to detention by offering its patients new '*individual, family and social conditions*" otherwise, it will be destined to succumb politically and socially, accepting to perform an exclusively normative function.

So, the culture of enquiry returns as a fundamental therapeutic factor not only for the residential TC represented by the RESM, but also for the whole social community, with its active agencies and those activated by the RESM. This therapeutic factor has as its objective, in accordance with the mandate assigned to it by both democratic institutions and the Italian social and political evolution, the emotional development and affective maturation of its service users, operators and all the stakeholders of a TC, so that they can actively collaborate in the planning of the therapeutic journey of its service users, as well as public services for all citizens.

Meaning of the community meeting in the RESM

An authentic democratic culture may be based on not only the psychotherapeutic organisation that takes place within the RESM, but also the organisation of the work that it is committed to co-constructing together with the other social institutions with which it interacts. Culture of care as a health practice, democratic culture as a practice of cohabitation/social coexistence, and service culture as a practice at the base of the professional choices of all operators involved, can be regarded as the three values that underpin the institutional ethos of the RESM in a democratic state, as constitutionally it is the one that conceived it (Bruschetta, 2018).

The process of the admission and discharge of patients presupposes a complex process, which requires collaboration between two powerful social institutions, that of health and that of justice, altering the theoretical model and the ideal work organisation of a TC conceived as psychotherapeutic setting. However, the culture of the TC can be inspired whenever it is possible to share or delegate decisional power (from administrators to operators to patients), and to apply or stimulate a more informal relational style, thus supporting the sense of belonging, participation, personal responsibility and collective treatment of patients in relation to the community, their choices and behaviours (Bruschetta et al., 2015a, 2015b).

This is only possible if service users and operators share the responsibility of building an emotionally safe, enabling and therapeutic environment for all, by establishing and actively participating in the most important therapeutic tool within the RESM, as for any other TC, a large community group open to all its members (service users, operators and administrators) defined by the tradition of the TC, the *community meeting*.[3] Within this community group, the most important decisions concerning the community are taken, the most burdensome tasks and the most demanding responsibilities are divided and finally, reflections on the most significant events that have occurred are shared. Through this TC group tool, the RESM can tackle the issues that most deeply affect the psychodynamic processes of that transitional space between healthy and juridical instances. That is the foundation of its institution. In this space the elements of an authentic democratic culture can take shape, which concern:

- the equality of rights among service users, even if the perpetrators of crimes that in other prisons would have been assigned to isolation, and in the collaboration of all to resolve conflicts between service users and between service users and operators; and
- justice concerning the correct use of power of the security operators and vigilance towards the patients, and in the use of the countervailing guarantee that the health institution ensures the well-being of its patients.

Within the *community meeting*, it becomes possible:

- for service users to take responsibility for their therapeutic and judicial journey, of which the RESM is only a starting point;
- for administrators, to liaise with all the necessary social and health authorities, in respect and to guarantee the rights of service users; and
- and for the operators, to develop, inside and outside the residential community, networking and work group practices that support the development of a democratic culture (first of all, programmes geared to recovery and employment developed by community mental health departments).

The correct use of *community meeting* remains one of the still problematic factors in RESMs in Italy, due to the difficulties in finding staff who have received training in DTC treatment (Pearce and Haigh, 2017), and management that recognises the value for the health and care issues, on a par with the legal and control ones. Development of community mental health services for users on probation now becomes the new challenge for the Italian NHS.

Conclusions

In conclusion, it is argued that the establishment of the RESM and its placement within the Italian judiciary system has allowed the reinforcement not only of the culture of care as a health practice, but also a democratic culture as a practice of social coexistence at the base of society, advocating values that are able to influence in return the whole health practices methodology in residential communities.

Cohabitation in RESM therapeutic environment, even if conflictual, just like coexistence of the different social instances in the local community that welcomes the RESM, is a democratic processes that can support development of new civilised principles of collaboration between individuals, groups and communities able to relaunch the values of the 'Basaglia' law (Basaglia, 1982) as a basis for mental health in Italy (Bruschetta, 2018), first of all the values of social participation and critique. If this happens, it will depend on the ability of all of us, health and/or judicial operators, to take up this new challenge, and not consider the RESM simply as a new form of the old FPH, but as the dismissal of the asylum institution still present in the folds of the Italian Penal Code and in Italian public society, despite 80 years having passed since the enforcement of the fascist code and 40 years since the passage of the law to close psychiatric hospitals.

From my experience in RESMs, I have understood that it is very important to devote energy and resources so that each new incoming user can develop at least a small sense of belonging to the TC environment and that at the same time each staff member can recognise in him at least one small presence of responsible agency. I learned that belonging and agency are two fundamental clinical aspects that characterise the settings of TCs for the treatment of users with serious mental disorders subjected to security measures. The promotion of a feeling of belonging is methodologically based on peer support, on time spent together informally and on group meetings to deal with emergencies and crises, while the promotion of responsible agency is based on the analysis of the meaning of the own actions, and on the infusion of confidence in the own ability to act, to achieve results and to be responsible for own behaviour.

The greatest difficulties are represented by the sharing, among all staff members and among all stakeholders, of an authentic democratic culture, as well as knowledge of the DTC treatment model.

Notes

1 Other provisions of the legislation instead respected the social function of the NHS and determined that,

the sole lack of individual therapeutic programs does not constitute appropriate evidence in support of the confirmation of social danger.

2 Foucault (1977) analysed the emergence of a 'micro-physics of power' (p.139) while the prison rose alongside other such homologous entities, like factories, schools, hospitals, and army barracks. These 'disciplinary institutions' shared common modes of organisation, intended to mould their members to the societal ends of the emergent capitalist system (Foucault, 1977, p.170). Normalising judgement depended upon a 'penal accountancy' which, following surveillance and examinations, established behavioural 'norms' by punishing divergence (Foucault, 1977, p.180). These common modes instated discipline within bodies, organising the modern penal system around small, seemingly insignificant techniques contrived to coerce behaviour.

3 This group, in my experience, meets regularly and frequently, under the direction of a staff in general made up of people with clinical and administrative responsibility in the RESM and by delegates of practitioners and users (these, democratically elected). This staff differentiates the supervision function of the psychodynamic processes assigned to an internal subgroup coordinated by the psychotherapist, from the functions of managing dialogue and group decisions assigned to a couple consisting of a user and a practitioner.

Bibliography

Basaglia F. (1968), L'istituzione negata, Milano: Baldini Castoldi Dalai.

Basaglia F. (1982), *Scritti II, 1968–1980*. Dall'apertura del manicomio alla nuova legge sull'assistenza psichiatrica, Collana: Paperbacks, Torino: Einaudi.

Bruschetta S. (2018), Il fattore democrazia nei Servizi di Salute Mentale delle società postmoderne. Presupposti Epistemologici e Costrutti Teorici del Progetto Visiting DTC. *Nuova Rassegna Studi Psichiatrici*, Vol 16 No 2. www.nuovarassegnastudipsichiatrici.it/index.php/

Bruschetta, S., and Barone, R. (2015b), Democratic therapeutic community in a network of 'enabling environments': Transformations of psychotherapeutic residential services in social postmodern crisis. *Academic Journal of Interdisciplinary Studies*, Vol 4, No 2 S2, pp.259–63. https://doi.org/10.5901/ajis.2015.v4n2s2p259

Bruschetta, S., Bellia, V., and Barone, R. (2015a), Manifesto per una psicoterapia di comunità. *RivistaPlexus*, Vol 12, pp.33–47. www.rivistaplexus.eu

Corleone, F. (2016), La Rivoluzione Gentile. La Fine degli OPG. Ed il Cambiamento Radicale. In *Fondazione Giovanni Michelucci 'La Nuova Città'*, Serie IX, N. 5, December 2016. Fondazione Michelucci Press.

Foucault, M. (1973–1974/2010), *Il potere psichiatrico. Corso al Collège de France*. Milano: Feltrinelli.

Foucault, M. (1977), *Discipline and punish: The birth of the prison*. London: Penguin.

Haigh, R. (2013), *The quintessence of a therapeutic environment: Five universal qualities*. In *Therapeutic communities past, present and future*, Vol 2. Eds. Campling, P., and Haigh, R. London: Jessica Kingsley.

Jones, M., Baker, A., and Freeman, T. (1952), *Social psychiatry: A study of therapeutic communities*. London: Tavistock.

Lees, J., and Manning, N. (2004), A culture of enquiry: Research evidence and the therapeutic community. *Psychiatric Quarterly*, Vol 75, No 3, 279–94.

Main, T. (1946), The hospital as a therapeutic institution. *Bulletin of the Menninger Clinic*, Vol 10, No 3, 66–70.

Main, T.F. (1989), *The ailment and other psychoanalytic essays*. London: Free Association Press.

Pearce, S., and Haigh, R. (2017), *A Handbook of democratic therapeutic community. Theory and practice*. London: Jessica Kingsley.

Pellissero, M. (2014), Ospedali psichiatrici giudiziari in proroga e prove maldestre di riforma della disciplina delle misure di sicurezza, *Diritto penale e processo*, 2014, 917 ss., 923 (l'evidenziazione grafica è dell'A.).

Rapoport, R. (1960), *Community as doctor*. London: Tavistock.

The therapeutic community in California prisons

A narrative

Rod Mullen and Naya Arbiter

11

Introduction

Therapeutic communities (TCs) in the United States began in 1958 with the establishment of Synanon, although Synanon never referred to itself as a TC. Shortly after Synanon incorporated as a California not-for-profit organization, it made its first attempt to establish an in-prison TC. While that effort failed, years later the New York based Stay'n Out therapeutic community provided the first solid empirical evidence of success in terms of recidivism reduction for an in-prison TC. This research eventually captured the attention of policy makers in California facing a dramatic increase in the prison population primarily driven by the "war on drugs" and increasingly harsh sentences; billions of tax payer dollars were spent on the largest expansion of prisons in US history. In 1990, California's Department of Corrections initiated a pilot TC in one of its state prisons. The documented successful outcomes of that first prison TC inspired the state to fund the largest initiative in the United States using the TC model to reduce the recidivism of criminal offenders. Thirty years later, however, there are no such programs using the TC model in California prisons—what follows is the story of the rise and fall of in-prison therapeutic communities in California.

Ozell Johnson Jr.

A 28-year-old African American man from Los Angeles is sentenced for robbery, sales of narcotics, and murder in 1984. After his conviction he is incarcerated in the Los Angeles County jail. Serving a life sentence, between 1987 and 1990, he is transferred from jail to state prisons, and in 1990 arrives at the R.J. Donovan Correctional Facility, adjacent to San Diego, just a month before an award is made to the Amity Foundation to begin the first prison therapeutic community in the state's history.

DOI: 10.4324/9780429317460-14

Ozell Johnson Jr., is one of the first "lifers"[1] selected by Amity to be a role model to the other 1,000 inmates on the yard of this new medium security prison. He gives the program credibility by demonstrating the tough emotional work needed to transform his life. Ozell works with Amity for 15 years as a peer mentor, becoming one of eight lifers in a program for 200 men. Ozell and his lifer colleagues are responsible for the "buy in" of other inmates, establishing a culture where honesty is respected, racism addressed, and stories shared. Serious incidents are reduced by over 80% compared to other units on the same yard. The use of "lifers," pioneered by Amity, becomes an important element in the recidivism reduction strategies of the Department of Corrections. In 2005, Ozell is transferred from R.J. Donovan and works in other prisons training other lifers how to effect change in prison treatment programs as he did. He is released on December 24, 2014. He was 58 years old and had been incarcerated continuously for 30 years.

Ozell is on parole, normally precluding him from being an employee working for an organization that provides services to other parolees, but the Department of Corrections makes an exception, allowing him to go to work immediately for Amity in Los Angeles. He reunites with the daughter he left when she was a baby and meets his grandchildren for the first time. He continues his career as a counselor and role model at a large campus devoted entirely to men on parole, almost all of whom were getting out of prison and many who had served lengthy sentences. His life begins to expand and grow. In 2018, in a beautiful ceremony, Ozell married his childhood sweetheart with 250 guests from many walks of life. Three of his "best men" are also former inmates with whom he had been incarcerated. Today, Ozell is a senior staff member at the first program in the United States for men who are being released from prison after serving 30 years or more.[2]

Early days

The first programs are born

The two persons most identified with the development of the TC method are Maxwell Jones and Charles "Chuck" Dederich. Jones' contribution began in the late 1940s, just after World War II, as he developed a methodology for treatment of neurotic soldiers in English hospitals that became known as the democratic therapeutic community. The approach reformed the hierarchical structure of hospitals, emphasizing shared leadership and social learning as well as open communication between doctors, nurses, and patients. In 1959, Jones came to the United States, accepting an invitation from Stanford University to be a visiting professor. In the early 1960s he was invited to be a consultant for the California Department of Corrections, where he shared his ideas about how the democratic TC could be incorporated into prison programs (Vandevelde, Broekaert, Yates, & Kooyman, 2004).

By the time Jones was working as a consultant, Synanon had come to national attention in part to a *LIFE magazine* profile (Life magazine, 1962). Many other stories appeared in the media, including testimony of Dederich and others from Synanon in front of Senator Thomas Dodd's committee on juvenile delinquency.[3] This was a time of social disruption in the United States: the war in Vietnam raged; civil rights protests filled newspapers and television screens; and the United States found itself also in the middle of a heroin crisis. Medical and other solutions had failed in dealing with drugs, so Synanon's apparent success stood out.

In 1961, Synanon began a pilot program at the Terminal Island Correctional Facility—a federal prison located just off the coast of Los Angeles. The program involved weekly visits by Synanon residents—ex-addicts and ex-inmates themselves—who engaged inmates in the Synanon "game" or encounter group. The project ran successfully for two years, but it was eventually terminated by institutional administrators who objected to Synanon's request to solidify and intensify the program by having the group of inmates involved housed together (Yablonsky, 1962; Clark, 2017).[4] Although Maxwell Jones and Charles Dederich were in close geographical proximity, and both interested in correctional policy, they met only once. Briggs reports that meeting fell apart when Jones criticized Dederich for his "autocratic approach"[5] (Briggs, 1963).

While the Terminal Island program failed, Synanon was invited to initiate a much larger project at the Nevada State Penitentiary in Reno in 1962. This project, which lasted for four years, was much larger. Inmates were housed together and Synanon was able to demonstrate not only successful recidivism reduction upon release but also significant improvements in inmate behaviors while incarcerated. This won the approval of the warden and correctional officers who were primarily concerned about institutional violence. This project can be characterized as the first fully developed and implemented prison TC in the United States. Unfortunately, a newly elected governor with a sharply conservative philosophy, terminated the Synanon project (Clark, 2017; Yablonsky, 1989).

In the early 1970s, Synanon made a final attempt to initiate a program for incarcerated men at the San Bruno jail in San Francisco. Like the Terminal Island project, this involved senior Synanon residents doing encounter groups at the jail. But, mirroring Terminal Island, jail administrators objected to

Synanon's suggestions for intensifying the program and Synanon eventually withdrew.[6] Although Synanon clashed with the California Department of Corrections[7] and was unsuccessful in developing any in-prison or community-based programs with them, individual parole officers who respected Synanon placed many men and women there throughout the 1960s and 1970s.

California Rehabilitation Center (CRC)

In 1963, as part of Maxwell Jones' consultancy to the California Department of Corrections, he had the opportunity to train correctional officers in his democratic TC methodology for several years (Vandevelde, Broekaert, Yates, & Kooyman, 2004). The largest state prison poject Jones worked on was the California Rehabilitation Center. The reviews on CRC's programs were mixed— many correctional officers considered the program a scam where inmates conned gullible correctional officers who staffed the program (Warden John Ratelle, personal communication, 1995). There were many problematic incidents, and even a murder in the prison, which damaged its credibility among officers and administrators as an effective approach. It was gradually weakened and abandoned as a failed experiment. However, Douglas Anglin, who was involved in the evaluation of CRC from its beginning, did a 25-year follow-up study that showed modest but positive outcomes. (Hser, Anglin, & Powers, 1993). CRC was best known for the implementation of the California Civil Addict Program (CAP)[8] that gave addicts an indeterminate non-felony sentence. The contribution of Jones was largely obscured, and CRC was not characterized as a TC.

"Nothing works"

The social turbulence of the 1960s and 1970s precipitated a social and political backlash. The Republican Party parlayed the turbulence and rise in crime rates to develop a "law and order" message, which was successful in displacing the Democratic Party in the Southern states and in promulgating state and national "tough on crime" policies. The new laws instituted by both parties paved the way for mass incarceration, an issue with which the United States is only now beginning to reckon (Alexander & West, 2012).

Robert Martinson's seminal 1974 article (Martinson, 1974), which stated that there were no measurable reductions in recidivism in the current correctional programs, was widely cited to support the swing to a much more punitive approach nationally, and the closure of all prison TCs (Cullen & Gilbert, 1982). California, which had been considered a leader in correctional reform in the 1960s, passed more than 1,000 severely punitive laws in the next decade, and closed most of its programs for inmates (Werth & Sumner, 2006). The hysteria over violent crime reached its apogee with the passage of California's "three strikes" law, giving any offender with three felonies, with at least one of them violent, a mandatory sentence of 25 years to life. It was proclaimed a panacea for violent crime, although many of those sentenced under that law were actually convicted of nonviolent crimes, including drug possession (Vitiello, 2002; American Bar Association, "Three Strikes Laws: A Real or Imagined Deterrent to Crime?", 2017)

California's first prison TC

Richard J. Donovan Amity Project

The 1980s saw California engage in a massive, multibillion-dollar prison expansion with 21 new prisons built in the state. But due to the harsh laws that had been passed, the prison population was growing so rapidly that even these prisons were overcrowded.[9] James "Jim" Rowland, the newly appointed director of corrections, said that California was "building prisons like there is no tomorrow, filling them with drug addicts, and we don't have a clue as to what to do with them" (Mullen, Ratelle, Abraham, & Boyle, 1996). Rowland was made aware of the success of the Stay'n Out program in New York, and decided to initiate a pilot project in one prison in California, with the intent of developing a successful model which could be expanded to other California prisons.

After nearly 30 years since Synanon's attempt to introduce a prison TC at Terminal Island, the first real in-prison therapeutic community in California began in 1990. This program involved 200 Level III[10] inmate volunteers housed together in the Richard J. Donovan Correctional Facility (RJD) near San Diego, a prison with a population of 4,600 inmates. This is where "lifer" inmate Ozell Johnson Jr. began his journey. Over 75% of the inmates in the Amity/R.J. Donovan TC had committed crimes of violence, in addition to drug use, drug trafficking, and drug-related crimes. Many of the inmates had histories of street gang involvement, and some had been affiliated with prison gangs.

Simultaneously, the National Institute on Drug Abuse had funded the Center for Therapeutic Community Research, headed by Dr. George De Leon. As part of the Center's portfolio, prominent criminal justice researcher Dr. Harry Wexler, initiated a five-year random design study of the Amity/ R.J. Donovan project—this proved critical in establishing the credibility of the outcomes (Wexler et al., 1999; Little Hoover Commission, 1998; Mullen, Ratelle, Abraham, & Boyle, 1996).

Critical elements of the Amity/R.J. Donovan TC were:

- It used staff consisting mostly of ex-addicts and ex-offenders trained extensively by Amity. (This was a break from prior California corrections programs that used mostly uniformed correctional officers.)
- It targeted a population characterized as being both unwilling to participate in treatment and unable to make significant changes in their well-established criminal lifestyles.[11]
- It pioneered a "joint-venture" approach with cooperative and collaborative relationships between corrections personnel and treatment personnel, including quarterly cross-trainings to maintain alignment.
- It paroled all inmates who completed the program immediately, with one-third paroling to a community-based program operated by the same treatment provider using the same philosophy, staff, curriculum, and practices.
- It implemented a TC curriculum incorporating both cognitive and behavioral elements that reflected the issues of this population of drug-involved violent offenders.
- It utilized "lifers," trained by Amity, convicted of violent crimes and serving life sentences, as mentors in the TC to enhance and maintain credibility and "buy-in" within the inmate population.

Outcomes

Successful drops in recidivism and violence

Wexler's research (Wexler, De Leon, Thomas, Kressel, & Peters, 1999) outcomes show a dramatic reduction in recidivism three years post-treatment for inmates who completed both phases of the program, contradicting the Rand study and the "nothing works" assertion, see Figure 11.1 "Three-year incarceration rates" below.

This was both unexpected and statistically significant. It had a major influence on changing the perception of treatment programs within the criminal justice system in California—and later in many other states. A secondary study was conducted on the institutional benefits of the TC. It showed an 87% drop in serious disciplinary incidents with the men in the Amity TC over six months compared to the general population (Deitch et al., 1998). This correlated with a reduction in sick leave by officers, an improvement in morale, and a significant reduction in both personnel costs to the institutions, and costs of medical care of inmates involved in violent incidents.

Three Year Reincarceration Rate

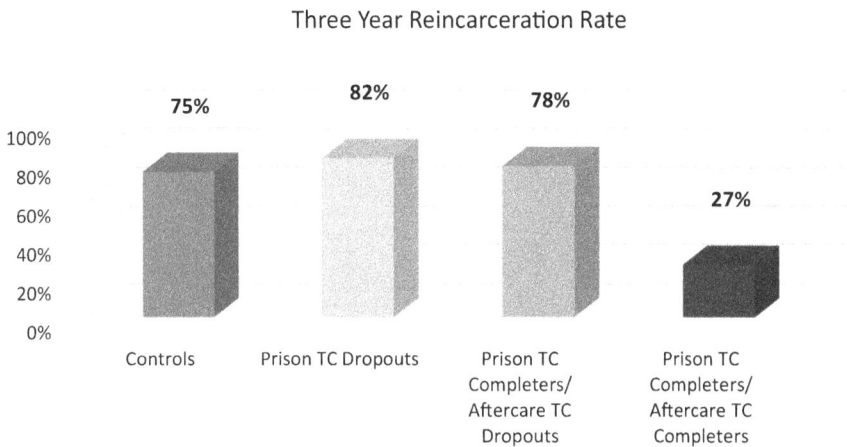

Wexler, H.K., Lowe, L., Melnick, G., and Peters, J. (1999)
Three-year reincarceration outcomes for Amity in-prison therapeutic
community and aftercare in California. *The Prison Journal, 79*(3), 321-336.

Figure 11.1 Three-year incarceration rates.

Expansion

The recidivism reduction results of the RJD/Amity TC came to the attention of policy makers in Sacramento at a crucial time (Little Hoover Commission, 1994). Predictions of continued increases in the prison population and projections by analysts of the need to build more prisons precipitated keen interest by legislators for implementation and replication of in-prison TCs as an important part of several proposed solutions to reduce the overcrowding of prisons. A year after the Amity/RJD TC was initiated, a TC was established in a women's prison, and then another for men at CRC. In 1993, the state legislature approved construction of the California Substance Abuse Treatment Facility at Corcoran (SATF), a rural community in central California and on the same site as an existing prison serving Level IV inmates.[12] A design charrette was held in 1994, which was instrumental in constructing a prison specifically for the TC treatment of 1,478 inmates simultaneously. The facility opened in 1997 and was the beginning of a very rapid expansion of both in-prison programs and community-based aftercare programs and administration. See Figure 11.2 which shows the dramatic growth of in-prison TCs in California.

In 1998, a seminal report was issued by the Little Hoover Commission, an independent, highly respected California state oversight agency that provides

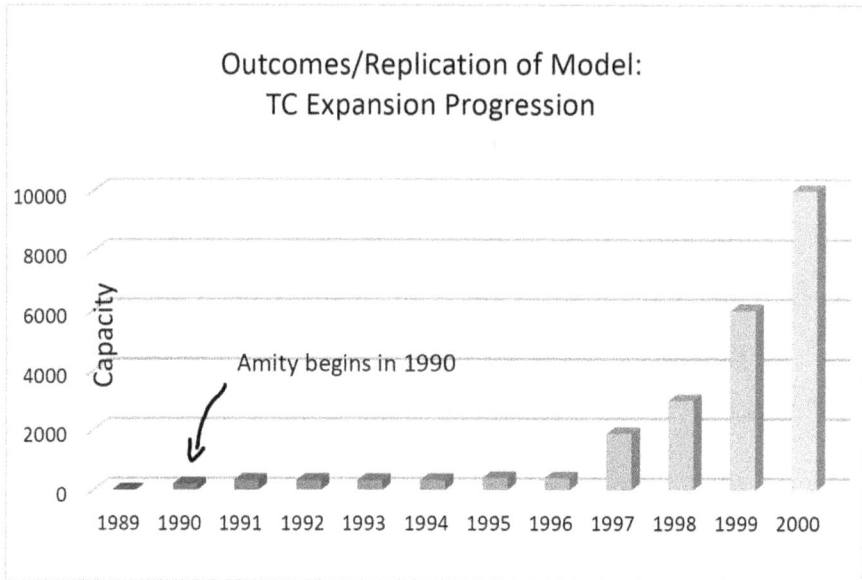

Figure 11.2 Dramatic growth of in-prison TCs in California.

reports, recommendations, and legislative proposals and investigates state government. This report specifically recommended the expansion of TC programs[13] stating, "The Legislative Analyst's Office estimated that extending treatment to serve an additional 10,000 inmates over those served today [using the Amity model] would increase savings to $80 million in annual operating costs and $210 million in one-time capital outlay" (Little Hoover Commission, 1998).[14]

Scaling up

The Office of Substance Abuse Programs (OSAP), established in 1988, was a suborganization within the CDC to develop, monitor, train, and evaluate the department's treatment programs. The OSAP staff developed a request for proposal (RFP) process for bidders who were competing to provide services. This process specifically required a TC program with a large portion of the bid devoted to the contractor's detailed proposal of how the "Eight Essential Elements" of the TC, developed by De Leon, would be implemented. But due to the legislative demand for rapid expansion of prison TCs, OSAP was quickly overwhelmed.

CDC's flagship program, the Substance Abuse Treatment Facility (SATF), with its dedicated design and large number of inmates, was the first to fall prey to some of the problems of expansion. In 1996, the SATF was the first program that used a "low bid" RFP process for determining successful bidders, something that has continued for the past two decades. While the maximum amount allowed in the bid was not generous, the two successful bidders, anxious to win the contracts, underbid significantly. As then-CDC director Jim Gomez noted later, this was a significant error, as it resulted in significant reductions in compensation for the contractor's employees, and reductions in training budgets (Gomez, personal communication, 1996).

At SATF, problems were exacerbated by being in a remote, rural location. The city of Corcoran at the time of the SAFT's opening had a population of 14,000, mostly involved in agriculture. There was virtually no qualified labor pool. So, in addition to very low wages offered, there were few qualified persons and little incentive for the appropriate diverse workforce from a more urban area to relocate. An evaluation revealed that inmates at SATF did no better than a matched sample of general population inmates who received no treatment (Office of the Inspector General, 2007). A later evaluation of the program revealed the following:

- Poor training for treatment staff
- Very high staff turnover
- Conflicts and lack of coordination between treatment and custody staff
- A program curriculum that was repetitive and dull
- Overcrowded sessions that countered a therapeutic community culture
- A disinterested group of participants who were mandated to participate[15]
- Low participation rates in residential and nonresidential aftercare
                      (Anglin, Prendergast, Farabee, & Cartier, 2002).

CDC supplemented the budgets at the SATF and provided technical assistance, but the results remained disappointing and became a major finding in a 2007 inspector general's negative report about the failure of treatment programs.

Community-based aftercare issues

By 1999, three major outcome studies of in-prison TCs, all funded by the National Institute on Drug Abuse, had been published. All showed that the greatest drop in recidivism was achieved when inmates leaving prison were enrolled in community-based services prior to reentry into the larger community (see Figure 11.3 "Evaluations of in-prison TCs").

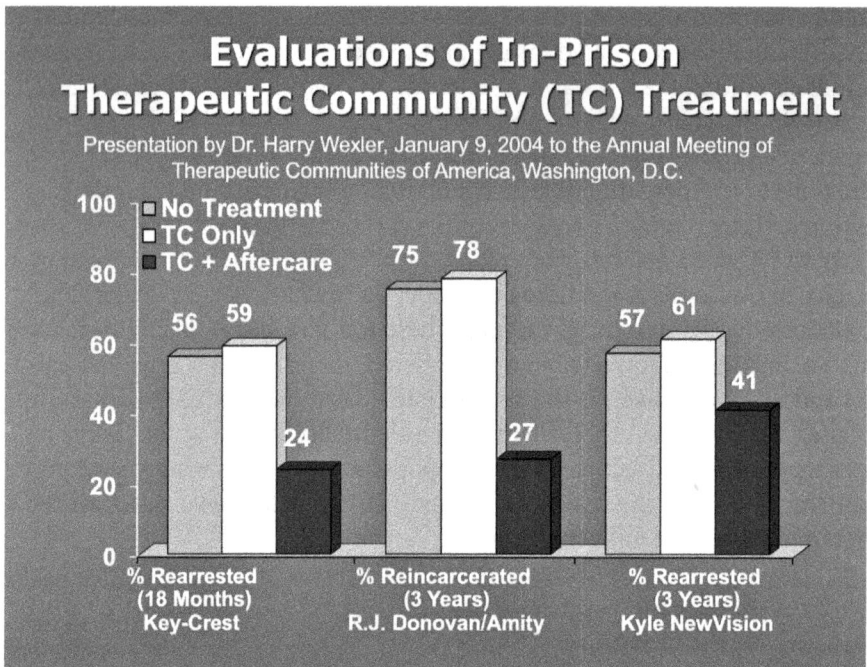

Figure 11.3 Evaluations of in-prison TCs.

Despite this compelling evidence, the development and funding of community-based services for inmates paroling from in-prison TCs never exceeded more than 50%). And for those who completed an in-prison TC, but did not participate in community-based services, at year post-release their recidivism was no better than general population inmates who received no treatment at all (Wexler et al., 1999).

TC treatment under fire

In the early 2000s, the word used most often to characterize the California Department of Corrections by media, legislators, and those within the department itself was "crisis." This was due largely to the continued overcrowding of prisons, multiple court actions against the CDC, opposition by the powerful correctional officers union, large budget overruns, and general political turbulence. In 2005, a new secretary was appointed.[16] He had a reform agenda but resigned a year later in frustration over the governor's lack of support, the increasing prison populations and overcrowding, the myriad of legal cases, and very concentrated opposition by the powerful correctional officers union.

Despite these multiple issues, up to this point, the TC prison programs along with community-based aftercare had enjoyed a collaborative working relationship with the CDC.

The first major change in the relationship with the California Department of Corrections came in the spring of 2005 when a state senator chaired a series of hearings over two years on waste in government programs. While the hearings covered a variety of issues, the spotlight was on the contractors providing TC treatment for state prisoners both in prison and in the community. The contractors were characterized in both the hearings and the press as inefficient, wasteful, and willfully squandering taxpayers' dollars (Select Committee on Government Cost Control, 2005).

The second event was a comprehensive audit of all of the contractors, with the intent of verifying the charges levied in the hearings. The audit was unusual in that expenditures previously approved by legitimate authorities were not only questioned but considered fraudulent. Many contractors were involved in prolonged legal proceedings, which concluded with some having to make reparations of hundreds of thousands of dollars to the state of California.

The third event was a 2007 report by the Inspector General which stated that "numerous studies show that despite an annual cost of $36 million, the Department of Corrections and Rehabilitation's in-prison substance abuse treatment programs have little or no impact on recidivism." The report characterized the cumulative dollars spent by the California Department of Corrections and Rehabilitation (CDCR, formerly CDC) on substance abuse programs for inmates and parolees as a

> billion dollar failure—a failure to provide an environment that would allow the programs to work; failure to provide an effective treatment model; failure to ensure that the best contractors are chosen to do the job at the lowest possible price; failure to oversee the contractors to make sure they provide the services they agree to provide; failure to exert the fiscal controls necessary to protect public funds; failure to learn from and correct mistakes—and most tragically, failure to help California inmates change their lives and, in so doing, make our streets safer.
>
> (Office of the Inspector General, 2007)

In response, the governor reorganized the California Department of Corrections and Rehabilitation and named a new head of its Division of Addiction and Recovery Services. The first decade and a half of this initiative to provide treatment to inmates and reduce recidivism had been characterized by a largely successful collaboration between the nonprofit treatment providers and the staff of CDCR, but by 2007 the attacks on the providers caused a breach in that relationship that continued for another decade.

End of the TC approach in prison

While the "billion-dollar mistake" became the headline of news stories throughout the state, a crucial fact was ignored. The CDCR's own data demonstrated that the programs that followed the model pioneered at the Amity/R.J. Donovan TC, where in-prison TC treatment was followed by continuing aftercare in the community, *did* produce a significant reduction in recidivism; see Figure 11.4 showing the results of the Department of Corrections own evaluation of the "Prison SAP" programs, which were based on the TC model.

Despite the myriad of problems in scaling-up this huge initiative, the recidivism rate decreased from approximately 40% in the non-treatment group to approximately 22% in the treatment group. Many of the findings of the inspector general's report were valid—but the "billion-dollar mistake"

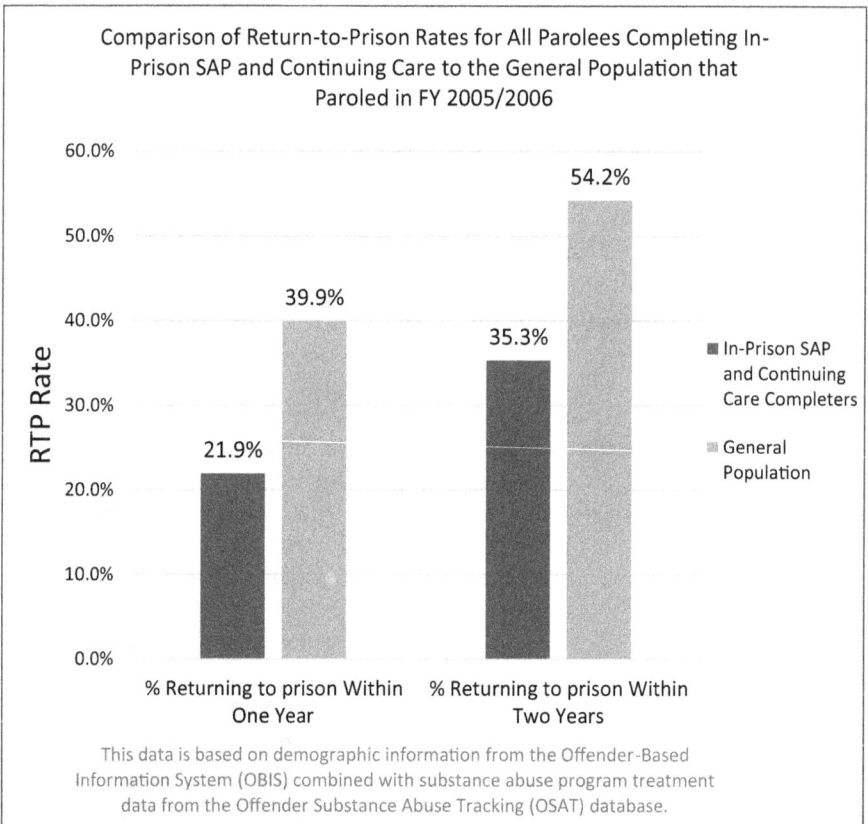

Figure 11.4 showing "Comparison of Return-to-Prison Rates for All Parolees Completing In-Prison SAP and Continuing Care to the General Population that Paroled in FY 2005/2006". RTP Rate values: % Returning to prison Within One Year — In-Prison SAP and Continuing Care Completers 21.9%, General Population 39.9%; % Returning to prison Within Two Years — In-Prison SAP and Continuing Care Completers 35.3%, General Population 54.2%. This data is based on demographic information from the Offender-Based Information System (OBIS) combined with substance abuse program treatment data from the Offender Substance Abuse Tracking (OSAT) database.

Figure 11.4 Results of Department of Corrections' own evaluation of "Prison SAP" programs, which were based on TC model.

headline completely obscured the success of those programs that had adhered faithfully to the TC model.

Given that the initiative had been declared a failure, CDCR initiated the Expert Panel on Adult Offender and Recidivism Reduction Programming. While this was a distinguished group of individuals both from academic institutions and those with significant correctional experience, it excluded any of the experienced practitioners or researchers who were knowledgeable about the TC, and particularly those who had intimate knowledge of the success of many of the in-prison TCs in California. This panel was responsible for the development of the California Logic Model, which focused on identifying the criminogenic needs of inmates and providing individualized treatment based on those needs (California Department of Corrections and Rehabilitation, 2007). See Figure 11.5, which is a summary of the criminogenic needs identified by the Expert Panel.

The report of the panel of experts resulted in the CDCR adopting a cognitive behavioral therapy model, which emphasized a classroom approach, in stark contrast to the "immersion" TC model, which combined both cognitive and behavioral elements in a holistic approach in which peer accountability was a key factor (California Department of Corrections and Rehabilitation, 2007).

The international financial crisis of 2008 caused major financial issues for California, as tax revenues decreased. State government required major reductions in spending throughout—but long-standing legal mandates prevented the California Department of Corrections from cutting costs in state correctional institutions. However, contractors providing services to inmates were not protected, and as a result all in-prison treatment programs

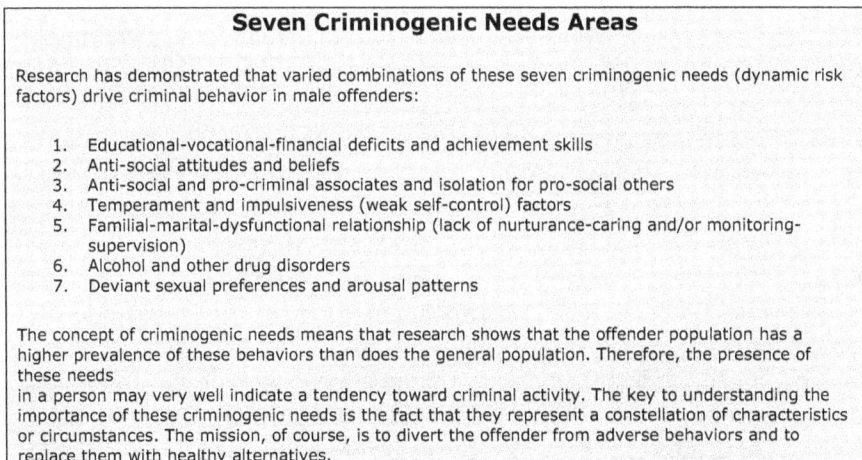

Seven Criminogenic Needs Areas

Research has demonstrated that varied combinations of these seven criminogenic needs (dynamic risk factors) drive criminal behavior in male offenders:

1. Educational-vocational-financial deficits and achievement skills
2. Anti-social attitudes and beliefs
3. Anti-social and pro-criminal associates and isolation for pro-social others
4. Temperament and impulsiveness (weak self-control) factors
5. Familial-marital-dysfunctional relationship (lack of nurturance-caring and/or monitoring-supervision)
6. Alcohol and other drug disorders
7. Deviant sexual preferences and arousal patterns

The concept of criminogenic needs means that research shows that the offender population has a higher prevalence of these behaviors than does the general population. Therefore, the presence of these needs
in a person may very well indicate a tendency toward criminal activity. The key to understanding the importance of these criminogenic needs is the fact that they represent a constellation of characteristics or circumstances. The mission, of course, is to divert the offender from adverse behaviors and to replace them with healthy alternatives.

Figure 11.5 Summary of criminogenic needs identified by Expert Panel.

were closed in October 2009. While implementation of the California Logic Model had significantly weakened the TC approach, the closing of programs in 2009 was the real end of TC treatment in state prisons.[17] In 2010, a few small prison programs were initiated using the CBT curriculums prescribed by the California Logic Model.

Realignment in California

For many years California unsuccessfully wrestled with its prison overcrowding issue without success. On May 23, 2011, matters came to a head when the US Supreme Court ruled that California needed to reduce its overcrowded prisons from its then 185%–200% of design capacity to 137.5% of capacity—a reduction of more than 50,000 inmates (*Brown v. Plata*, 2011). Later that year, the state legislature passed two important bills. Under these new laws, low-level, nonviolent offenders would be housed in county jails rather than state prisons. And, upon release, many would be on county probation rather than state parole supervision. Within 15 months, 24,000 offenders who would have gone to CDCR prior to realignment were incarcerated in county jails, and the parole population dropped significantly (Owen & Mobley, 2012). As intended, this did two things: first, it significantly reduced the state prison population, and second, it concentrated the most serious and violent population of inmates in state prisons.

California progression

In the past few years, California's citizens and legislators have increasingly supported liberalizing criminal justice reforms. In 2014, a ballot measure, Proposition 47, was passed. It was known as the Safe Neighborhoods and Schools Act. This new law converted many nonviolent offenses (particularly drug and property offenses) from felonies to misdemeanors, and allowed those presently convicted to petition to have their felony convictions retroactively reduced. California's infamous "three strikes" law was amended as well with Proposition 36, enabling an estimated 3,000 offenders to petition for release, and allowing many new offenders to avoid the 25 years-to-life sentences imposed by that law. Additionally, Proposition 64, which legalized marijuana, aided in decreasing prison populations since illegal possession was the cause of many strict sentences in years prior. Finally, Proposition 57, the last of Governor Jerry Brown's reforms before he stepped down, allowed inmates to earn more "good time" credits for participating in programs and also allowed people convicted of nonviolent crimes to go before the parole board,

Recent Policy Changes Impacting the Inmate Population

In recent years, the Legislature and voters enacted various constitutional and statutory changes that significantly impacted the composition of the state's inmate population. Some of the major changes include:

- 2011 Realignment. The 2011 Realignment limited who could be sent to state prison. Specifically, it required that certain lower-level offenders serve their incarceration terms in county jail. Additionally, it required that counties, rather than the state, supervise certain lower-level offenders released from state prison.
- Proposition 36 (2012). Proposition 36 reduced prison sentences for certain offenders subject to the state's existing three-strikes law whose most recent offenses were nonserious, nonviolent felonies. It also allowed certain offenders serving life sentences to apply for reduced sentences.
- Proposition 47 (2014). Proposition 47 reduced penalties for certain offenders convicted of nonserious and nonviolent property and drug crimes from felonies to misdemeanors. It also allowed certain offenders who had been previously convicted of such crimes to apply for reduced sentences.
- Proposition 57 (2016). Proposition 57 expanded inmate eligibility for parole consideration, increased the state's authority to reduce inmates' sentences due to good behavior and/or the completion of rehabilitation programs, and mandated that judges determine whether youth be subject to adult sentences in criminal court.

Figure 11.6 Summary of several major changes in California law regarding criminal offenders.

requesting mitigation, before serving their entire sentence. See Figure 11.6 which summarizes several major changes in California law regarding criminal offenders.

And regression

As California's revenues rebounded from the dark days of the financial collapse, an expansive implementation of CDCR's recidivism reduction programs occurred, including vocational training, education, and cognitive behavioral therapy. In 2017, the Legislative Analyst's Office wrote a report evaluating the effectiveness of CDCR's efforts. The report cited three principles that they identified as the mainstays for successful recidivism reduction programs. First, programs need to be based on evidence-based treatment models; second, they need to be cost effective; and finally, treatment should be focused on the inmates that are the highest risk to recidivate and cause harm in the community. The report found CDCR failing in all three areas (Legislative Analyst's Office, 2017). During the same period, one contractor wrote a memo to the secretary of corrections, which stated:

It is time for CDCR to really examine the model of treatment adopted after the Inspector General's "Billion Dollar Mistake" report in 2007. The model which is currently being used began poorly and continues to drift swiftly from the "best practices" that have been identified here in California and around the country. There have been no evaluations of the current programs—if there were, they would be found to be ineffective.

(Mullen, June 26, 2017)

In January 2019, the California state auditor issued a report to the legislature stating, "inmates who completed in-prison cognitive behavioral programs (CBT) recidivated at about the same rate as inmates who did not complete the programs." This is a significant finding for CDCR, the governor, and the legislature—all of whom supported and encouraged the often-hasty expansion of these types of programs into all of California's 36 prisons without evaluating effectiveness early on.

A crossroads

The 2019 state auditor's report pointed out many of the same findings as in the inspector general's 2007 report regarding CDCR's failure in implementing and supporting programs. However, the report is significantly flawed. It makes the erroneous assumption that if CDCR implemented its current CBT programs correctly, there would be a major drop in recidivism. This is incorrect for several reasons. First, a National Institute of Justice report states, "there is good evidence that CBT, in the controlled setting of a prison therapeutic community, can reduce the risk of reoffending" (National Institute of Justice, 2016). Essentially, that is a definition of the TC programs that CDCR has jettisoned. Second, the "evidence-based" curricula[18] that are available, and which CDCR is mandating, were not designed for violent felons, which is the population that CDCR now has after the realignment. The report also ignores the fact that no matter how well a prison program is delivered, recidivism will not be significantly affected unless it is followed by a continuation of aftercare services in the community, also a fundamental weakness in CDCR's present programs. Finally, the report completely ignores what prior programs accomplished regarding substantially reducing the recidivism of violent offenders (Wexler, Burdon & Prendergast, 2005). Despite the evidence that the CBT curricula were not effective, the California legislature interpreted the state auditor's report to mean that the California Department of Corrections and Rehabilitation had failed by not being assertive enough that the CBT curriculums being used were evidence based according to the US Department of Justice website (CrimeSolutions.gov). So instead of examining the failure of these programs, CDCR was instructed to "double down" on them in the expansion of addiction treatment programs in every institution.

Discussion

In 1995, the Department of Corrections bid out the first treatment program in a Level IV prison, the California State Prison, Los Angeles County, located in Lancaster. The 200 men in this TC program were quite different from those in the many other TC treatment programs in the state. They were younger, mostly minority, with longer sentences, less legal employment pre-incarceration, more opioid addiction but less overall addiction. Their criminal careers began much younger than other inmates, and they had many more suicide attempts, many more arrests, and more violent felony convictions. An evaluation of the program found surprising results: this extraordinarily challenging population were as successful in reducing their recidivism as lower-level inmates *as long as they* completed at least 90 days of community-based aftercare (Wexler, Burdon, & Prendergast, 2005). When inmates with multiple convictions for violent felonies return to prison, they typically are arrested and convicted for another violent crime. Unsurprisingly, they are at much greater risk for violence both in prison and in the community when they are released, compared to other lower-level inmates. The significance of this finding, identified at both the R.J. Donovan and CSP Los Angeles TCs, was that these programs could be accurately characterized as violence reduction programs. This is exactly what CDCR needs with its current inmate population of violent offenders serving long sentences.

A mile wide and an inch deep

The current CBT programs[19] contradict many of the findings from evaluations of successful programs:

- Inmates are not housed together.
- There are no services in the housing unit.
- The program is classroom style.
- It does not involve the inmates in taking responsibility for themselves or each other.
- People are often released back into the general population and not sent directly into community-based aftercare upon program completion.

This situation is further exacerbated by the realignment, with a significant proportion of those released from state prison not paroled through the state, where they might receive effective aftercare. Instead they are sent to 56 independent counties that deliver aftercare (or not) in no regulated or coherent manner. One of the failures of realignment was no accountability for the counties, which received millions of dollars, to provide effective community-based services for those released from state prisons. Also, Proposition 57 gives "good time" to inmates who participate in programs, helping to keep the population under the Supreme Court mandated limit. But the unintended consequence in many cases was "watered down" programs that have little or no ability to reduce recidivism.

Quality over quantity

There are many ways to evaluate an effective program for hard-core offenders, but one shortcut might be D + I + F = RR (Duration + Intensity + Fidelity = Recidivism Reduction). See Figure 11.7 which diagrams out this relationship.

Short, non-intensive programs delivered poorly are not going to get the job done. There are many studies demonstrating the effectiveness of TCs working with correctional populations, particularly with the populations that have the most difficulty when in other modalities, even if they are considered "evidence based." (Aslan, 2018; Wexler & Prendergast, 2010; Martin, O'Connell, Paternoster, & Bachman, 2011). Effective TCs, however, are not the kinds of programs that can be scaled-up rapidly. They require a substantial investment in workforce development; a bid process with a focus on quality and results; fidelity to the model, which has proven to be effective; and a massive investment in developing community-based aftercare facilities available for all who complete the in-prison program component. This challenge creates a logical rationale for CDCR to reconsider its current programs in every prison. Most of the current CBT programs could be delivered through tablets used by inmates, which is committment to have common in correctional programs. For intensive, immersion TC type programs, it would make more sense to have several large treatment prisons in or near urban centers where there is total support and buy-in for the treatment program from the warden, to the sergeant, to the inmates themselves. This also avoids the staffing problems inherent since the majority of prisons are located in remote rural areas where attracting and retaining compent staff is near impossible.

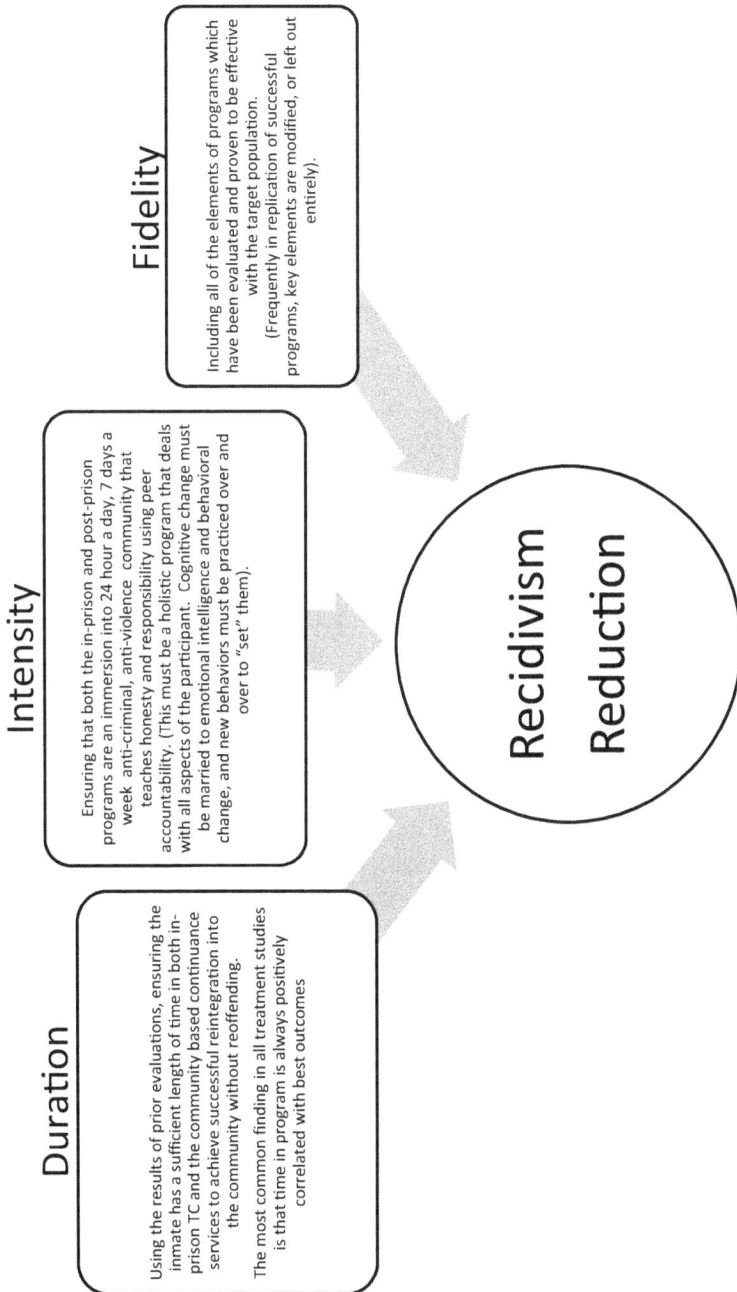

Figure 11.7 Critical elements for recidivism reduction.

Fidelity

Including all of the elements of programs which have been evaluated and proven to be effective with the target population. (Frequently in replication of successful programs, key elements are modified, or left out entirely).

Intensity

Ensuring that both the in-prison and post-prison programs are an immersion into 24 hour a day, 7 days a week anti-criminal, anti-violence community that teaches honesty and responsibility using peer accountability. (This must be a holistic program that deals with all aspects of the participant. Cognitive change must be married to emotional intelligence and behavioral change, and new behaviors must be practiced over and over to "set" them).

Duration

Using the results of prior evaluations, ensuring the inmate has a sufficient length of time in both in-prison TC and the community based continuance services to achieve successful reintegration into the community without reoffending.

The most common finding in all treatment studies is that time in program is always positively correlated with best outcomes

Recidivism Reduction

Pay for Success

In reviewing the history of prison TCs in California, it becomes clear that those that substantially reduced recidivism are the ones that were given appropriate support and displayed fidelity to the essential components of the model. The ones that failed were largely a result of political factors that ignored the actual compromised the program; had poor implementation by the contractor; or received a lack of support by the institutional staff. How could this be addressed in the future? Pay for Success (PFS) is a funding approach to contracting. It ties payment for service delivery to the achievement of measurable outcomes. If applied to correctional TCs, that would be a specific recidivism reduction target. The government (or private funder) is assured that they do not have to pay for the services if the agreed-upon outcomes are not achieved. The contractor signs on to a high-fidelity approach with confidence because the payer must provide the support and the critical elements needed for success. A credible independent evaluator determines if the results have been achieved (Hawkins, McClure, & Paddock, 2017). This type of performance-based contracting is a "win-win-win-win"[20] if implemented properly, with the ultimate "winner" being the man or woman paroled and the concentric circles of success around him or her.[21]

Conclusion

While correctional policies and practices are often argued from the "30,000 foot level" in either abstract or financial terms, it is important to remember that these inmates are people who hit the lottery of bad breaks. They are generally from dysfunctional families embedded in crime-ridden neighborhoods. They are disproportionally black or brown and as such victims of systemic racial discrimination and bias. They have had few educational opportunities or job prospects while combating other factors such as homelessness, racism, sexism, addiction, and poverty. Not very long ago the conventional wisdom was that they were incapable of changing their lives and rejoining society as responsible citizens, part of a societal self-fulfilling narrative.

Fortunately, the last six decades has proven that within a TC that is faithful to the model now well established by decades of research and evaluation, change is not only possible but probable. Many of these men and women are able and willing to do the hard personal work to break out of the shackles of their prior experience. They are willing to take risks and assume responsibilities in order to achieve lives that are productive and honorable. They become productive workers, responsible parents, taxpayers, and contributors to the social fabric of their communities. But since men make up the bulk of prisoners, frequently the women inmates are ignored—a mistake. Since they are the primary caregivers, providing help to women often reaps the greatest public benefits, as the woman who is successful is most often the person who has the greatest effect on preventing children from being the next generation of societal failures, and inmates. And a small, but critical segment of the inmates, like Ozell, become the most effective catalysts for change as they are willing to commit the rest of their lives to helping others as they were helped.

Notes

1 "Lifers" are inmates serving a life sentence, some with and some without the possibility of parole. Until recently, time served averaged in excess of 25 years.

2 A sad note is that Ozell contracted Covid-19 in the summer of 2020. Although he recovered from the infection, he died in September 2020 from a massive heart attack. Since he had an underlying coronary condition, it is likely that the aftermath of the virus was responsible for his untimely death.

3 "Mr. President, there is indeed a miracle on the beach of Santa Monica, a man-made miracle that I feel can benefit thousands of drug addicts." Excerpt from Senator Dodd's speech on the floor of the US Senate, September 6, 1962.

4 James "Jimmy" Middleton, Synanon resident and formerly incarcerated at Terminal Island and other prisons, wrote, "It is conceivable to me as an ex-inmate myself that someday Synanon could become an established part of the prison program throughout the United States." His statement was prescient, but it would be Synanon's offspring that would spread the TC in prisons.

5 Dederich had been a minor executive with Gulf Oil and brought some of the hierarchical structure of the corporate world to Synanon, along with the more democratic approach of Alcoholics Anonymous.

6 Naya Arbiter worked in the Synanon research department and reported this information.

7 At one point, Dederich had signs posted in Synanon's Santa Monica facility explicitly stating that no member of the CDC was allowed on Synanon's properties. Some of the various conflicts are detailed in Clark's 2017 *Recovery Revolution*.

8 This program entailed a seven-year court commitment to treatment for primarily heroin addicts that included an intensive and lengthy initial confined period (providing drug treatment, job training, and educational advancement) with transition services and further treatment on release to the community for a lengthy parole period. Detected relapse to drug use resulted in a return to confinement, typically for short periods, and re-release with enhanced services and monitoring.

9 The inmate population in California state prisons increased from 23,000 in 1980 to 154,000 in 1997, with over 60% of parolees returning to prison within three years.

10 California has a point system for classifying prisoners based on their risk to harm others within the prison, and their risk for harm in the community upon release. Levels 1 and 2 are low security, often housing inmates in dormitory settings; Level III is medium security with inmates (who may have committed violent crimes) housed in two-person cells; Level IV are inmates who pose the greatest threat and are housed in high-security institutions, and often in single cells with little time outside those cells.

11 The widely distributed 1982 RAND Corporation study, *Varieties of criminal behavior*, specifically singled out this population as unamenable to treatment.

12 "One of the most important aspects of the CDC/Amity collaboration was the confidence that it gave the Legislature and the Governor to authorize over $100 million dollars to build the largest dedicated prison drug treatment program in the world. It is clear that Amity results are going to help shift the public debate here in California about corrections to a more treatment-oriented approach." James Gomez, director of the California Department of Corrections, 1996 (Mullen, Ratelle, Abraham, & Boyle, 1996, p. 122).

13 "The prison based drug treatment should be greatly expanded. Certain high-level offenders should be targeted for therapeutic community drug treatment in prison and aftercare programs following their release" (Little Hoover Commission, Beyond Bars, 1998, p. vii).

14 Little Hoover Commission, 1998, p. 67.

15 This in contrast to the Amity/RJD TC in which all participants were volunteers, with a large waiting list of inmates who wished to participate.

16 A reorganization occurred that combined the position of the director of corrections and the secretary—eliminating the position of director, and which changed the name of the agency to the California Department of Corrections and Rehabilitation.

17 While a program at R.J. Donovan has continued, it is not a TC.

18 The mistake here is a fundamental misunderstanding of what "evidence based" actually means. A curriculum that was found to be "evidence based" in reducing the recidivism of low-level nonviolent offenders is not "evidence based" for a population of extremely criminal violent offenders any more than an evidence-based curriculum for second graders is evidence based for high school students.

19 The CDCR programs initiated in 2020 addressed some of these issues.

20 Four wins: funder, contractor, inmate, public

21 Amity has been part of a PFS project in Los Angeles providing case management, services, and affordable housing for the highest utilizers of the Los Angeles County jail. Because of its demonstrated success in saving millions of county dollars, the project has grown from a small pilot project to over $100 million annually.

References

Alexander, M., & West, C. (2012). *The new Jim Crow: Mass incarceration in the age of colorblindness* (rev. ed.). New Press.

Anglin, M.D, Prendergast, M.L., Farabee, D., & Cartier, J. (2002). *Final report on the Substance Abuse Program at the California Substance Abuse Treatment Facility (SATF-SAP) and State Prison at Corcoran: A report to the California legislature.* California Department of Corrections, Office of Substance Abuse Programs.

Aslan, Laura. (2018). Doing time on a TC: how effective are drug-free therapeutic communities in prison? A review of the literature. *Therapeutic Communities: The International Journal of Therapeutic Communities, 39*(1), 26–34. https://doi.org/10.1108/TC-10-2017-0028

Bird, M., Grattet, R., & Nguyen, V. (2017). *Realignment and recidivism in California.* Public Policy Institute of California. www.ppic.org/publication/realignment-and-recidivism-in-california/

Briggs, D.L. (1963). Convicted felons as social therapists. *Corrective Psychiatry and Journal of Social Therapy 9*, 122–127.

Brown v. Plata (2011, May 23). www.supremecourt.gov/opinions/10pdf/09-1233.pdf)

California Department of Corrections and Rehabilitation. (CDCR). (2007, June 29). *Expert Panel on adult offender reentry and recidivism reduction programs.*

California Department of Corrections and Rehabilitation. (CDCR). (2007). *A roadmap for effective offender programming in California*. Report to the California State Legislature. http://sentencing.nj.gov/downloads/pdf/articles/2007/July2007/document03.

California Department of Corrections and Rehabilitation. (CDCR). (2008). Court upholds Corrections' finding that contractor misused one million in taxpayer dollars". Sacramento, CA. www.cdcr.ca.gov/news/2008/01/03/court-upholds-corrections-finding-that-contractor-misused-one-million-in-taxpayer-dollars/

California Department of Corrections and Rehabilitation. (CDCR). (2012). *2012 outcome evaluation report*. www.cdcr.ca.gov/Adult_Research_Branch/Research_Documents/ARB_FY_0708_Recidivism_Report_10.23. 12.pdf

California Department of Corrections and Rehabilitation. (CDCR). (2019, January). *Several poor administrative practices have hindered reductions in recidivism and denied inmates access to in-prison rehabilitation programs*. California State Auditor Report. Report Number 2018-113.

Chaiken, J., & Chaiken, M. (1982). *Varieties of criminal behavior*. RAND Corporation.

Clark, C. (2017). *The recovery revolution*. Columbia University Press.

Cullen, F., & Gilbert, K. (1982). *Reaffirming rehabilitation*. Anderson Publishing.

Dannenberg, J. (2007, April 15). California DOC substance-abuse contractor audits reveal $5 million in overcharges. *Prison Legal News*. www.prisonlegalnews.org/news/2007/apr/15/california-doc-substance-abuse-contractor-audits-reveal-5-million-in-overcharges/

Deitch, D., Koutsenok, M., McGrath, P., Ratelle, J., & Carleton, R. (1998). *Outcome findings regarding in-custody adverse behavior between therapeutic community treatment and non-treatment populations and its impact on custody personnel quality of life*. University of California San Diego, Department of Psychiatry, Addiction Technology Transfer Center.

Farabee, D., Prendergast, M., Cartier, J., Wexler, H., Knight, K., & Anglin, D. (1999). Barriers to implementing effective correctional durg treatment models. *The Prison Journal, 79*(2), 150–162.

Hawkins, R., McClure, D., & Paddock, E. (2017). *Using Pay for Success in criminal justice projects*. Urban Institute in conjunction with the US Department of Justice, Bureau of Justice Assistance. www.urban.org/research/publication/using-pay-success-criminal-justice-projects/view/full_report

Hser, Y.-I., Anglin, M.D., & Powers, K. (1993). A 24-year follow-up of California narcotics addicts. *Archives of General Psychiatry, 50*(7), 577–584.

Legislative Analyst's Office. (2017). *Improving in-prison rehabilitation programs*. https://lao.ca.gov/Publications/Report/3720

Life magazine (1962, March 9). Synanon House: Where drug addicts join to salvage their lives.

Little Hoover Commission. (1994). *Putting violence behind bars: 1994*. Report #124.

Little Hoover Commission. (1998). *Beyond bars: Correctional reforms to lower prison costs and reduce crime*.

Martin, S., O'Connell, D., Paternoster, R., & Bachman, R. (2011). The long and winding road to desistance from crime for drug involved offenders: The long-term influences of TC treatment on re-arrest. *Journal of Drug Issues, 41*(2), 179–196.

Martinson, R. (1974). What works? Questions and answers about prison reform. *National Affairs, 48* (summer 2021), 22–54. www.nationalaffairs.com/public_interest/detail/what-works-questions-and-answers-about-prison-reform

Mullen, R. (2017, June 26). Letter to the Secretary of the Department of Corrections and Rehabilitation.

Mullen, R., Ratelle, J., Abraham, E., & Boyle, J. (1996). California program reduces recidivism and saves tax dollars. *Corrections Today, 58*(5), 118–123.

Mullen, R., Rowland, J., Arbiter, N., Yablonsky, L., & Fleishman, B. (1999). *Building and replicating a successful recidivism reduction program: The Amity Therapeutic Community for Level III inmates in the California Department of Corrections.* https://static1.squarespace.com/static/6050e8e53cea454e57494a2d/t/60de43cc4dd79f540d491098/1625179087482/1999-09-Rowland-et.-al.-Building-Replicating-In-Prison-TC.pdf

Mullen, R., Rowland, J., Arbiter, N., Yablonsky, L., & Fleishman, B. (2001). California's first prison therapeutic community: A 10-year review. *Offender Substance Abuse Report, 1*(2), 17–18, 26–30.

Mullen, R., Schuettinger, M., Arbiter, N., & Conn, D. (1998). Reducing recidivism: Amity Foundation of California and the California Department of Corrections demonstrate how to do it. In Tekla Miller (Ed.). *Frontiers of justice* (Vol. 2). II. Biddle Publishing Company.

Myers, R.R., & Goddard, T. (2018). Virtuous profits: Pay for success arrangements and the future of recidivism reduction. *Punishment & Society, 20*(2), 155–173.

National Institute of Justice, Office of Justice Programs. (2016). *NIJ Journal, 277.*

Office of the Inspector General. (2007). *Special review into in-prison substance abuse programs managed by the California Department of Corrections and Rehabilitation.* California state government report.

Owen, B., & Mobley, A. (2012). Realignment in California: Policy and research implications. *Western Criminology Review, 13*(2), 46–52.

Prison Journal (1999). Special issue: Drug treatment outcomes for correctional settings, Part 1, 79(3).

Select Committee on Government Cost Control. (2005). California State Senate. [Video]. www.senate.ca.gov/media-archive

Supreme Court of the United States. (2011). *Brown, Governor of California, Et Al. v. Plata, Et Al.* No. 09–1233. Decided May 23, 2011.

Vandevelde, S., Broekaert, E., Yates, R., & Kooyman, M. (2004). The development of the therapeutic community in correctional establishments: A comparative retrospective account of the 'Democratic' Maxwell Jones TC and the hierarchical concept-based TC in prison. *The International Journal of Social Psychiatry, 50*, 66–79. Ttps://doi.org/1177/0020764004040954

Vitiello, M. (2002). *Three strikes laws: A real or imagined deterrent to crime?* American Bar Association. www.americanbar.org/groups/crsj/publications/human_rights_magazine_home/human_rights_vol29_2002/spring2002/hr_spring02_vitiello/

Werth, R., & Sumner, J.M. (2006). *Inside California's prisons and beyond: A snapshot of in- prison and re-entry programs.* University of California Irvine, Department of Criminology, Law and Society, Center for Evidence-Based Corrections.

Wexler, H., Burdon, W., & Prendergast, M. (2005). Maximum-security prison therapeutic communities and aftercare: First outcomes. *Offender Substance Abuse Report, 5*(6), 81–96.

Wexler, H.K. (2004). Evaluations of in-prison therapeutic community (TC) treatment prison based therapeutic community treatment: history and research update. Presentation to Annual Meeting of Therapeutic Communities of America, January 9, 2004.

Wexler, H.K., & Prendergast, M.L. (2010). Therapeutic communities in United States' prisons: Effectiveness and challenges. *Therapeutic Communities, 31*(2), 157–175.

Wexler, H.K., De Leon, G., Thomas, G., Kressel, D., & Peters, J. (1999). The Amity Prison TC evaluation: Reincarceration outcomes. *Criminal Justice and Behavior, 26*(2), 147–167. https://doi.org/10.1177/0093854899026002001

Wexler, H.K., Melnick, G., Lowe, L. & Peters, J. (1999). Three-year reincarceration outcomes for Amity in-prison therapeutic community and aftercare in California. *The Prison Journal*, 79(3), 321–36.

Yablonsky, L. (1962). The anticriminal society: Synanon. *Federal Probation, 26,* (pp. 50–61).

Yablonsky, L. (1989). *The therapeutic community: A successful approach for treating substance abusers*. Gardner Press.

Yates, R., De Leon, G., Mullen, R., & Arbiter, N. (2010). Straw men: Exploring the evidence base and the mythology of the therapeutic community. *International Journal of Therapeutic Communities, 31*(2), 95–99.

The KETHEA PROMITHEAS TC in Greece

12

Apostolos Tsirgoulas

In this chapter we will have a glimpse at the philosophy, the therapeutic aims, the day-to-day living, as well as the profile of the members of one of the first TCs within the detention system of Greece, the KETHEA PROMITHEAS TC in the Thessaloniki Detention Center. First, however, we take a look at how Greek legislation evolved regarding drug addiction, then we provide an overview of services for drug addiction within the prisons in Greece, and finally we identify the available options for treatment for an inmate with addiction issues.

Background

In 2013, a major change took place in Greece regarding legislation for drug-addicted people. By law, for the first time, drug use was not considered a criminal act. On the contrary, an addicted person is considered as someone who should be treated more favorably in a court of law. Also for the first time, drug addiction therapy has been recognized as a way to deal with antisocial behavior. Although the actual aim was to decongest the prison population, for the first time by government law, there was an admitted connection between drug use and delinquent behavior (Apostolou, 2016).

This new legislation also recognized the right of prisoners with addictions to participate, should they wish to, in one of the state-recognized programs for addicted people. In other words, we have by law, recognition of the right to treatment and therapy. With this new legislation, a prisoner is given the right to seek help, even after conviction. Paraskevopoulos and Kosmatos, commenting on this last point, argue that, even implicitly, we now have a governmental admission that imprisonment may push a person toward overuse and misuse or even addiction (Paraskevopoulos & Kosmatos, 2013).

The new legislation is more forgiving for people selling small amounts of drugs, recognizing that it is part of an addicted person's daily routine, in order to make ends meet. However, it became stricter regarding selling large amounts of drugs.

DOI: 10.4324/9780429317460-15

Table 12.1 General statistical data of prisoners – convictions at 1 January each year (2015–2019).*

	01/01/2015	01/01/2016	01/01/2017	01/01/2018	01/01/2019
Number of Inmates	11798	9611	9560	10011	10654
Waiting Trial	2470	2510	2829	3260	3317
Number of Foreign Prisoners	6882	5289	5195	5291	5822
Number of Women	572	486	527	551	553
Number of Juveniles	358	245	250	139	173
Convictions Related to Drugs	2872	1827	2034	2159	2372
Death Sentence	0	0	0	0	0
Life Imprisonment	982	960	941	933	960
Long-Term Imprisonment					
From 5–10	2887	2013	1798	2027	2154
From 10–15	1827	1360	1150	1031	1191
15 and above	2244	2093	2142	2054	2219
Short-Term Imprisonment					
Up to 6 months	66	63	46	43	62
From 6 months up to 1 year	126	78	84	73	82
1–2 Years	178	137	150	157	150
2–5 Years	446	326	366	391	469
Debt-Related Imprisonments	23	56	10	17	16
Non-Convicted Residents	549	15	44	25	34

*Translated from the official Justice Department site (2019)

Finally, the 4139/2013 law gave prisoners the right to early discharge, upon completion of one-fifth of their sentence, should they register with a recognized drug addiction program as a prisoner, under the condition that they continue therapy upon discharge (Apostolou, 2016).

According to the Ministry of Justice, Transparency and Human Rights (2019), of the total 10,645 inmates, 2,159 of them were convicted for drug-related offenses. Since 2003 there has been a steady 20% to 30% of inmates, with drug-related convictions. Please refer to Table 12.1.

Looking at the Figure 12.1 the first line refers to charged people and the dotted line refers to the cases related to drugs from 2000 up until the year of 2018 (REITOX, 2018)

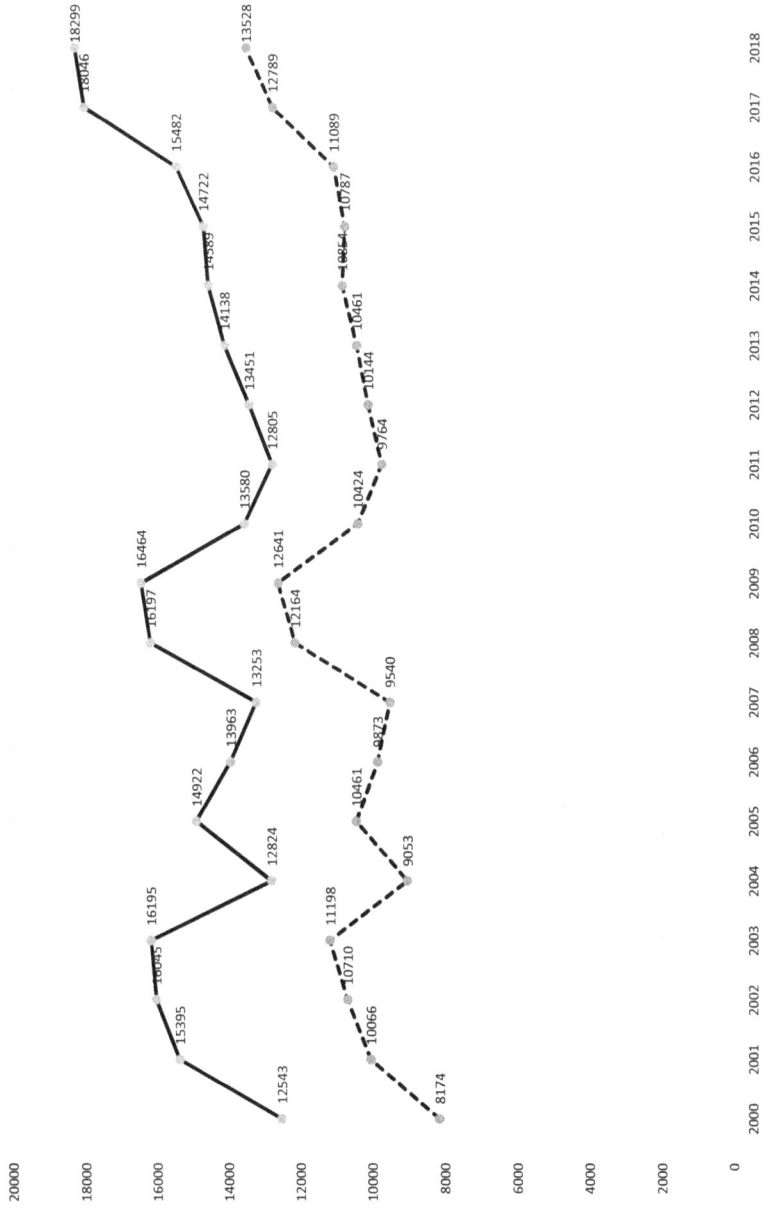

Figure 12.1 REITOX Focal Point collects annually data from the Greek Drug Enforcement Agency regarding arrests and charges related to drugs. REITOX reports an increase in charged people from 2011 to 2016 (REITOX, 2018).

It is clear that drug-related arrests and convictions are a major issue in Greek society. However, as stated, in almost each annual report of the Greek Reitox Focal Point, drug-addicted people within the prison system are an extremely vulnerable social group, with very specific needs (REITOX, 2015, 2016, 2017, 2018). Meeting these needs is the primary aim of each intervention developed during the past years within the prison system in Greece, by providing counseling and therapy as well as harm reduction and social reintegration. The organizations that intervene within the prison system in Greece are: KETHEA, OKANA, the Ministry of Justice Transparency and Human Rights, and 18 ANO (Psychiatric Hospital of Attica).

Although we will focus here on KETHEA PROMITHEAS, we will briefly outline all the recognized interventions that are established within the Greek prison system.

OKANA

OKANA is a Greek abbreviation and is used in the international literature to stand for, in English: Organization Against Drugs. OKANA was established by the 2161/1993 law. Its main aims are described as: a) planning and implementing prevention programs, as well as therapy, career counseling and social reintegration programs; b) conducting research on a national level into the factors that lead to the use of drugs; c) informing the public about the consequences of drug use, as well as promoting private initiatives for people who wish to participate in dealing with the problem; d) collaborating with international organizations promoting coordination with the European Union and international community; e) publishing research data on the drug problem nationally and internationally and submitting to the Ministry of Health suggestions for measures that need to be taken (OKANA, 2018a).

The OKANA network comprises 75 prevention programs, 57 pharmaceutical substitution treatment programs, four drug-free treatment therapeutic programs, three in-prison units, one rehabilitation unit, one social and vocational reintegration center, and one unit for immediate help as well as a help line.

Providing substitutes to illicit drugs is OKANA's main intervention tool. OKANA provides pharmaceutical substitutions, that is, methadone, as well as psycho-social support. With the aid of such a substitute, and as people reduce their use of heroin, their health improves. In 2014, the first such programs within the prison system started, one in Patra (Agios Stefanos Prison) and another one in Athens (Koridalos Prison) (OKANA, 2018b).

18 ANO (Psychiatric Hospital of Attica)

Since 1961, under the auspices of the Psychiatric Hospital of Attica, 18 ANO unit started treating people addicted to drugs and alcohol. Its services are free of charge for both their clients as well as their families. The therapeutic model is an eclectic, person-centered one. The intervention is psycho-social, without the aid of pharmaceutical substitutes (18 ANO, 2018).

The therapeutic tools implemented are individual and group therapy, gymnastics, art, and participation in social events. Those with a dual diagnosis may also be treated, even if they are under prescribed medication. 18 ANO aims to help people become completely free of drugs, by changing their ways of living, and move towards becoming an autonomous person. Through introspection, people are guided to investigate the roots of their addictive behavior, and to form a new identity, to aid reintegration into society (18 ANO, 2018).

Therapy consists of three basic phases. In the first three months, the focus is on encouragement, motivation, and sensitization. This is the initial stage that leads to the formation of a therapeutic contract. The second phase, the TC, focuses on psychological recovery and lasts around seven months. It is the time that group and individual therapy takes place as well as drama and art therapy. People are supported in understanding their addictive behavior that led to drug addiction, and in finding new ways of living. The third phase, usually around a year, involves social reintegration. During that time, apart from group and individual therapy, participants may participate in art, music, theater, photography, dance, cinema groups, and so on.

Within the Greek detention system, 18 ANO runs an intervention at the Women's Prison of Korrydallos Correctional Facility, Athens, as well as at the State Detention Psychiatric Hospital. The only requirement for someone to participate in treatment is a written statement declaring they have an addiction issue, as well as a written request to the prison social services, stating their wish to participate in 18 ANO groups. These group sessions within the prison aim to motivate addicted prisoners to reconsider their way of living, to help look at possible causes that led them to imprisonment, and to enhance their determination toward recovery. The groups are open, and participation may lead to the 18 ANO ex-prisoners program, upon discharge..

The Therapeutic Center for Prisoners with Drug Addictions. Ministry of Justice Transparency and Human Rights

The Therapeutic Center for Prisoners with Drug Addictions opened at the beginning of September 2002 at Eleonas, Thebes, Greece. It is a specialized therapeutic detention center under the auspices of the Greek Ministry of Justice, Transparency and Human Rights. Within this establishment, addicted prisoners serve their sentence while they follow a therapeutic multistage program.

The Center adopts the therapeutic philosophy of the drug-free TC programs: voluntary participation; abstinence from drug use, violence, and sexual relations with other members ; in all activities of the program (therapeutic sessions, work, educational schemes and so on); respect for each other; and mutual help among its members. The program is a multistage one: It begins with counseling sessions at the central prison in Athens, and an initial preparation stage (A stage) as a new prisoner is moved to the premises of the Center. Following the first stage, and after an evaluation, the inmates enter the second stage (B stage) in which work and therapy coexist. The goal is to uphold the therapeutic commitment and to reject prison and drug culture. A pre-community stage helps more advanced members move to the next stage. The third and main stage (C stage) is community based, where they live, work, and share daily life along with intense therapy. After at least six months and upon discharge, ex-inmates are allowed to move to the final stage (D stage): rehabilitation and social reintegration into the social milieu. People receive help with accommodations and participate in group therapy sessions and various organized leisure activities.

The supervision of the program is provided by a psychiatrist responsible for overseeing these individuals: four psychologists, four social workers, a music therapist, a nurse, and a criminologist-sociologist, along with security and administrative staff. All are trained in drug addiction interventions and also receive external supervision by an expert on the subject.

Upon enrolment, members meet once a week as a group. The next phase involves twice weekly group therapy sessions. During the main counseling stage, members participate in daily morning and evening individual sessions, once-a-week group therapy, music therapy, literature lessons, athletics, theater, cinema, and various other educational and therapeutic schemes.

During the pre-community stage, there are two therapeutic group meetings every week, along with daily individual sessions. The main therapeutic stage involves daily morning sessions, three group therapy sessions every week, art therapy (painting, theater), educational sessions, peer sessions, encounter groups, daily work structure sessions, cinema, and extra-therapeutic schemes.

At the final stage, inmates meet twice a week in a group. All members of the program may also have individual sessions with either psychologists or social workers. Finally, family members are supported by social workers. A group meeting takes place every month for family members and relatives (KATK, 2018).

KETHEA

KETHEA is the abbreviation used to refer to the organization within the international literature. It comes from the Greek abbreviation *ΚΕΘΕΑ*, which is translated: Therapy Center for Dependent Individuals. KETHEA is the largest rehabilitation and social reintegration network in Greece. Under the auspices of the Ministry of Health, it has been providing services to people with drug addictions and their families since ITHAKI, the first Greek TC, which was set up in 1983. Some of the key features of KETHEA's intervention are the following:

People receiving its services do not need to pay any fee and their attendance is voluntary. They attend either a day center or a residential TC, and all their expenses for food or cleaning are covered. People are only asked to pay their personal expenses for tobacco and leisure activities. However, these expenses may also be covered, if they are able to provide proof that they have no income or financial support from family.

There are no pharmaceutical substances or substitutes in treatment. Therapy is mainly provided through counseling and psychotherapy. The goal of treatment is to identify and address the psychosocial factors that contribute to addiction. The individual participating in the program is treated not as a patient passively undergoing treatment, but as an active participant in the therapy who accepts responsibility for changing they behavior in relation to the abuse of drugs, and who examines its causes. Participation in the therapeutic programs is not mandatory, and the individuals undergoing treatment are free to leave at any time. From the moment an individual decides to enter a therapeutic program, they are obliged to actively participate in their treatment, as well as all other activities in order to remain in that program (KETHEA, 2019).

Addiction is approached as a multifaceted phenomenon and family cannot be excluded from this approach. The treatment process involves taking the individual into account, along with their family and interpersonal network and the broader social context. Families are encouraged to participate in the whole process, and they are also provided counseling and support, whether parents, siblings, or partners.

Health care is considered to contribute to the quality of life and in this multifaceted approach it cannot be excluded. All therapeutic programs closely collaborate with hospitals and major health institutes, and clients are supported in and expected – as part of the therapeutic process – to take care of their health issues. Many therapeutic programs even employ part-time dentists, as oral hygiene is a major issue among drug addicts.

Education and training are considered important in an addicted person's rehabilitation, so it is highly regarded. Vocational trainers and teachers are hired to help clients either complete their basic education or acquire skills and knowledge, in order to be more favored applicants upon reentering the world of work.

Legal support is also provided. Lawyers exclusively associated with KETHEA help clients with their legal issues or even represent them in court.

Finally, all KETHEA's work is closely monitored and evaluated quantitatively and qualitatively by researchers who exclusively collect data from the field, either residential TCs or day centers. All this accumulated knowledge is communicated through training programs, not only for KETHEA's staff but also other professionals who wish to further enhance their knowledge of the addictive personality's characteristics.

With all this accumulated knowledge and experience in the treatment of drug addiction, KETHEA cannot ignore the need for counseling within the prison system. The official reports of drug use mentioned above may not reflect the actual drug use within prisons, which is probably much higher. In an unpublished study conducted by KETHEA PROMITHEAS in 2016, 42% of the prisoners in the Thessaloniki Detention Facility were found positive for a variety of substances.

The way KETHEA responded was, first, with counseling programs. Counseling groups of five to six people, to up to 20 people meet on a regular basis, either weekly or every fortnight. These interventions are usually part of another, larger therapeutic program, with the only exceptions of KETHEA PROMITHEAS and KETHEA EN DRASI, both of them created specifically for interventions within the prison system. Each program adopts its unique approach to counseling, depending on the needs of the inmates, the therapist's background and training, as well as the therapeutic program's philosophy, which is partly independent, although close to the organization's basic approach to drug addiction. There are currently 20 counseling programs run by KETHEA within prisons throughout Greece, and they include two major phases, simple referred to as "phase A" and "phase B."

The first one, phase A, provides people with awareness and understanding of the organization, its main aims, and philosophy. At this time, people are motivated, assessed, and assisted to express an initial therapeutic goal. The later phase B is more demanding regarding self-awareness about addiction and delinquency, as well as commitment toward changing drug-related habits. Completion of "phase B," leads to admission for intense therapy, either upon discharge or within the prison.

Intense therapy within the prison system is introduced with the TCs. Three of them, which are part of the KETHEA EN DRASI program, run more like a day center from nine to five. In August 2021, KETHEA EN DRASI inaugurated a secluded cell block section, within Korydallos Prison, solely for its TC members. TC members at the end of the day return to prison blocks, with the rest of the inmate population. All of these TCs run in the south of Greece close to the capital, and two of them are for female inmates. There is a fourth TC in the north of Greece, part of the KETHEA PROMITHEAS program. Its members are completely secluded from the rest of the population, and it runs on a 24-hour basis. The approach endeavored within this TC will be elaborated later in this chapter.

A drug-addicted client discharged from a TC or from a counseling program is eligible for admission to the two, semi-residential reception and reentry centers for ex-prisoners. One runs in the capital of Greece, Athens, as part of the KETHEA EN DRASI program, and the second in Thessaloniki, in the north of Greece, under KETHEA PROMITHEAS. These TCs provide housing and food as well 24-hour care to ex-inmates during the particularly delicate first days upon discharge. However, as time passes, particularly if there is a supportive family environment, people are encouraged progressively to participate on a non-residential basis. During this time, rehabilitation is the main focus, and the treatment evolves from residential to semi-residential. TC members are supported toward their financial independence and the structure of a drug-free social network.

KETHEA PROMITHEAS is a therapeutic program that has offered services in central and northern Greece officially since October 2012. The services provided are:

- counseling to four prisons in central and northern Greece;
- a 24-hour TC in Thessaloniki Detention Center;
- semi-residential reception and reentry center for ex-prisoners;
- family support;
- educational and vocational training; and
- research.

The TC of KETHEA PROMITHEAS was the first TC in Greece, within a prison, in a completely secluded block. The members of the TC have minimal to no interaction with the rest of the prison population, with their own private dining and rest areas as well as a yard for their outdoor time and activities. Their three-bed sleeping cells are also secluded, and the whole prison block complex is guarded by a single four-shift guarding post. The cells open at 8:30 a.m. and members return to them at 7:30 p.m.. The maximum capacity of the TC is 40 people. The staff team comprises a psychologist, a sociologist, a social worker, and a former member of a TC. The morning to midday hours are usually for group therapy, which is the main tool of intervention. After lunch-time, there is free time as well as vocational training time, with tutors running courses on grammar, literature, and computers, as well as physical activities. Finally, from time to time, volunteers run various projects and activities such as theater, music, and art.

After completion of the counseling phase, a member is eligible for referral to the TC. The manager of the TC, in collaboration with the manager of the counseling unit, evaluates a member's inquiry, and a day for admission is set. In coordination with the warden, the potential member is sent to the TC and goes through the intake group. This is actually a group interview, where the candidate is given the opportunity to introduce himself to a small represen-tative group of the community, express an initial therapeutic goal, as well as learn about the community. Members at this stage have the responsibility to either accept the candidate or refuse their admission, setting specific steps and goals for a later admission. Should the candidate be accepted, they are asked to sign a contract, where all the rules and responsibilities are clearly stated. Some rules are labeled "basic" ones, meaning in practice that breaking them would lead to immediate discharge from the TC. These rules forbid the use of violence or threat of violence, the use of drugs, breaking the law, and breaking confidentiality. Another set of guidelines sets the framework of the intervention:

- Participation: it is a model that requires members' active participa-tion from day-to-day living to therapy.
- Cooperation with the staff and other members, and a general openness.
- discussion about drugs or their life in crime is strictly limited during therapy.
- Taking care of themselves and being responsible for their living space.
- Not to borrow anything between each other.
- Consenting to drug testing whenever required by the staff or other members of the community.

The Model of the TC: Key Points.

- **Responsibility**. The community is self-organized into work groups for administration, ordering supplies, cleaning, preparation of food, health issues, and even the care of plants. Being responsible is a crucial step of treatment, as usually people with addiction issues abstain from taking on responsibilities and they need to re-enhance such abilities.

- **Self-help**. All members are involved in each other's well-being, meaning that everybody actively participates, to enhance growth and self-awareness, not only for oneself but also for every other member and the community as a whole.
- **Group Therapy**. It is the basic tool for therapy and members are expected to actively participate. A group session may be:
    - Encounter Group: During this group deviant or disturbing behavior either towards self or others is challenged by the group members.
    - Thematic Groups: People are given time to share traumatic experiences in order to see how these are projected onto the here and now of their day-to-day living or how they may have affected decisions and a way of living that led to drugs and crime.
    - Family Group: With the TC manager as the conductor, issues of the therapeutic approach and the philosophy of the TC are discussed.
    - Marathon Group Sessions: Throughout the year, there are times of emotional upheaval: Christmas or other religious significant dates, absence of staff members for holidays, newcomers introduced to the community, acting out, and so on. "Marathons" help the community deal with these strong feelings. As tension builds up, the community pauses from any other activities for one or two days and focuses inward on its dynamics. During those days, a set of consecutive two- to three-hour group sessions, either in small groups or the whole community, from morning until evening are strategically planned by staff in order to overcome crisis, conflict, or emotionally intensity; regain trust within the community; and redefine personal and communal therapeutic aims.
- **Education and Vocational Training**. As part of their first steps toward rehabilitation, members take grammar and basic Greek classes, information technology, and literature.
- **Openness to Outside Community**. The TC remains as open as possible to people from outside who can provide positive role modeling or even be a distraction from the inmates' day-to-day routine. Volunteers, sports clubs, and literary people, are invited to give lectures, participate, and interact with the members of the TC.
- **Short Leaves**. Inmates with long sentences in Greece, after some years, are by law entitled to a "short leave," every three months, and up to six days each time. During their short leave, the members of the TC in prison are escorted to the KETHEA PROMITHEAS Reception and Re-entry Center for Ex-Prisoners TC in Thessaloniki city center,

which is where they will enroll upon discharge. Thus they become more familiar with the setting that eventually they will integrate into toward their rehabilitation after imprisonment.

- **After Treatment**. Clients may take advantage of their therapy time in prison and become eligible before the court for early discharge. Should this be the case, usually courts require a mandatory admission to the Reception and Re-entry Center for Ex-Prisoners. This seems to minimize the risk of relapses and delinquent behavior, and helps people rehabilitate within a secure setting and with professional support.

Social demographic data

The profile of TC clients during the last two years is described below. This data is collected by the KETHEA PROMITHEAS research department and is part of the annual report of KETHEA.

Seventy-eight per cent of the clients had never received any drug addiction treatment before. The average age is 37 years (ranging from 24 years to 63 years of age). Regarding domicile, 28.6% were living with their parents and a third were living with other addicted people. Most of them are Greek citizens. Regarding employment, 21.4 % were mainly unemployed, 50% had a regular job and 28.6% were working part-time before imprisonment. Thirty-nine per cent never completed basic education, dropping out of school at the age of 17; 7.1% completed secondary school; and 25% entered higher education.

Drug use

Half of our clients stated heroin as the main substance of misuse, 28.6% cannabis and 14.3% cocaine. Regarding method of drug use, 32.1% preferred oral intake of the drug, 32.1 % inhaling the drug and 35.7% intravenous use. The average age when the primary drug use started was 19.1 years. All reported a secondary substance use apart from the primary one, with 71.4% reporting cannabis as their first substance. The average age reported for the first use of cannabis was 16 years. Secondary substances that were reported are: 32.1% cannabis; 39.4 % cocaine, amphetamines and stimulants; and 18% sedatives or tranquilizers.

High-risk habits

A total of 71.4% reported intravenous use sometime in the past. The average age for first intravenous use was 23 years, and 46.4% reported using a shared needle sometime in the past. Regarding transmissible diseases, 39.3% reported that they are positive for hepatitis C; 7.1% reported that they have never had a test for HIV; and 3.6% have never had a test for hepatitis B.

Family history

A quarter of clients reported alcohol use/misuse by the father and 14.3% drug use by the father as well, while 7.1% reported drug use/misuse by the mother, and 14.8% reported substance use/misuse by siblings.

Health issues

Half of clients have reported serious health issues. Thirty-seven per cent reported history of mental health issues, with mainly depression being reported.

Legal issues

More than a third had served a previous sentence. Forty-six per cent had convictions related to drug use, 28% for violent behavior (assault, robbery, murder, arson), and 18% for theft and breaking and entering. The average age for first arrest was 19.2 years and the average number of arrests was eight.

During the three years that this pilot project was running, 90 people accessed its services. The average length of stay was 266 days. Twenty-six members were part of the TC at the time of writing. The average number of TC members is 23. Twenty-nine people were referred to the KETHEA PROMITHEAS Reception and Re-entry Center for Ex-Prisoners after discharge.

Conclusions: thoughts

Drug addiction is definitely a major issue among the prison population in Greece, and only relatively recently has it been treated as such. Most of the people found in prisons with addiction issues never sought help before, seem to have spent most of their productive years in and out of detention establishments, and have a variety of health issues and highly risky health habits. They are low educated and usually come from families with alcohol or drug issues. It is safe to assume that these people, without any kind of intervention towards rehabilitation, would most likely end up having issues with the law at some point after discharge. Although is not safe to conclude how effective the interventions are so far, the fact that people remain in therapy upon discharge is encouraging. But it is not an easy job and the obstacles to this sort of intervention are numerous.

With the exception of The Therapeutic Center for Drug Addict Prisoners Ministry of Justice Transparency and Human Rights in Eleona Thebes, all of these interventions are units that run within a larger establishment, that is, a prison. Staff from KETEA PROMITHEAS are hired by KETHEA, which is funded by the Ministry of Health. However, the TC is literally situated in the middle of the Thessaloniki Detention Center, which was until recently under the Ministry of Justice and lately under the Ministry of Citizen Protection, that is, the police department.

It is as if the ongoing debate of whether to punish or to rehabilitate, to blame or to forgive is revived day after day, as staff have to pass seven control doors in order to reach the TC and share their time, emotions and professional knowledge with people living on the outskirts of society.

Communication and collaboration seem to have helped address these extremely delicate dynamics between KETHEA staff and detention officers. Before even the inauguration of the TC in the Thessaloniki Detention Center, the prison warden, the chief officer and a team of detention officers participated in seminars jointly organized by KETHEA and the Law School University of Thessaloniki. The chief detention officer as well as the warden have a clear idea of KETHEA's intervention aims, tools and methodology. On the other hand, staff from KETHEA started to be more aware of safety issues that would not have troubled them in any other setting before.

Apart from trust, what seems to have complemented this delicate balance is clear boundaries between responsibilities. Safety issues and rules are non-negotiable and TC members have to comply, without exception. On the other hand, detention officers have to respect therapy and confidentiality. There is only one detention officers' post in the facility, situated at the cell blocks where TC members sleep. Within the TC's premises there isn't any guard, even on Sundays, when there is no staff member on duty, but only on-call. Through time the TC has managed to convince and introduce officers and the warden to the values and the principles of the therapeutic contract. As the wider prison developed trust, belief and confidence in the TC, there was more space for it to be autonomous and for its therapeutic culture to thrive. This space is vital in order for TC members to trust their feelings, thoughts and experiences and for it to feel more like home and less like a penitentiary.

Is it worth it? Definitely yes. With the crisis of the closed TC as a method and intervention to addiction, there is a vast population that definitely seeks this accumulated expertise within prisons. Drug-addicted inmates have many reasons to seek help as Court of Appeal judges will see them more favorably as TC members, their living conditions will dramatically improve as they do their time and certainly, they will be given a chance to make good use of their sentence towards rehabilitation.

There were a lot of problems along the way. Inmates with no drug addiction issues may pretend to be addicted in order to have the privileges of being in a TC during their sentence. Having those people mixed in a TC with people who do actually have an addiction issue, most definitely will have a negative impact on therapy. When individuals have such a hidden agenda in a TC, it can trigger dynamics such that there is more likely to be a negative impact on inmates with actual addiction issues, who are often more dramatic and definitely more vulnerable. There are significant challenges to how non-addicted people can be screened during counselling or in a TC. What is more difficult to cope with, and to reframe therapeutically, is the situation where a whole therapeutic community repetitively challenges an inmate for not being addicted, while they stubbornly declare that they are. It is a simple paradigm. A more delinquent personality will most likely blame others, while addicted people usually need to learn cope with guilt.

Furthermore, people with very long sentences end up staying in therapy longer than an average TC member would have stayed. Due to lack of any other alternative, these people are eventually asked to return to the main prison population with minimal support. It is unlikely that one or two private sessions per month could support an inmate who has to return back to the rest of the prison population after therapy. These people are vulnerable and their therapy experience is usually frowned upon by other inmates.

KETHEA has accumulated vast experience in the field of addiction for almost four decades; however, within the detention system, issues have emerged that even the most experienced counselor never dealt with before. Research seems to be more vivid on the other side of the Atlantic, while here in Europe we seem to struggle to communicate good practices and the research seems scarce. The value of expanding the evidence base will be to draw attention, government funds and to expand their provision. Moving away from detention and from recycling criminal behavior, and aiming toward rehabilitation seems a measure that down the road would certainly be more cost effective for governments and will have a positive impact on society as a whole.

References

18 ANO. (2018). www.18ano.gr/profil-18ano

About KETHEA. (2019). www.kethea.gr/kethea/einai-kethea/

Apostolou, T. (2016). *Sentencing of drug offenders: Legislators' policy and the practice of the courts in South Eastern Europe*. Sakkoulas Publications SA.

KATK. (2018). www.katk.gr/therapeutic-center-for-drug-addict-prisoners/

Ministry of Justice, Transparency and Human Rights. (2019, January). General statistical data of prisoners – convictions at 1st January each year. www.ministryofjustice.gr/site/en/PenitentiarySystem/Statisticaldataondetainees.aspx

OKANA. (2018a). http://okana.gr/2012-01-12-13-11/ti-einai-o-okana

OKANA. (2018b). http://okana.gr/2012-01-12-13-29-02/deltia-typoy/item/601-koridallos

Paraskevopoulos, N., & Kosmatos, K. (2013). *Drugs*, N.4139/2013 (3rd ed.). Sakkoulas Publications SA, Athens Thessaloniki.

REITOX. (2015). *Annual report 2014 of drug problem and alcohol in Greece*. Reitox National Focal Point, Athens.

REITOX. (2016). *Annual report 2015 of drug problem and alcohol in Greece*. Reitox National Focal Point, Athens.

REITOX. (2017). *Annual report 2016 of drug problem and alcohol in Greece*. Reitox National Focal Point, Athens.

REITOX. (2018). *Annual report 2017 of drug problem and alcohol in Greece*. Reitox National Focal Point, Athens.

Hosting nurseries in prisons
13
Prison-based 'mothers with babies' units as therapeutic communities

Jacqui Johnson and Andrew Frost

Introduction

Arrangements for placing infants with their incarcerated female parent to achieve rehabilitative and social goals is not a new idea (Bauer, 2019; Smith, 2014). In New Zealand, prison-based Mothers with Babies Units (MBUs) were formally established through the Corrections (Mothers with Babies) Amendment Act in 2008. Prior to the late 1980s, New Zealand prison regulations gave scant consideration to women who entered prison at a time they had young children in their care. Due to concerns about unsuitable conditions, fear of criminal influence, increased cost, and disturbance to the prison system, there was reluctance to allow even newborn babies to remain with their mother (Dalley, 1993b). It was not until a 1989 Committee of Inquiry into the Prisons System, which acknowledged the critical importance of the role of the primary caregiver in the life of the infant, that the matter was seriously confronted. The subsequent report recommended children up to two years of age be allowed to reside in prison with their mothers. Conditions for mothers and babies began to change towards allowing incarcerated mothers to be with their children over the subsequent few years. By 2002, purpose-built units for bonding, breastfeeding, and housing day visits for women and their babies were established in New Zealand's three women's prisons. Provision was subsequently made for the babies of eligible mothers to reside with them in self-care units until the babies were six months old (Clayworth, 2012). The 2008 Act then extended this age limit to two years, and to provide a more suitable environment. It was intended to allow extended opportunity for contact between mother and child, thus enhancing bonding and relationship development. These dedicated facilities were to incorporate parenting support (Department of Corrections, 2017a). By providing spaces resembling self-contained homes for a mother and her child to live independently, these units were established to prevent mother-child separation at this critical time,

DOI: 10.4324/9780429317460-16

and to support 'healthy' attachments and continuity in the relationship with their children.

The incarcerated parent/infant: ideology, social policy, and well-being

Socially, there is a tradition of idealisation surrounding the role of the female parent in the life of her child. The expectations that follow this gendering tradition are reflected in recent New Zealand statistics for parents facing incarceration. According to a report prepared for the Quaker United Nations Office in 2012, at the time of incarceration, 47 per cent of females in New Zealand were at the time caring for children, compared to 26 per cent of males. Furthermore, 35 per cent of female prisoners were sole carers, compared to 12 per cent of males (Robertson, 2012). When a father goes to prison, children most often remain in the care of their mother (Berry & Eigenberg, 2003; Ferraro & Moe, 2003). Yet, when a mother goes to prison, children are likely to be cared for by female relatives (Chesney-Lind & Brown, 2016; Ferraro & Moe, 2003). Statistics such as these reaffirm the ideology of motherhood and society's gendered expectations that childcare is the primary concern of the female parent. This results in serious implications for families when they face maternal imprisonment (Freitas, Inácio, & Saavedra, 2016; Pollock, 2003). Perhaps reflecting these expectations, there is considerable attention in the academic literature highlighting the social and emotional implications of nurturing infant bonds and preserving mother/child relationships (Ainsworth, 1979, 1989; Bowlby, 1980; Perry, 2013). Imprisoned mothers contend with the stigma of failing these normative sociocultural expectations (Snyder, Carlo, & Coats-Mullins, 2002). Furthermore, in all these ways, the children of mothers in prison are also recognised as being particularly vulnerable to disrupted attachment in their development (Byrne, Goshin, & Blanchard-Lewis, 2014; Craig, 2009; Kanaboshi, Anderson, & Sira, 2017).

Given this reality for the imprisoned mother/infant, it is clear that for initiatives such as the MBU, to effectively support well-being there is a range of interests to consider and challenges to face, including the needs of the child, and the needs of the parent in 'mothering' the child. For these 'good-life' imperatives (Ward & Salmon, 2009), the development of human goods such as a sense of mastery, competence, self-determination, intimacy, and belonging (Ward & Salmon, 2009) are considered axiomatic.

In a recent study, Johnson (2019) considered the experiences of New Zealand MBUs through the eyes of 12 women during the time of their period of incarceration and their simultaneous residence in one of these units, as well as subsequent experiences upon their release from prison. To build a picture of this lived experience, the research took the form of a qualitative enquiry, based on a series of in-depth interviews, participant observations, and journaling. Thematic analysis was applied to these raw data. This study revealed that, while there were clear indications of progress towards meeting the goals of the MBUs, there were also significant obstacles. Further analysis suggested that these shortcomings were associated with a complex set of contradictions, inherent in the fundamental paradox represented by inmates raising infants in a prison setting. While socially progressive in its physical arrangements, this new setting retained some traditional elements of carceral culture that proved antithetical to the intentions of the policy and significantly hampered its realisation.

Contradiction, ambiguity, and paradox

The functional merging of the two forums – the nursery and the prison – holds both obvious challenges (Ward & Salmon, 2009), but also latent opportunities. The complexity of the contradictions became apparent in the course of Johnson's (2019) study. In this section of our chapter we draw attention to two key aspects of this paradoxical tension between setting and purpose. Firstly, we consider the challenges participants faced parenting within the restricted prison system and in negotiating relationships with prison officers in their seemingly dual role; secondly, we consider how the milieu and arrangements of the MBU contributed to the level of parental involvement participants experienced, and their persistent struggle to take up autonomy in the role of parent. Ultimately, participants' stories were found to reflect the lack of self-determination they experienced over their own lives and those of their children, with implications for the development of the mother-child relationship.

'Officer Nana': the ambiguous role of frontline prison staff

One of the most noticeable ways this research reflected the contradictory intention of the MBU was in the direct relationships between officers and prisoners. On the one hand, the MBU provided the opportunity for members of the two groups to develop unique and supportive relationships that were different to the way they were conducted in mainstream prison settings. Participants shared stories of everyday moments that revealed officers and prisoners effortlessly relating. Officers were observed holding babies, helping with toddlers, and spending apparently 'informal' time in the units, chatting in a relaxed and familiar way. One officer attended the birth of a child and, in a symbolic moment, cut the umbilical cord. In another incident, a previous inmate returned to prison on her child's birthday to visit some of the staff that she referred to as the 'nanas'. These opportunities for displays of humanity demonstrated mutual respect, and encouraged connections and meaningful relationships between mothers, children, and staff. The predominant characterisation by participants in this research of officer-prisoner relationships, however, was that they were tense. As well, officers clearly were expected to resolve a conflicting role, as they were both advocate for the parent/infant and representative of what is a total institution (Craig, 2009; Goffman, 1961; Liebling & Arnold, 2004; Silverman, 2005). The challenging nature of this dual role required officers to conduct traditional tasks of monitoring and disciplining prisoners, while simultaneously providing respectful, meaningful, and supportive relationships to mothers (Hannah-Moffat, 1995, Liebling & Arnold, 2004). In drawing attention to the daily reality faced by prison staff, Crawley and Crawley (2008) highlight how officers who carry out additional specialist roles must 'challenge long-established entrenched occupational norms' (p.149). Other research notes how the conduct of prison staff is fundamental to the operation of Department of Corrections programmes, with relationships between officers and prisoners and the use of authority determining how well any institution functions (Crewe, 2011; Dowden & Andrews, 2004; Liebling, 2011).

Participant stories illustrated how having officers so intimately involved in daily parenting was difficult and sometimes created a challenging space within which to perform the role of mother. Because of the power relations implicit, they often experienced this presence as oppressive intrusion, limiting their ability to parent autonomously and influencing their perception of how they viewed themselves in their mothering role. Participants spoke of difficulty managing what appeared to be conflicting responsibilities where officers switched between operating in a responsive and compassionate manner, and imposing authority. Western ideals of parenthood, particularly, imply that the ability of a mother to parent successfully requires a certain level of autonomy (Luther & Gregson, 2011). Participants in the (2019) Johnson study, however, expressed distress at times when surveillance and control by officers extended to monitoring and instructing their mothering. Some participants struggled with officers directing them in their parenting role, by means of what they considered to be unqualified advice. One participant opined that, to intervene in this way, staff should have 'some kind of paper that says you can know these things.' Most apparent throughout this research was participants' continual struggle for autonomous mothering and their freedom to exercise legitimate parental authority.

Moran and colleagues noted that the fragile nature of the officer-inmate relationship in a prison nursery was exacerbated by the predominance of its system of privileges and punishments (Moran, Pallot, & Piacentini; 2013). Baradon and others found that where parent/prisoners violated institutional rules, they were made accountable in ways that impacted on the children (Baradon, Fonagy, Bland, Lénárd, & Sleed, 2008). Such regimes have the potential to disempower prisoners in the MBU more than the mainstream prison population, as they experience additional control through punishments directly involving their children. Linking children's opportunities to prisoner misconduct was a mechanism of social control unique to the MBU, with most participants in Johnson's (2019) research voicing concerns about what they believed to be a realistic threat of having their child removed due to their own misconduct. Furthermore, mothers taking on the often-contradictory status of both parent and prisoner resulted in confusion around both identity and role, resulting in constant stress (Berry & Eigenberg, 2003; Eloff & Moen, 2003; Goffman, 1969). The requirement of prison officers to record case notes and document non-compliant conduct in the context of apparent compassion and concern towards participants further highlighted the contradictory nature of the officer-prisoner relationship. Case notes used in the prison provided a further means through which women's behaviour was scrutinised and documented daily to maintain up-to-date information about prisoners. Indeed, the content of case notes extended beyond documenting participants' individual behaviour to monitoring and noting a parent's involvement with her child. On one occasion recorded, case notes seemed to have been used as a method to control behaviour when the observation of one participant's lack of engagement with her child at playgroup was noted by an officer as possible inclusion in a file considered by a parole hearing. Coupled with this, the practice of officers addressing prisoners by surname only stood out at the time of this research as a mechanism of distancing and reinforced power relations.

Mother/prisoner: the lived experience of residents of the MBU environment

The accounts of the women who participated in this research reflect the complex dynamics involved in bringing the nursery into the prison. Essentially, the MBU attempts to merge two settings that differ dramatically in function. The fundamental concern of the correctional facility (the prison), is with safely and humanely containing its inmates, while also conducting the traditional functions of criminal justice, such as retribution, incapacitation, and rehabilitation (Eloff & Moen, 2003). The nursery is a nurturing space, intended to facilitate basic and fundamental physical, psychological, and social needs by means of a supportive set of close – generally intimate – relationships. Initial analysis of the data in Johnson's (2019) study revealed that the merged (prison/nursery) environment gave rise to constant ambiguity, as officers and prisoners sought to negotiate their paradoxical relationships. Furthermore, such negotiations are carried out in an environment that is characterised by power relations and in a setting that can appropriately be described as a total institution (Goffman, 1961). Such an environment, in sociological terms at least, represents a gradient heavily in favour of the correctional system and its capacity to discipline the conduct of inmates by means of continual surveillance and overt power. Nevertheless, closer examination of the data revealed several ways in which inmates engaged in acts of resistance to correctional authority (Crewe, 2007; Foucault, 1977, 1980). As well, it was apparent that – beyond their formal roles – parents, children, and officers often engaged in moments of family-like intimacy, and that often these encounters developed into relational habits around the care of the children that reinforced these qualitative relationships.

The struggle for self-determined motherhood

In prison, the philosophies of the penal tradition shape the experience of motherhood (Craig, 2009; Haney, 2013). The arrangement of the regulatory environment of the MBU limited a mother's choice in prison and arguably undermined parental authority. In this section we consider the impact of these ambiguous and contradictory features of MBU on the routines and everyday experience of its residents, with particular regard to the intended outcomes of these units. Although the explicit purpose of the MBUs was to offer mothers the opportunity to parent by taking responsibility and making decisions for their child (Department of Corrections, 2017a), participants experienced their preference to parent independently (and the self-determination that requires) as struggle in the constrained and structured environment of the prison facility. Their stories illustrated constant negotiation, as they navigated an environment in which their autonomy as mothers was challenged by custodial requirements that were consistent with traditional correctional imperatives. Elements of mothers' decision-making were continually redirected and absorbed by the correctional facility.

While residents were encouraged to parent and interact with their children in appropriate and socially acceptable ways, this was always secondary to consistency with prison regulations. In this way, procedures and regulations specific to the prison environment ultimately determined conduct. Despite the presence of children, residents were still subjected to regular pat-downs, room searches, prison lockdowns, and curfews overseen by uniformed officers. As noted in research from other custodial-based mother and baby units, struc-tural regulations placed restrictions on the way in which the women could be parents while incarcerated (Jensen & DuDeck- Biondo, 2005; Luther & Gregson, 2011). The presence of these disciplinary technologies meant some aspects of the prison routine appeared to contradict the intention of the MBU to provide a nurturing space (Johnson, 2019).

Restricting movements within the prison environment meant that ultim-ately participants' activities with their children around the prison were limited. Limitations on behaviour and choices such as when to sleep, when to wake, and what can and cannot be eaten, made it difficult for a mother to exercise choice and to represent authority in the life of her child (Clarke, 1995; Haney, 2013; Luther & Gregson, 2011). Although prison policy states 'a prisoner is responsible for the preparation of meals for herself and her child whilst in the self-care unit' (Department of Corrections, 2018), residents argued against being restricted in what food they could choose for their child. Furthermore, a mother's choice around sleeping with her child was not permitted for reasons of safety (Department of Corrections, 2017a, p.10), based on concerns around research into sudden infant death syndrome (SIDS; Ministry of Health, 2019; Plunket, 2019; Tipene-Leach, Hutchison, Tangiora, Rea, White, Stewart, & Mitchell, 2010). This policy, however, discounts research with Māori com-munities relating to co-sleeping, bed-sharing, and parent responsivity, which associates such practices with outcomes of more confidence and independ-ence in children (Horiana, Barber, Nikora, & Middlemiss, 2017; Jenkins, Harte, & Ririki, 2011). Because participants felt keeping time commitments was an aspect of their fitness as a parent, punctuality was important to them. Yet, because most outside arrangements were made for them, they had little control in this respect. Participants spoke about how they felt helpless as a mother in these situations.

A false paradise: life in 'the bubble' of 'Mother Prison'

While the living environment inside the MBU provided security, structure, and shelter within the MBU and the ability to spend dedicated time with their child without the influence of any of the daily realities from their lives outside, there was a risk that the MBU created a 'false paradise'.

Bosworth (2016) makes the counter-intuitive suggestion that prisons might provide a false sense of security for prisoners. This was evident for some participants in Johnson's (2019) research who became distanced from the reality of their lives on the outside. This was found to have implications for their reintegration success. Some participants were found to experience significant difficulty adjusting to life after release and struggled without the comfort and safety they found in the routine prison environment. Almost all participants felt they had limited support from community agencies when leaving prison and were distressed by their constrained capacity to manage their own lives. The transition from a secure and closed environment to the wider community was experienced as a sudden increase in the pace of life, with one participant stating, 'getting out was overwhelming cause everything just happened so fast'. Stories of institutional dependency emerged from two participants who reported they were unable to cope on the outside and, they claimed, intentionally breached parole to return to prison within a year of their release. Both of these participants spoke enthusiastically about their decision to return to the place where they found shelter, routine, security, and had discovered their own 'prison family'. Without the necessary skills to handle the multiple demands of reintegrating and resettling, women are unlikely to succeed in attempts to avoid recidivist offending (O'Brien & Bates, 2005; Richie, 2001).

In an ironic twist, the restrictive and limiting environment of the MBU symbolised, for some participants, the parental authority and control they sought in relation to their children. Indeed, some participants appeared to develop a sense of dependency and reliance on the institution, which came to be personified as 'Mother Prison'. The compelling nature of this relationship seemed to be borne out in the subsequent admissions of two residents who acknowledged breaching parole conditions in an attempt to return to prison. In a sense, the MBU represents a space to parent within a system where prisoners are essentially parented themselves: being told when to sleep, eat, and when to be confined to their units. Distrust accompanied prisoners, who were watched, monitored, and escorted, similar to the supervision afforded to a toddler from their caregiver or parent figure. Consistent with the findings of Crewe (2009), some participants implied that, paradoxically, the more restricted and confined they were, the freer they felt. When decisions were made for them and they were told what to do and when to do it, prisoners experienced less responsibility or accountability (Crewe, 2009). As highlighted in other international research, prison for mothers in this study was as a place offering shelter, routine, comfort, and community and, for some, respite from their lives outside (Clarke, 1995; Ferraro & Moe, 2003). This level of provision experienced was described by one participant as the 'bubble', where the burden of responsibilities was limited by 'not dealing with or worrying about the rent, not getting places, just looking after [child], there was nothing else'. Another participant explained that when needing attention for her child, she 'just went up to the officers, then they would organise the trip, organise the vehicle, organise everything and it's done that day'. In this way, the parentified institution might inadvertently help create an unrealistic level of dependency, further undermining the autonomy and self-reliance needed for successful reintegration (Morash & Schram, 2002).

Although some participants experienced a relative sense of psychological security and freedom from responsibility inside the prison, others referred to the demands and stress they felt in parenting alone. 'Intensive mothering' is the term coined by Hays (1996) that refers to the culturally informed notion of a good mother as one who invests considerable time, money, energy, and emotional labour into the role of motherhood (Elliott, Powell, & Brenton, 2015; Reich, 2014). Within the MBU, the parents' role is primarily as primary caregiver for their children (Department of Corrections, 2017a). Staff and other mothers in the unit were able to help care for children for short periods; however, mothers were expected to be responsible for their child at all times when in the unit (Department of Corrections, 2017a, p.10). This meant motherhood for some was experienced as demanding and lonely. Participants commonly spoke about having no one to pass their child to when the child was upset, teething, or just hard to settle. Participants commented on the resentment they felt about experiences that could have been shared with partners or families when new babies arrived but were dealt with alone. One participant reported that she felt exasperated when unable to hand her baby over and move to a space where she was not able to hear the child cry to create some temporary relief. Some participants had family members regularly involved in the care of their children when they were on the outside and were not used to parenting alone. Further difficulty arose when participants reported admitting to needing support would be interpreted as a sign of incompetence and a failure to cope in motherhood. Some participants did not want to ask officers for help, as they did not want to appear incapable.

Although participants acknowledged that the demands associated with 24-hour parenting were challenging, they also appeared to appreciate the uniqueness of this opportunity to individually engage with their child without the stress of competing demands in the typically chaotic circumstances of their outside lives. Life in the MBU was described as structured and predictable, which enabled time to be spent in a slow-paced and stable environment. Although participants' stories reflected the impact of incarceration, having this time with their child was for some the first time they had been able to prioritise their child's needs. Despite having three children on the outside, one participant said that this 'kind of feels like my first baby'. Having the opportunity to be this invested and focused on their child's development meant participants had time to 'just notice the little things that you take for granted in your child's growth'. Comments were also made on the additional health benefits for their child in having 'the opportunity to breastfeed longer' than they did with their other children, promoting positive psychosocial development and mother-child attachment (Cargo, 2016; Elliott- Hohepa, & Hungerford, 2013).

Furthermore, participants commented that their children who experienced the value of time with them in the MBU were more advanced than their siblings at a similar age. Most participants felt the structured environment of the MBU encouraged good mothering, with one participant describing herself on the inside as a 'superstar mum'. When participants were able to spend time with their child, and when the quality of that time was sensitive, responsive, engaging, and stimulating for the infant, secure attachment and healthy development became more likely.

This substantial role expected of participants solely responsible for the care of their child within the MBU, was at times at the expense of furthering themselves in practical skills or qualifications that might benefit them when reintegrating. Although the prison tried to help balance parenting responsibilities and programme obligations, this was not always the case. For example, some participants were unable to take their children to certain programmes, which limited their course involvement. One gave up her place in a computer course to provide for her child, on the basis that being a mother was her primary responsibility. Such an emphasis on being the sole provider for the child when in prison may have implications for the future of both mother and child when attention is not paid to assisting the mother to develop knowledge and resources needed to successfully manage their post-release life. If participants are not supported in gaining skills that will benefit them on release, they are at risk of being even more underprepared and under-resourced when reintegrating than mainstream prisoners.

Clearly, the contradictions inherent in the MBU nursery/prison concept became apparent through these insights into the lives and experiences of its principle members – the parents. These contradictions played out in the roles and functions: in rehabilitation versus control; in support versus surveillance. They also played out in the ambivalence of these participants: in privacy versus intrusion; in autonomy versus security; in appreciation versus resentment; in formality versus formality; in intimacy versus distance. It occurred to us that the opportunities implicit in these contradictions – and the paradox they collectively represent – might be resolved through enhanced internal consistency and role clarity. We further considered that these enhancements, and indeed that MBU goals more generally, might be promoted with the introduction of principles inherent in features of the therapeutic community (TC). In order to be explicit in conducting a thought experiment around this thinking, in the next section we describe the characteristics of a TC in its democratic variant. We then go on to carefully consider what potential benefits the introduction of this format might confer on the MBU, in terms of helping to resolve the contradictions, ambivalence, and conflicts encountered in the 2019 research.

The therapeutic community: concept and features

In the course of a large-scale systematic review of TCs, Lees and colleagues proposed the following working definition of the TC concept:

> A consciously designed social environment and program within a residential or day unit in which the social and group process is harnessed with therapeutic intent.
>
> (Lees, Manning, & Rawlings, 1999, p.1)

A TC is typically established alongside a specific programme of treatment. It is based on the recognition of the potential benefits gained in attending to the social-emotional climate of closed environments. In a review, Ware and colleagues (Ware, Frost, & Hoy, 2010) concluded that the TC represents 'a systematic and purposeful method of psycho-social treatment, where community is the method of change' (p.724), and is ideally characterised by the following features:

- Responsibility is devolved to residents where their full immersion in the community is desirable in order that they absorb and adopt its culture.
- The entire social order, including the institution's organisation, is used purposefully for therapeutic purposes.
- The ultimate goal is the enhanced ability of clients to function appropriately in the 'outside world' upon release or reintegration.
- Residents' experiences occur against a background of consistent and predictable values and principles designed to facilitate comprehensive resocialization.
- The environment is characterised by a positive and rehabilitative subculture, developed and maintained with the active participation of both staff and residents.
- Common elements are the provision of a communal living experience, encouraging open communication, and promoting psychological and social adjustment.
- All relationships are considered potentially therapeutic, and attention is directed in all social experience, interaction, and activity towards therapeutic goals.
- The arrangement generally requires the creation of a bounded and relatively autonomous environment.
- It provides a balance between autonomy and dependence (i.e. interdependence)

- While residents are accorded the liberties and opportunities to act relatively freely, the environment must also be responsive, confronting actions that are inconsistent with therapeutic goals.
- There is a strong emphasis placed on teams: within and between staff and residents, balanced with a good measure of self-responsibility.
- Treatment is not provided as such, but is *made available* to residents of the TC.

(Ware, Frost & Hoy, 2010)

Key social features of the 'democratic' form of TC are collaboration, democratisation, permissiveness, confrontation, and a prospective orientation (Kennard, 1983; Lees, Manning, & Rawlings, 2004; Rapoport, 1960). Typical submodalities and forums within this variant of TC are:

- group therapy;
- regular and frequent resident-led community meetings (involving staff and residents);
- committees and subcommittees, mentoring programs, structured activity days;
- therapy-related employment opportunities; and
- other arrangements where conduct and practices are openly raised and processed.

These authors also concluded that the TC format had proved to have value in forensic rehabilitation when applied to settings such as prisons (Ware, Frost, & Hoy, 2010). We will go on to consider this application, and specifically to units such as the MBU, in the following section.

Mothers with Babies Units as therapeutic communities

In seeking to address contradictions that appear as obstacles to the intention of prison-based mothers with babies units, the following section considers how establishing a TC might provide a setting more conducive to achieving their goals.

Research into group treatment supports the idea that 'group cohesiveness is essential to achieving treatment gains' (Marshall & Burton, 2010, p.143). This echoes features found in the TC model, which emphasises a collaborative approach to relationships between members of the community, be they community residents or those employed to provide service in that community (i.e. the staff; Gowing, Cooke, Biven, & Watts, 2002). Penehira and Doherty (2013) found that the 'sharing of struggles' created a group environment more conducive to change. In addition to the group experience, the quality of the relationship between the individual and the programme provider appears to have more impact than any single therapeutic technique, and is a critical factor for successful rehabilitative programmes (Andrews, Bonta, & Wormith, 2011; Marshall & Burton, 2010). The majority of the participants in the first author's (2019) study had undertaken a group-based programme (Kowhiritanga; Department of Corrections, 2017b) emphasising relationship enhancement through collaboration. These participants consistently commented that the collaborative style of facilitators was a key factor in neutralising the hierarchy between staff and prisoner, thereby impacting favourably on their experience of programme engagement. They spoke of this experience as a powerful approach to programme provision, which encouraged a sense of belonging through recognition of similar problems shared within a trusted group environment. The appeal of this programme for the participants in this research was due to the prominence of relationship-enhancing activities such as group work, group support, cultural discourse, facilitator style, and the personal connections on the programme. Kowhiritanga recognised participants as part of a wider system of family-like connections, related to extended family and community.

The explicit expectation of a prison-based TC is that prison officers play an active role in contributing towards individual and community well-being. The positive attributes of officers as highlighted in mothers' stories illustrate their unique involvement with the children within the MBU. Within a TC, all institutional staff are considered community members and central to the functioning of the group through their supportive involvement and contribution (Alcohol Advisory Council of New Zealand, 2010). Staff become role models, encouraged to 'offer personal experience as part of the therapeutic interaction' (Gowing et al., 2002, p.9) presented in a non-threatening and non-authoritarian manner.

A TC may be able to provide participants with increased responsibility and management over their own lives and those of their children. By providing legitimated forums such as regular and frequent resident-led meetings where outcomes are in essence supported by the institution, a TC may be conducive to an environment in which residents are able to parent more autonomously. By being able to make more of their own decisions around their child's eating and sleeping arrangements, and being responsible for their child's needs outside of the prison, parents gain experience more likely to increase their confidence and to attain a sense of mastery and competence (Ward & Salmon, 2009). In this way the unit model may be able to address these aspects of developed dependency found in the stories of the participants in this research. Moreover, this environment may be more able to mirror the community environment residents will return to, minimising the disparity between the provision participants experience within the prison and what they return to in their lives outside.

A TC framework may be a way to address the isolated and demanding experiences participants shared in their role as sole parent within the MBU. The benefits of using this community dynamic through sharing experiences and contributing to the well-being of the group, may encourage shared care and communal collaborative practice to assist participants to parent in a supportive group environment. A TC framework draws on the strengths of those more experienced group members, mirroring a more collective approach to childcare rather than an isolated individualistic one. In this way, residents are supported to draw on each other as resources in increasing their own self-determination, while contributing to this community ideal. Using TC foundations, the MBU could provide the 'village' that it anecdotally takes to 'raise a child'. Extending on the concept of collaboration through the framework offered by principles of a TC, family and community networks might be strengthened and relationships developed. More emphasis could be placed on involving fathers and family in this community model, with more 'community' days and organised family events. These fundamental relationships have the potential to impact on long-term outcomes for families (Alcohol Advisory Council of New Zealand, 2010). Establishing family support while in prison may provide the opportunity for these connections to continue and to promote *whanaungatanga* between the mother/child and their wider family, with a view to enhancing these relations on release.[1]

Parents in Johnson's (2019) study referred to the importance to them of marking significant events in the lives of their children – developmental milestones, such as naming and birthdays. With limited access to recording equipment (such as cameras) and a general lack of authority to organise social events, they are often frustrated in commemorating these occasions. They also valued opportunities to be seen in the role of host and the sense of pride this brought. The anthropological term 'definitional ceremony' (Myerhoff, 1986; Moore and Myerhoff, 1977) describes a social event intended to bring members of a community together in order to focus its attention in valorising an important individual or family event. Definitional ceremonies have the integrative benefit of enhancing community cohesiveness and a sense of belonging in the individual, thus reinforcing social capital. They enable 'opportunities to be seen and in one's own terms' (Myerhoff, 1986, p.267). A TC framework provides for the authority to honour such intentions and the organisational apparatus to schedule the events that could bring them to life.

We suggest that the strengths-based approach of TCs may add value here in their 'communitarian orientation' of facilitating and supporting connectedness between individuals and communities (Fortune, Ward, & Polaschek, 2014, p.95). Research highlights the valuable role community connections and comprehensive reintegration services could play in reducing the likelihood of women reoffending (Richie, 2001). International prison nursery programmes typically encourage women to widen their focus from being primarily responsible for their child. These facilities provide early childhood nursery services within the prison to care for the child for part of the day, while the mother fulfils course obligations or employment in the community or the correctional facility. Emphasising features of normalisation, these international jurisdictions attempt to mirror the circumstances women face when in the reality of their lives outside of the prison (International Centre for Prison Studies, 2008). These programmes support women to bridge the connection between MBUs and community reintegration, involving themselves outside of the prison before they are released. For participants of this research leaving the security of 'Mother Prison', it was clear that these established relationships to networks within their communities before release was vital to facilitate reintegration.

Conclusion

Nursery prisons have been established in several jurisdictions internationally, with the intention of addressing the intergenerational social harms resulting from the separation between infant and its primary caregiver. Recent research has recognised, however, that the unmediated operation of a nursery within a prison raises issues that severely limit this purpose being realised. Based on qualitative inquiry into the lives of participants in a prototypical facility in this study, we suggest that establishing a TC as the organising principle for these facilities holds promise in resolving the contradictions in role and function that underlie these limitations. By introducing a format based on community participation and mutual support and by enhancing legitimacy and empowerment, the TC framework may encourage the development of parental autonomy and self-determination among its community members, supporting parent-child attachment. A TC model encourages collaboration and investment in mutual well-being by supported opportunities to assert claims, to contribute to shared goals, and to engage productively. Skills acquired, relationships established, and a general sense of self-confidence, competence, and mastery over their own lives as parents may then translate to participants' lives on release.

Note

1 Whanaungatanga: relationships through shared experiences together, providing people with a sense of belonging and family connection.

References

Ainsworth, M D. (1979). Infant–mother attachment. *American Psychologist, 34*(10), 932–937.

Ainsworth, M. (1989). Attachment beyond infancy. *American Psychologist, 44*(4), 709–716.

Alcohol Advisory Council of New Zealand. (2010). *An evaluation of Moana House residential therapeutic community.* Wellington: Alcohol Advisory Council of New Zealand. www.hpa.org.nz/sites/default/files/imported/field_research_publication_file/Moana_House_Evaluation.pdf

Andrews, D., Bonta, J., & Wormith, J. (2011). The risk-need-responsivity (RNR) model: Does adding the Good Lives model contribute to effective crime prevention? *Criminal Justice and Behaviour, 38*(7), 735–755.

Baradon, T., Fonagy, P., Bland, K., Lénárd, K., & Sleed, M. (2008). New Beginnings – an experience-based programme addressing the attachment relationship between mothers and their babies in prisons. *Journal of Child Psychotherapy, 34*(2), 240–258.

Bauer, E. (2019). Infant inmates: An analysis of international policy on children accompanying parents to prison. *Michigan State International Law Review, 27*(1), 93–128.

Berry, P., & Eigenberg, H. (2003). Role strain and incarcerated mothers: Understanding the process of mothering. *Women & Criminal Justice, 15*, 101–119.

Bosworth, M. (2016). *Engendering resistance: Agency and power in women's prisons.* London: Routledge.

Bowlby, J. (1980). *Attachment and loss: Loss, sadness and depression.* (Vol. 3). New York: Basic Books.

Byrne, M. W., Goshin, L. S., & Blanchard-Lewis, B. (2014). Preschool outcomes of children who lived as infants in a prison nursery. *The Prison Journal, 94*(2), 139–158.

Cargo, T. (2016). Kaihau waiū: Attributes gained through mother's milk: The importance of our very first relationship. In W. Waitoki & M. Levy (Eds.). *Te manu kai i te matauranga: Indigenous psychology in Aotearoa / New Zealand* (pp.243–269). Wellington, NZ: The New Zealand Psychological Society.

Chesney-Lind, M., & Brown, M. (2016). Women's incarceration and motherhood: Policy considerations. In T. G. Blomberg, J. Mestre Brancale, K. M. Beaver, & W. D. Bales (Eds.). *Advancing criminology & criminal justice policy* (pp.370–380). London: Routledge.

Clarke, J. (1995). The impact of the prison environment on mothers. *The Prison Journal, 75*(3), 306–329.

Clayworth, P. (2012). Prisons. In *Te Ara: The Encyclopedia of New Zealand.* www.teara.govt.nz/en/prisons

Craig, S. C. (2009). A historical review of mother and child programs for incarcerated women. *The Prison Journal, 89*(1), 35s–53s.

Crawley, E., & Crawley, P. (2008). Understanding prison officers: Culture, cohesion and conflicts. In J. Bennett, B. Crewe & A. Wahidin (Eds.). *Understanding prison staff* (pp.134–152). Devon, UK: Willan.

Crewe, B. (2007). Power, adaptation and resistance in a late-modern men's prison. *British Journal of Criminology, 47*(2), 256–275.

Crewe, B. (2009). *The prisoner society: Power, adaptation and social life in an English prison.* Oxford: Clarendon Press.

Crewe, B. (2011). Soft power in prison: Implications for staff – prisoner relationships, liberty and legitimacy. *European Journal of Criminology, 8*(6), 455–468.

Dalley, B. (1993b). Prisons without men – The development of a separate women's prison in New Zealand. *Journal of Social History, 27*(1), 37–60.

Department of Corrections. (2017a). *New beginnings – Mothers with Babies Unit.* www. corrections.govt.nz/resources/newsletters_and_brochures/new_beginnings_-_mothers_ with_babies_unit.html

Department of Corrections. (2017 b). *Kowhiritanga for Women (Service Description).* Author.

Department of Corrections. (2018). *Prison Operations Manual. M.03.02.09 Management of prisoner with resident children general standards.* www.corrections.govt.nz/resources/ policy_and_legislation/Prison- Operations-Manual/Movement/M.03-Specified-gender- and-age- movements/M.03-2.html

Dowden, C., & Andrews, D. A. (2004). The importance of staff practice in delivering effective correctional treatment: A meta-analytic review of core correctional practice. *International Journal of Offender Therapy and Comparative Criminology, 48*(2), 203–214.

Elliott, S., Powell, R., & Brenton, J. (2015). Being a good mum: Low income, black single mothers negotiate intensive mothering. *Journal of Family Issues, 36*(3), 351–370.

Elliott-Hohepa, A., Hungerford, R. (2013*). Report on phase three of the formative evaluation of the Mothers with Babies Units.* www.corrections.govt.nz/__data/assets/pdf_file/0014/700313/ Evaluation_of_the_implementation_of_the_Mothers_with_Babies_Policy_final_.pdf

Eloff, I., & Moen, M. (2003). An analysis of mother–child interaction patterns in prison. *Early Child Development and Care, 173*(6), 711–720.

Ferraro, K. J., & Moe, A. M. (2003). Mothering, crime, and incarceration. *Journal of Contemporary Ethnography, 32*(1), 9–40.

Fortune, C., Ward, T., & Polaschek, D. (2014). The Good Lives Model and therapeutic environ- ments in forensic settings. *Therapeutic Communities: the International Journal of Therapeutic Communities, 30*(3), 95–104.

Foucault, M. (1977). *Discipline and punish: The birth of the prison.* London: Allen Lane.

Foucault, M. (1980). *Power/knowledge: Selected interviews and other writings, 1972–1977.* New York: Harvester Press.

Freitas, A., Inácio, A., & Saavedra, L. (2016). Motherhood in prison: Reconciling the irreconcil- able. *The Prison Journal, 96*(3), 415–436.

Goffman, E. (1961). *Asylums: Essays on the social situation of mental patients and other inmates.* Chicago: Aldine Publishing.

Goffman, E. (1969). *The presentation of self in everyday life.* London: Allen Lane.

Gowing, L., Cooke, R., Biven, A., & Watts, D. (2002). *Towards better practice in therapeutic com- munities.* Victoria: Australasian Therapeutic Communities Association.

Haney, L. (2013). Motherhood as punishment: The case of parenting in prison. *Signs: Journal of Women in Culture and Society, 39*(1), 105–130.

Hannah-Moffat, K. (1995). Feminine fortresses: Woman-centered prisons? *The Prison Journal, 75*(2), 135–164.

Hays, S. (1996). *The cultural contradictions of motherhood.* New Haven: Yale University Press.

Horiana, J., Barber, C. C., Nikora, L. W., & Middlemiss, W. (2017). Māori child rearing and infant sleep practices. *New Zealand Journal of Psychology, 46*(3), 30–37.

International Centre for Prison Studies. (2008). International profile of women's prisons. www. prisonstudies.org/sites/default/files/resources/downloads/wom   ens_prisons_int_review_final_report_v2.pdf

Jenkins, K., Harte, H., & Ririki, T. K. (2011). Traditional Maori parenting: An historical review of literature of traditional Maori child rearing practices in pre-European times. Auckland: Te Kahui Mana Ririki. www.ririki.org.nz/wp- content/uploads/2015/04/TradMaoriParenting.pdf

Jensen, V., & DuDeck-Biondo, J. (2005). Mothers in jail: Gender, social control, and the construction of parenthood behind bars. In S. Lee Burns (Ed.) *Ethnographies of Law and Social Control* Bingley, UK: Emerald Group, pp.121–142..

Johnson, J. (2019). *Monitored mothering: The experience of mothers who parent within New Zealand women's prisons.* [Unpublished doctoral dissertation]. University of Canterbury, New Zealand. https://ir.canterbury.ac.nz/handle/10092/100061

Kanaboshi, N., Anderson, J., & Sira, N. (2017). Constitutional rights of infants and toddlers to have opportunities to form secure attachment with incarcerated mothers: Importance of prison nurseries. *International Journal of Social Science Studies, 5*(2), 55–72.

Kennard, D. (1983). *An introduction to therapeutic communities.* London: Routledge and Kegan Paul.

Lees, J., Manning, N., & Rawlings, B. (1999). *Therapeutic community effectiveness: A systematic international review of therapeutic community treatment for people with personality disorders and mentally disordered offenders* (CRD Report no. 17). York: NHS Centre for Reviews and Dissemination, University of York.

Lees, J., Manning, N. & Rawlings, B. (2004). A culture of enquiry: Research evidence and the therapeutic community. *Psychiatric Quarterly. 75*(3), 279–294.

Liebling, A. (2011). Moral performance, inhuman and degrading treatment and prison pain. *Punishment & Society, 13*(5), 530–550.

Liebling, A., & Arnold, H. (2004). *Prisons and their moral performance: A study of the values, quality and prison life.* Oxford: Oxford University Press.

Luther, K., & Gregson, J. (2011). Restricted motherhood: Parenting in a prison nursery. *International Journal of Sociology of the Family, 37*(1), 85–103.

Marshall, W., & Burton, D. (2010). The importance of group processes in offender treatment. *Aggression and Violent Behavior, 15*(2), 141–149.

Matua Raki. (2012). *Supporting New Zealand's therapeutic community workforce: An investigation of current needs.* A scoping report developed by Matua Raki for the Ministry of Health. www.matuaraki.org.nz/uploads/files/resource-assets/therapeutic-   communities-scoping-report.pdf

Ministry of Health. (2019). Keeping baby safe in bed: 6 weeks to 6 months. www.health.govt.nz/your-health/pregnancy-and-kids/first-year/first-6-weeks/keeping-baby-safe-bed-first-6-weeks

Moore, S. F., & Myerhoff, B. G. (1977). *Secular ritual.* Amsterdam: Van Gorcum.

Moran, D., Pallot, J., & Piacentini, L. (2013). Privacy in penal space: Women's imprisonment in Russia. *Geoforum, 47*, 138–146.

Morash, M., & Schram, P. (2002). *The prison experience. Special issues of women in prison.* Long Grove, IL: Waveland Press.

Myerhoff, B. (1986). Life not death in Venice. Its second life. In V. Turner & E. M. Bruner (Eds.). *The anthropology of experience* (pp.261–286). Chicago: University of Illinois Press.

O'Brien, P., & Bates, R. (2005). Women's post-release experiences in the US: Recidivism and re-entry. *International Journal of Prisoner Health, 1*(2), 207–221.

Penehira, M., & Doherty, L. (2013). Tu mai te oriori, nau mai te hauora! A kaupapa Māori approach to infant mental health: Adapting mellow parenting for Māori mothers in Aotearoa, New Zealand. *A Journal of Aboriginal and Indigenous Community Health, 10*(3), 367–382.

Perry, B. D. (2013). Bonding and attachment in maltreated children. *The Child Trauma Center, 3*, 1–17. https://childtrauma.org/wp- content/uploads/2013/11/Bonding_13.pdf

Plunket. (2019). Sleep – Plunket. www.plunket.org.nz/your- child/newborn-to-6-weeks/sleep/

Pollock, J. M. (2003). Parenting programs in women's prisons. *Women & Criminal Justice, 14*(1), 131–154.

Rapoport, R. (1960). *Community as doctor.* London: Tavistock.

Reich, J. A. (2014). Neoliberal mothering and vaccine refusal: Imagined gated communities and the privilege of choice. *Gender & Society, 28*(5), 679–704.

Richie, B. E. (2001). Challenges incarcerated women face as they return to their communities: Findings from life history interviews. *Crime & Delinquency, 47*(3), 368–389.

Robertson, O. (2012). *Collateral convicts: Children of incarcerated parents: Recommendations and good practice from the United Nations Committee on the rights of the child: Day of general discussion.* www.quno.org/sites/default/files/resources/ENGLISH_Collateral%20C onvicts_Recommendations%20and%20good%20practice.pdf

Silverman, S. W. (2005). When the state has custody: The fragile bond of mothers and their infants on the prison nursery. In L. Gunsberg, & P. Hymowitz (Eds.). *A handbook of divorce and custody: Forensic, developmental and clinical perspectives* (pp.245–58). Hillsdale, NJ: Analytic Press.

Smith, P. S. (2014). *When the innocent are punished: The children of imprisoned parents.* London: Palgrave Macmillan.

Snyder, Z. K., Carlo, T. A., & Coats-Mullins, M. M. (2002). Parenting from prison. *Marriage & Family Review, 32*(3–4), 33–61.

Tipene-Leach, D., Hutchison, L., Tangiora, A., Rea, C., White, R., Stewart, A., & Mitchell, E. (2010). SIDS-related knowledge and infant care practices among Māori mothers. *New Zealand Medical Journal, 123*(1326), 88–96. www.nzma.org.nz/__data/assets/pdf_file/0003/37515/tipene- leach.pdf

Ward, T., & Salmon, K. (2009). The ethics of punishment: Correctional practice implications. *Aggression and Violent Behavior, 14*(4), 239–247.

Ware, J., Frost, A., & Hoy, A. (2010). A review of the use of therapeutic communities with sexual offenders. *International Journal of Offender Therapy and Comparative Criminology, 54*(5), 721–724.

Collaboration, cohesion and belonging

Can prison therapeutic communities provide a framework for imprisonment?

14

Richard Shuker

The harmful consequences of imprisonment are well documented (See Sykes, 1958, Scott, 2015). Whilst a minority view holds that 'prisons work', there has been little consistent evidence cited to uphold this position (Crewe & Levins, 2019). The numerous and wide-ranging adverse outcomes associated with imprisonment are instead those which are most evident. Loss of rights of citizenship, autonomy and disenfranchisement are perhaps the most overt and intended consequences of imprisonment. However, significant negative, more unintended consequences associated with imprisonment have also been well documented. These include the erosion of the individual's sense of identity and personal meaning, constraining relationships, competitiveness for limited resources, and a veneer of compliance which tacitly creates an unhealthy prison sub culture; where those incarcerated have little or no alignment with the goals and values of the organisation, these have greater potential to emerge (see Crewe, 2009, Crewe & Liebling, 2015). Others have cited the potential of prisons to be complicit in the re-traumatisation of a population who have already lived through and experienced significant psychological physical and emotional hardship, where violence, self-harm and suicide, threat and lack of safety are ever present (Jones, 2015).

This chapter will explore the social and organisational structures which can lead to separation and mistrust and how this can lead to individual and group conflict. It will argue however that even within the context of imprisonment, group belonging and collaboration are fundamental drives which can be harnessed to create a culture of collaboration and cooperation. It will go on to explore how prisons do have a capacity to enable positive social identities and how these, instead of causing conflict, can lead to cohesion. It will focus on how group processes can empower and how the structures of a therapeutic community (TC) can have wider relevance for other forensic settings.

DOI: 10.4324/9780429317460-17

Psychological disorder, culture and social context

Dominant psychological models have largely adopted an 'individualistic' approach to how individual responsibility, well-being and personal distress are conceptualised; these have often been regarded as existing independently from the cultural and social context from which they emerge (Sampson, 1988). Attempts to understand and change human behaviour have often reflected the social, cultural and political climate (of predominantly Western cultures) with limited reference being made to their complex interaction in behaviour viewed as 'problematic'. This has been evident in the clinical status given to cognitive behavioural therapy (CBT) over the past 20 years or so, reflected in policy and practice developments (Layard & Clark, 2014). Some have also argued however that approaches to treating psychological disorder as a personal and individual problem, rather than been a collective and social phenomenon, are heavily influenced by prevailing political (Summerfield, 2012) and economic ideologies (Warner, 2004); others have suggested that the expansion of CBT-based approaches has neglected the role that adverse experiences and economic and social impoverishment have on emotional, psychological and interpersonal problems. The dominance of the biomedical model has contributed to an entrenched position where the basis of physical and psychological health has been overwhelmingly regarded as genetic or biological. A far-reaching but inevitable consequence of this position is that attempts to understand psychological disorder from a sociocultural perspective have received far less attention, reflected in the observation that psychological theory and research has explored 'individual selves', disconnected from the social and natural world (Moloney & Kelly, 2008).

The potential and power of groups

Reicher (2017) has observed how psychological research has generally approached the study of group behaviour from a perspective which sees group processes and group influence as unhealthy, having little to offer in providing any positive impact and potential. Conclusions drawn from the study of groups have focused on their propensity to promote conformity, aggression, irrational judgement and poor decision-making, concluding that the drive to group membership is at the cost of impaired judgement and behaviour. The capacity of group membership to provide any positive influence has generally been overlooked.

The limitations of viewing psychological disorder as something located primarily within individual psychology are however becoming recognised.

The immense importance of social and societal structure in understanding and changing behaviour and in promoting or alleviating distress is increasingly acknowledged (Platow & Hunter, 2014). The British Psychological Society (Johnstone & Boyle, 2018), developing a framework for conceptualising psychological problems, has recently argued that 'the individual does not exist, and cannot be understood, separately from his/her relationships, community and culture; meaning only arises when social, cultural and biological elements combine; and biological capacities cannot be separated from the social and interpersonal environment' (p.9). This centrality of social factors also becomes apparent when considering how variations in societal culture (e.g. whether individualistic or collective) have an impact on our personal values, self-concept, the nature of relationships and cognitive processes (Oyserman et al., 2002). As well as the particular culture we inhabit shaping our goals and sense of self, this also provides a framework for how we make meaning of the world, and shapes our motives and influences our values and priorities (Oyserman & Lee, 2008).

What is also becoming evident from the study of social context, groups and communities is the importance of the identities these provide people. Haslam et al. (2018) suggest that the extent to which 'we understand, treat and engage with other people depends very much on the degree to which we see them as sharing a social identity with us' (p.15). Furthermore, groups and group processes characterised by connection and belonging have the potential to promote, nurture and sustain personal change and are central factors to the process by which people come to desist from offending (McNeil, 2006); in mental health recovery the importance of having shared social identities with valued groups has also been recognised (Leamy et al., 2011).

What is emerging is a body of evidence to suggest a revised, repositioned view on the value of social and group membership. This highlights their importance in psychological and physical health, personal change and well-being. This also has implications for the way in which social arrangements are structured, and the relationships which emerge from this, in creating a healthy social environment characterised by cohesion rather than conflict. The following section will outline some of ways in which groups offer such potential.

Health, well-being and belonging

It is recognised that people understand themselves and adapt their behaviour according to social dynamics and group relationships of which they are a part (Baumeister & Leary, 1995); personal identity is shaped by the communities to which people belong (Gilmore, 1990). Mental health, social adjustment and treatment outcomes have also consistently been found to be associated with a sense of belonging (Baumeister et al., 2005, Hawksley et al., 2003, Dingle, 2018).

The power of group membership has also been made strikingly evident in its capacity to promote health and an increased length of life. Holt-Lunstad et al. (2010) demonstrated that social connectedness and group membership make a contribution to mortality that is independent of other health factors, observing that group membership and social connection are a powerful component in recovering from ill health, more so than factors like drugs or diet. Haslam (2018) goes on to make the case for the importance of group and community belonging. He argues that the social identity this provides, forms the basis for connection, meaning and purpose, suggesting that

> The internalisation of social identity provides the essential platform for a range of attitudinal, perceptual and behavioural phenomena. These include a sense of similarity, commonality and connectedness [...] and the ability to influence and coordinate the thinking and behaviour of those in-group members.
>
> (p.31)

Relationships and values

Membership of a group also has the capacity to determine and influence personal values and norms (see Moos, 2008). Where people identify with a particular group, the way in which they anticipate and interpret the world is likely to be shaped by the values the group holds. This is evident from within the field of addictive behaviour where the mutual support, affirming relationships, abstinence norms and group-based values of honesty and openness are key factors in treatment outcome.

Studies of group behaviour have also consistently found that having knowledge about an individual's attributes does not help us predict their behaviour (Turner et al., 1987). What determines how people relate are the identities established from being a member of a group. It is this which has the capacity to create personal meaning and determine behaviour. What is further apparent is that where people categorise their group as being distinctive and separate from others, the impact on personal identity, beliefs and behaviour becomes all the stronger. As powerfully demonstrated by Tajfel (1972) in his studies of group behaviour, 'distinction from the "other" category provided an identity for their own group, and thus some kind of meaning to an otherwise empty situation' (p.39).

The 'social identity' we hold is significant in determining how people relate and has implications for their psychological health. In studies replicating the

Stanford prison experiment (Haney et al., 1973), it was observed that as prison officers' sense of identity became eroded, their mental health deteriorated and stress, paranoia and depression increased (Haslam 2018). He argues that the personal and collective identity that group membership provides is critical to how we behave. Group belonging can promote 'a sense of trust and support, control and agency, and a sense of purpose, direction and meaning [and] the way we interact with other people: whether we love them, whether we lead them, whether we help them' (p.32).

This has implications for the social arrangements of organisations where there are clear differentiations in power, status and influence; the extent to which people identify with the organisation and with specific groups within it, has a profound impact on the relationships, behaviour and values of its members.

Empowerment and motivation

Membership of a social group can have a powerful effect on how we understand ourselves and our personal aspirations. It can provide support, shape values and provide a reference point for how we understand and define ourselves. Reicher (2017) identifies two transformations that can mobilise people to achieve positive goals, which become possible when people see themselves as part of a group. Firstly, he suggests the world can be seen in common terms where goals and priorities are agreed; secondly, people can collaborate, align their efforts and become empowered to reach common goals. Group membership can also have a motivating influence which promotes personal agency. For example, adhering to messages about health behaviour is motivated by the social identities which group membership gives (Oyserman, 2008). The extent to which people identity as having a 'recovery' over a 'substance misuser' identity has also been shown to be key in successful outcomes and abstinence (Dingle et al., 2018).

The potential of group membership to exert a powerful influence on how people view, understand and relate to each has become evident in events surrounding the Holocaust. An analysis of the repeated failed attempts by the Nazis to deport Bulgarian Jews has shown how the Bulgarian people felt a sense of cohesion and attachment which galvanized efforts to protect and help the Jewish community. This collective concern and action occurred because they saw them as part of their own community (Bar Sohar, 1998). They were not regarded as a separate or distinct social group but a group possessing the same shared identity, with whom they felt a sense of connection. It was this sense of connection and shared experience which drove care, compassion and concern (Todorov, 2001).

Desistance, belonging and social factors

Although the bio-psychosocial model intended to give equal significance to biological, psychological and social factors (Engel, 1977), it is the biological approaches which still predominate (Jonstone & Boyle, 2018). The compelling evidence from studies which explore why people desist from offending is that this is a process significantly tied into social factors including a sense of belonging and connection, social groups and social networks (Weaver, 2016, McNeil, 2006). Such evidence however appears not be reflected in practice. Psychological interventions aimed at rehabilitation continue to emphasise the importance of changes in individual factors such as attitudes, beliefs, emotional and behavioural regulation, and a focus on the 'treatment' of these individual factors has predominated (Mews et al., 2017). When social elements (norms, culture) are recognised as important in changing behaviour, they are set apart from the complex interaction involved in psychology, cognition and personality, and there is limited awareness of their role in shaping our sense of and understanding of who we are (Farrow et al., 2017).

Social context, group relationships and cooperation

Given the capacity that social context has to shape identities and exert a powerful impact on well-being, attitudes and behaviour, we need to consider what it is about forms of social arrangements that provides the backdrop for cooperation rather than conflict to develop.

Separation and division

Explanations for prejudice have often focused on an analysis of individual psychology and personality (Allport, 1958). However, studies of group behaviour have told us something rather different about the nature of conflict and division. The work of Sherif and Sherif (1969) has been pivotal in highlighting how conflict depends very much on the relationships and interdependencies between groups within the wider social context in which they exist. To a large extent, it is the *context* in which groups function that provides the mediating influence determining whether rivalry and hostility predominate or whether they become a force for cooperation and collective good; it is changes in social context and structures which lead to changes in intergroup relationships and behaviour rather than the attributes of group members. Platow and Hunter (2014) argue, for example, that rivalry and conflict can only be understood at the group and intergroup rather than individual level, and can be accentuated where social arrangements allow 'intergroup competition for limited and valued resources [which] can produce negative stereotypes, prejudice and discrimination' (p.840).

Categorisation

The social categorisation which membership of a particular group or community provides can unite, empower and motivate. Aligning oneself with a particular social category can provide meaning, bring people together and shape behaviour (Reicher & Hopkins, 2001). In many ways this aspect of group membership can inspire and motivate action towards positive goals. However, it can also have the potential in certain contexts and circumstances to lead to rivalry (Oakes et al., 1994).

Sofsky (1993) in his analysis of concentration camps during World War II tells us something important about social processes and how the wider social context has the capacity to determine group behaviour. He suggests however that attempts to understand the atrocities committed by looking at the individual motivations and psychologies of the perpetrators provides only an inadequate and incomplete explanation, arguing that:

> individual psychopathology or ideological blindness necessarily leads to banalisation of the concrete deeds. The organised crime was monstrous – not the perpetrators. The alternative to criminology or psychology is not a general theory of society. Between these two poles lies a true and distinctive field for the analysis of power: the organisation of the camp, and situated actions.
>
> (p.9)

The process of rigid social categorisation, that is, the 'asocial', the 'criminal', the 'Jew', the 'homosexual', the 'political' prisoner, the 'gypsy' and so on both caused and perpetuated social inequality and division within the camp, where, 'the system of categorisation acted as a mechanism for differentiation. It created distances, intensified antagonisms' (p.112). Where people are unable to form social bonds, become emotionally disconnected and remain separated, they lost the identity and capacity to take positive action. What the above analysis tells us is that where categories are created, they intensify difference, distance and separation, and dictate perceptions and judgements.

Empathy, rivalry and shared values

There is substantial evidence that the experience of group membership has the capacity to bring about shared values and associated empathy as well as having the capacity to cause rivalry. This has become powerfully demonstrated in research looking at neural activity which has shown how individuals can feel more empathy for those in their group. Empathic response can however be mediated by perceptions regarding group status (Feng et al., 2016), and racial categorisations (Avenanti et al., 2010). Empathy is dependent on the relationships which exist between groups. For example, whether people are regarded as a possible rival to the in-group is a strong mediating variable dictating empathic response (Chang, 2016). Within a context of rivalry and envy towards an 'out-group', an empathic bias occurs. Richins et al. (2018) found that a rival group's experience of pain did not activate the neurobiological responses associated with empathy, with the authors arguing that empathy and compassion vary depending on the relationships between groups concluding that empathy is reserved for 'us' and not 'them'. What this demonstrates is that 'imposing a social categorisation in the absence of other social relations is sufficient to elicit intergroup bias' (p.12). What seems to matter here is both the social context in which the groups exist and the relationships between the groups.

An example of the capacity of belonging and connection to promote shared values and concern has been demonstrated by Bishop (2018) in her study of heavy metal culture. She observed the ability of group culture to bind people together in a way which created a sense of order and rules governing conduct. Exploring the way people behaved in the apparent chaos of the festival 'mosh pit', she found the heavy metal community to be global and inclusive, where the shared values and shared identity as music lovers saw social norms both emerge and be observed. These norms dictated prosocial conduct and a collective positivity. Even within the context of seeming disorder, values and a shared identity can create rules promoting altruism and concern for others.

The above discussion raises a number of important questions concerning how positive and empowering relationships between groups can be established and how this can become possible within prisons. Under what conditions do people come together so that they are able to work together collaboratively? Under what circumstances do conflict and antagonism emerge, and in what contexts do cooperation and harmony emerge? How can the wider social system in which groups operate, influence the formation of positive group norms and values? Furthermore whilst groups have been regarded by many as a means by which people lose reason and morality, in what circumstances do they have the capacity to empower, motivate and galvanise, and allow individual members to develop a clear sense of self, meaning, personal values and purpose? The next part of the chapter will consider and address these questions.

Prison social climates

Whilst the focus on prison climate and culture has predominantly been through the lens of the social and psychological harm they present, more recent work has started to consider the extent to which prisons can have the potential to be experienced as positive to those who live within them, where imprisonment does not have to be harmful or painful and is not necessarily 'distortive and wholly negative' (Wacquart, 2002).

Two important interlinked developments have in part influenced this thinking. Firstly, there has been a change in the understanding of crime and, more importantly, the processes by which people come to desist from or move away from criminal behaviour. It is now recognised that this is usually a gradual process rather than one where a sudden change in temperament and outlook leads to a radical change in behaviour. Secondly, criminality and behaviour are seen to be strongly influenced by the nature of the social context; social, community and psychological support have all been shown to have a strong bearing on offending and desistance from offending. As argued by Auty and Leibling (2020), the starting point for this can be finding one's place in a 'moral community'. The nature of the prison social climate is strongly related to violence, disorder and reconviction. However, where features such as safety and fairness are present, these can 'bind' people together in a way where positive values and engagement emerge. The importance of supportive relationships where social interactions and social structures help prisoners engage, become involved and participate in their imprisonment is a hugely important variable in providing prisoners with a revised, desistance-orientated outlook. Liebling et al. (2019) found that where prisons have an ethos 'of community spirit, clear boundaries, and deeply humane relationships founded on "intelligent trust"' (p.107), they have a capacity to be a positive force where personal change indeed becomes a reality.

Crewe and Levins (2019) cautiously suggest that despite the well-documented evidence of the psychological, emotional and social harms which prisons can cause, they do have, at the best, the capacity to be 'reinventive'. Certain regime elements seem important in this process: prisoners' experience of kindness, trusting friendships, and revised identities established through respectful social relationships. Where these factors are present, they observed 'a voluntaristic commitment to the regime, [and] active engagement in the process of identity reconstruction' (p.1), arguing that the experience of imprisonment has the potential to be a positive intervention.

What studies like these tell us is that social context matters. Where the context is right, prisoners can develop their potential and engage collaboratively and positively with the regime and in their incarceration. What this also tells us is something about the capacity of relationships. Where the quality of relationships is positive, what we see is the inherent capacities of those imprisoned to emerge (Auty & Liebling, 2020). As important however as the *quality* of relationships is, where the relationships between groups serve to establish categories which create rivalry, competition and mistrust, the social climate of prisons is unlikely to be one which promotes health and well-being.

The questions of under what conditions are people more inclined to work together constructively, and in what context are cohesion and cooperation likely to occur, will now be considered.

Therapeutic communities and social arrangements

TCs have emphasised that it is the relationships and the organisational values and culture on which they are based that have the capacity to bring about change (Pearce & Haigh, 2017). Relationships which create cohesion, trust and accountability can only thrive where there are certain social arrangements in place. Relationships offer means of support, connection and belonging. They can instil ownership, involvement and empowerment which can reshape identity; they can reframe how people view and experience self and others.

Those who refer themselves to prison-based TCs often have histories of persistent, serious offending (Shine, 2000, Newberry, 2010) and their experience during custody has often been marked by significant disruptive behaviour (Newton, 2010). The consistent evidence suggesting that the behaviour of prisoners within TC regimes is characterised by high levels of engagement and low rates of rule breaking (Cullen, 1997, Newton, 2010) is therefore of interest and deserves further consideration. Likewise, if the premise is accepted that the radically improved behaviour of TC residents is to a large degree on account of their social arrangements rather than the individual attributes of their residents, the central question of whether TC structures and practices are relevant to other custodial settings needs to be addressed.

An exploration of the experiences of those participating in TCs has addressed two questions: the first, what is it about the TC experience that has the capacity to engage people, many with significant antisocial backgrounds, within a prison setting which requires high levels of emotional and personal investment; the second, what is it about this regime which provides participants with an experience which is personally meaningful, valuable and fulfilling. Residents' narratives of what 'hooks' them into and engages them within the regime suggests four main themes: the presence of a safe place to discuss and explore problems from the past that contribute to their offending, the experience of supportive, caring and trusting relationships, the opportunity to connect with others who have shared experiences, and the experience of collaboration and shared goals (Stevens, 2013, Genders & Player, 1995).

Similar themes also emerge in how residents understand their own personal journeys of change. Psychological vulnerability and change are inextricably linked by residents and made possible where there are trusting, caring and genuine attachments to others (Rhodes, 2010). Being given real and genuine responsibility within a climate of accountability and empowerment (Dolan, 2017) is also regarded as instrumental in the process by which residents' identities become redefined and enabled by the roles they embrace (Stevens, 2013). Finally, the insight and personal meaning established from the group therapeutic experiences are also experienced as particularly significant in the process of change and desistance (Dolan, 2017).

Establishing a prison community

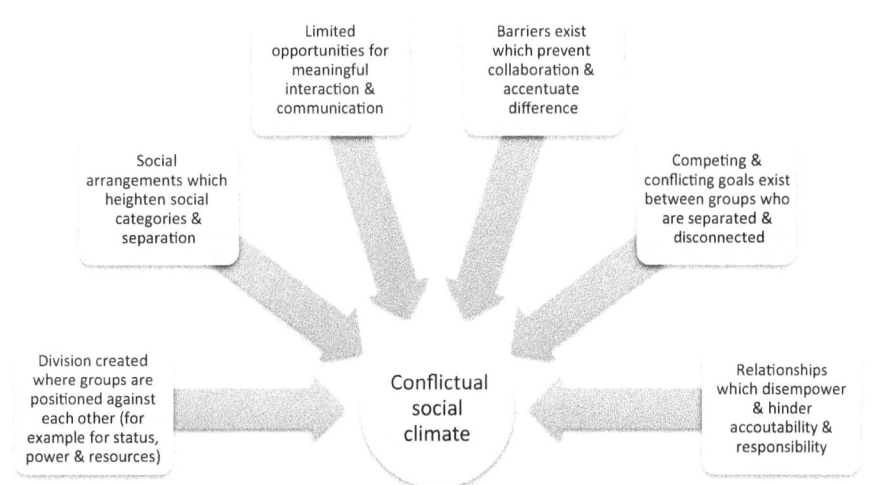

Figure 14.1 Social context and conflict.

As has been seen, the wider systemic context in which people form relationships plays a crucial role in how individuals understand and experience each other; the social arrangements have an overwhelming impact on how people relate to each other. Figure 14.1 highlights the nature of the social context likely to create the context for conflict. What is clear is that rivalry and hostility are more likely to be seen in specific circumstances. Where groups are positioned against each other for resources or status, divisions which foster suspicion and mistrust are more likely to be created. The conditions for conflict become more pronounced where arrangements create distinct social categories which heighten division. Lack of opportunities for interaction and communication lead to a sense of disconnection, and where barriers encourage or accentuate differences between groups, hostility and mistrust become prevalent and pronounced. Furthermore, where competing goals exist between already socially disparate and disconnected groups, the conditions for conflict become more established.

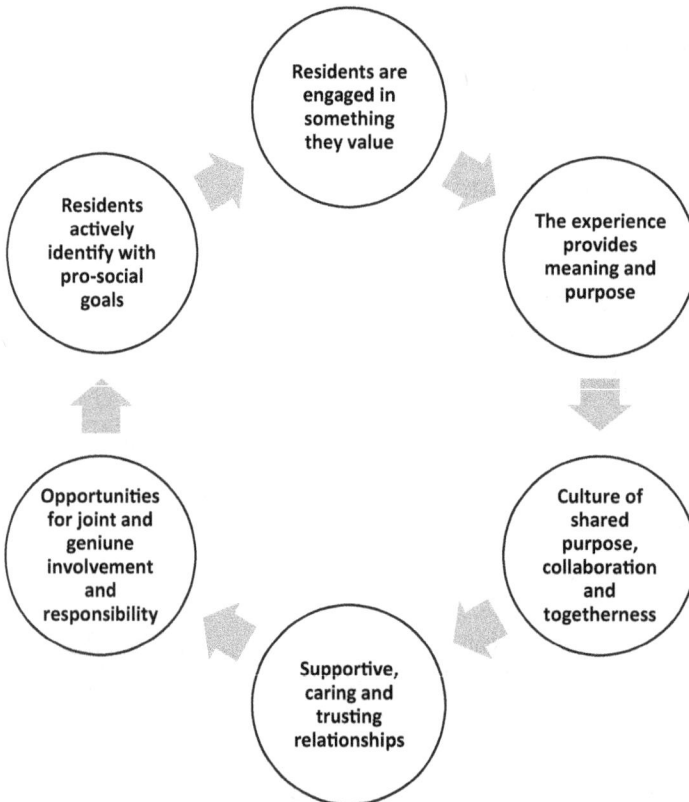

Figure 14.2 Social structures promoting cohesion and engagement.

The structures and practices within prison democratic TCs demonstrate that an alternative set of social arrangements can be put in place which have the potential to safely contain and support those with the highest risk and complex personality needs. Figure 14.2 outlines the arrangements and organizational structures which are more likely to promote cohesion and cooperation. Where residents can be part of an experience they value and are invested in, they can become psychologically engaged and involved. It is this sense of ownership which cultivates meaning and purpose; collaboration becomes more enhanced where a set of shared goals (such as safety or decency) becomes established which people actively identify with as playing a joint role in their pursuit. Collaboration can be brought about by social arrangements which engender cooperation rather than separation. Where relationships are characterized by trust and respect and are able to empower and foster responsibility, the context for cohesion becomes strengthened. This suggests a framework for a social context which can actively and positively engage its residents.

A framework for relationships

The compelling evidence derived from the study of group processes, and the experiences seen in organisations such as TCs, tells us that the social arrangements within prisons can be structured either to mitigate or elevate the risk of conflict; violence and disharmony are not inevitable outcomes. Relationships can be established where collaboration rather than hostility can predominate. The work of Ashworth (2001) suggests that identity, belonging, meaning and personal agency are not only fundamental human needs in any personal transition; they are also central in personal recovery in mental health (Leamy et al., 2011) and desistance from offending (McNeill, 2006). This also lends itself to a framework outlined for the collaborative relationships which emerge where the social arrangements of prison-based TCs are in place.

Identity Research from the desistance literature suggests that changes in identity often precede reductions in offending. Positive contextual influences can lead to changes in identity (Needs & Stantiall, 2018). Residents strongly identify with the shared, prosocial goals of TCs and become invested in the communities and their ethos. Stevens (2013) argues that positive, validating relationships can lead to a redefined identity and sense of who people are and their personal capabilities.

Belonging Social and evolutionary psychology suggest the drive for belonging is strong, as is the need to connect and build relationships with groups (Veale et al., 2014). People have an engrained drive to establish significant and long lasting interpersonal relationships. Survival and group membership are intrinsically linked (Blackhart et al., 2006). Group cohesiveness and the quality of relationships formed within the group have been found to be more important to outcome than the specific therapeutic methods adopted (Hubble et al., 2010), and psychotherapeutic approaches which have the capacity to create belongingness have the potential to be effective across a number of outcomes (Pearce & Pickard, 2013). Nurturing therapeutic experiences, fostering attachment and belonging, can promote changes in the prefrontal cortex, associated with emotional regulation and empathy (Fonagy & Adshead, 2012).

Empowerment and agency Haigh (1999) argues that psychological development comes where the individual can see themselves as empowered, having the capacity to make autonomous decisions and where they are accountable and responsible for actions and behaviour. Authentic relationships can be experienced where openness, accountability and genuine responsibility are present, and within this context personal agency will develop. Empowerment and ownership is seen as an important factor in change (Adler et al., 2008), and a belief about one's ability to change is an important predictor of outcome (Pearce & Pickard, 2013).

Meaning Needs and Stantiall (2018) argue that patterns of inflexible and self-defeating behaviour are maintained to prevent invalidation. Personal meaning can however be established from the relationships developed (Woodward, 2011). In circumstances where people may become preoccupied with self-preservation, trust is lost and meaning and personal validity become lost. Establishing personal meaning is often both a drive for entering into and an outcome of psychotherapy where the relationships established with the group members or individual therapist are often regarded as the salient factors in helping clients regain or establish a sense of personal meaning (Yalom, 1985).

Prison cohesion and the relevance of the TC social climate

A frequently asked question about how far the practices of TCs are relevant to the wider prison community clearly needs consideration. TCs have sometimes been criticised on account that only a minority of prisoners with particular attributes, personal goals and expectations would be prepared to engage in their processes, and for this reason lack wider relevance. Whether they have wider applicability beyond the small number of prisons which adopt this approach indeed remains an important question. In response to this,

Bennett and Shuker (2018) have reflected that 'although there is a good case for increasing the availability of therapeutic interventions and units, the DTC approach in its entirety would not be appropriate or suitable for all prisons and all prisoners' (p.52).

There are however some aspects of TC regimes which could have broader applicability and have the potential to inform wider prison practice. It is evident though that in order for these to become meaningful and relevant, they need to be implemented as part of a wider approach to developing and sustaining a positive social climate. Shared goals need to be negotiated, staff supervision needs to be a priority, a consensus needs to be reached on organisational structure and practice, and a service-wide clarity of purpose and role needs to be agreed. Importantly, prisoners need to be at a particular stage in their own lives, personal development and often their prison sentence where they are ready to engage and participate in this prison environment and social climate.

The following, outlined in Figure 14.3, provides a summary of how the culture and values of a TC are reflected in the practices, activities and social arrangements adopted. A number of themes emerge where the culture and values of TCs become embedded within the wider routines of the prison. Whilst not all may be relevant to wider prisons, some may have the potential to offer something to the culture and practices within other penal settings.

Opportunities for genuine involvement

An analysis of the experiences of residents participating in prison TCs highlights that being given genuine responsibility has a profound effect on shaping their relationship with the wider prison. It also is a symbolic act which conveys belief and trust and encourages people to reappraise how they approach their incarceration. Residents are elected into genuine and meaningful voluntary positions within their community, they chair meetings, organise events and engage with universities and charities. More importantly, they are given a key role in decision making, the maintenance of a safe environment, resolving conflicts and supporting others.

Hope, affirmation and empowerment

Residents arrive at Grendon with a hope that the therapeutic experience will provide value and meaning, and a belief that personal change and recovery will be reality. They have a sense of optimism. The aims and ethos of the

Culture and Values	Organisational Practices, Structures and Activities
Opportunities for genuine involvement, participation and responsibility	All residents have a valued voluntary role within their community Joint meetings between staff and residents which allow dialogue, accountability, conflict resolution and community planning Active engagement with external agencies such as universities, charities
Hope, affirmation empowerment	Expectations and responsibilities invested in the resident community Key events, achievements and success recognised acknowledged and celebrated Clearly established organisational values, culture and ethos affirming values of respect, decency and a belief in personal change Welcoming and engaging culture in prison visits
Shared goals and collaboration	Shared activities (including meals), Opportunities for joint participation and activities such as hosting drug awareness, diversity, staff selection Resident role in staff interviews and selection Peer involvement in treatment planning and reviews of progress Resident involvement and representation in policy meetings
Prioritising and investing in key events	**Family days** – spend all day on a wing eating together, visiting cells **'Therapy' visits** – facilitated meetings with family members **Visits with a Difference** – Children and families spending the day together
Trusting, collaborative and respectful relationships	Structured and spontaneous opportunities for connections Formal joining and leaving events and rituals Informal time between staff and residents prioritised Working together in shared social activities ie meals, sports events, games, quizzes Routine use of first name terms Hand shake on arrival
Safety	Staff and peer established rules and constitution governing behaviour and expectations Shared access to social spaces such as offices, meal times Community involvement in support and accountability process following conflict or rule breaking

Figure 14.3 Creating cohesion with a prison.

therapeutic regime are communicated prior to their arrival. Many residents report hearing of TCs and their values and culture earlier in their sentence and how this has captivated their interest. This optimism is also created and sustained, in part, by the sense of responsibility and belief invested in the resident community; a jointly written 'constitution' which establishes a set of principles for respectful, decent and community-minded behaviour conveys a sense of meaning and purpose.

Shared goals

The regime emphasises and prioritises opportunities for shared activities and participation. Residents and staff eat meals together and are involved in jointly organising and hosting events such as drug awareness or victim empathy conferences. Their clear and established role in the staff selection process creates attachment and furthers a culture of collaboration. They actively engage in reviewing and revising the wing constitution. What is clear is that residents and staff value many of the same things; the experience of TCs suggests that meaning and purpose, rewarding relationships and a sense of safety are goals of shared importance.

Significant, key and symbolic events

Prioritising key events has a significant impact in shaping culture and values. These include 'family days' in which families experience a day on the prison wing, see where residents live and sleep, and get to know the staff team and come to understand more about the regime and its goals. Events such as these allow families to develop an attachment and affiliation to with the prison and the therapeutic work the residents are involved in.

'Therapy' visits are held for residents needing to build relationships with family members. These are facilitated by uniformed and non-uniformed staff. These events promote a culture which is supportive and containing, and where residents are able to reaffirm and rebuild relationships with loved ones and foster a greater understanding of their experiences.

Collaborative relationships

Creating collaborative relationships has always been at the core of TC practice. These have been essential to both therapeutic outcomes and the social climate within TCs. The learning from TCs suggests that establishing trusting and respectful relationships is made possible where opportunities for connection and interaction, both formal and informal, are deliberately prioritised. TC practice demonstrates that a culture of cooperation and trusting relationships are closely linked and suggests how opportunities to build relationships can be found within institutions and organisations. Where groups are not seen as a threat, shared goals and values are more likely to be established. TCs tell us that practices can be put in place which have a significant impact on relationships between people. Open communication and dialogue influence the nature of the relationships, with authority being seen as legitimate and dependable.

Safety

The experience of safety is valued and sought after by residents who refer themselves to therapeutic communities. The safe social climate engages residents and staff and is experienced as a prerequisite in the conditions for change. A culture of safety is established where residents and staff are involved in agreeing a set of social norms which all have a role in creating and maintaining. What TCs also suggest is that where residents have ownership of the rules and constitution, they have an alignment and attachment to the organisation and are more likely to work within these rules. The collaboration and connection where residents identify strongly with the organisation rather than see themselves as separate and disconnected promotes a culture of safe practice.

Conclusion

When considering the reasons why prisoners wish to participate in a therapeutic programme, it is apparent that these are not particularly unusual or remarkable in themselves. Safety, connection, finding meaning and purpose, and working through life's difficulties are, in varying degrees, all important for those referring themselves to a TC. In some ways this reflects the notion of a desire for a 'good life' (see Ward & Maruna, 2007). It also reflects a fundamental desire prisoners have to live in a community with a sense of morality. Something else which becomes apparent is the hope residents have for an experience which will be restorative and nurturing, that will lead to personal change, and which they have the capacity to achieve, after many repeated cycles of failed attempts to do so. What TCs show us is that those considered disturbed and antisocial have similar aspirations and hopes, to the rest of us. They also show that conflict and violence are not inevitable, and that prisons can have the capacity to be both safe and restorative. TCs also show us that where a prison has a clear set of values reflecting respect, safety, meaning and purpose, they provide an alternative to other forms of imprisonment which prisoners find compelling and engaging.

Prisoners' experiences of TCs suggest that renewed identities can be established where people wish to collaborate and connect and work together in creating something they value and take pride in. Although it is recognised that TCs cannot be exported in their entirety to other prisons, they do suggest something positive and hopeful about prisons, the possibilities they offer, and the experiences of those who both live and work in them. TCs may also suggest something else. Even for those with the most pervasive and deep-rooted difficulties, the experience of imprisonment can be helpful, valuable and meaningful.

There is a set of practical and pragmatic issues which arise when considering the wider applicability of TCs to prisons. They tend to be smaller and more resource intensive than other prisons. They also require staffing by those with a particular set of skills, training and personal attributes; whilst these practical considerations clearly cannot be overlooked what TCs suggest is that prisons have a potential which is perhaps unrecognised. Relationships can thrive within a context of humane containment, safety and decency, and people within prisons can work alongside each other and become personally invested in establishing considerable meaning and benefit out of the experience of incarceration.

References

Adler, J. M., Skalina, L. M., & McAdams, D. P. (2008). The narrative reconstruction of psychotherapy and psychological health. *Psychotherapy Research, 18*, 719–34.

Allport, G. W. (1958). *The nature of prejudice.* Garden City, NY: Doubleday.

Ashworth, B. E. (2001). *Role transitions in organisational life: An identity-based perspective.* Mahwah, NJ: Lawrence Erlbaum Associates.

Auty, K., & Liebling, A. (2020). Exploring the relationship between prison social climate and reoffending. *Justice Quarterly, 37*(2), 358–81. https://doi.org/10.1080/07418825.2018.1538421

Avenanti, A., Sirigu, A., & Aglioti, S. M. (2010). Racial bias reduces empathic sensorimotor resonance with other-race pain. *Current Biology, 20*, 1018–22.

Bar Zohar, M. (1998). *Beyond Hitler's grasp. The heroic rescue of Bulgaria's Jews.* Holbrook, MA: Adams Media.

Baumeister, R. F., & Leary, M. R. (1995). The need to belong – desire for interpersonal attachments as a fundamental human motivation. *Psychological Bulletin, 117*, 497–529. https://doi.org/10.1037/0033-2909.117.3.497

Baumeister, R. F., DeWall, C. N., Ciarocco, N. J., & Twenge, J. M. (2005). Social exclusion impairs self-regulation. *Journal of Personality and Social Psychology, 88*, 589–604.

Bennett, J., & Shuker, R. (2018). Hope, harmony and humanity: Creating a positive social climate in a democratic therapeutic community prison and the implications for penal practice. *Journal of Criminal Psychology, 8*(1), 44–57. https://doi.org/10.1108

Bishop, L. (n.d.). *Smoke, smell and skins: Hierarchy in heavy metal* [Unpublished PhD dissertation]. University College London.

Blackhart, G. C., Baumeister, R. F., & Twenge, J. M. (2006). rejection's impact on self-defeating, prosocial, antisocial, and self-regulatory behaviors. In K. D. Vohs and E. J. Finkel (Eds.). *Self and relationships: Connecting intrapersonal and interpersonal processes.* (pp.237–53). New York, NY, US: Guilford Press.

Chang, L., Krosch, A. R., & Cikara, M. (2016). Effects of intergroup threat on mind, brain, and behavior. *Current Opinion in Psychology, 11*, 69–73.

Crewe, B. (2009). *The prisoner society: Power, adaptation, and social life in an English prison.* Oxford: Oxford University Press.

Crewe, B., & Levins, A. (2019). The prison as a reinventive institution. *Theoretical Criminology, 24*, 1–22.

Crewe, B., & Liebling, A. (2015). Staff culture, authority and prison violence. *Prison Service Journal, 221*, 9–14.

Cullen, E. (1997). Can a prison be therapeutic? The Grendon template. In E. Cullen, L. Jones, & R. Woodward (Eds.). *Therapeutic communities for offenders* (pp.75–100). Hoboken, NJ: John Wiley & Sons.

Dingle, G. (2018). Addiction and the importance of belonging. *Psychologist, 31*, 36–8.

Dingle, G. A., Haslam, C., Best, D., Chan. G., Staiger, P. K., Savic, M., Beckwith, M., Mackenzie, J., Bathish, R., & Lubman, D. I. (2019). Social identity differentiation predicts commitment to sobriety and wellbeing in residents of therapeutic communities. *Social Science & Medicine, 237*, 112459. https://doi.org/ 10.1016/j.socscimed.2019.112459

Dolan, R. (2017). HMP Grendon therapeutic community: The residents' perspective of the process of change. *The International Journal of Therapeutic Communities, 38*(1), 23–31.

Engel, G. L. (1977). The need for a new medical model; A challenge for biomedicine. *Science, 196*, 129–36.

Feng, C., Li, Z., Feng, X., Wang, L., Tian, T., & Luo, Y.-J. (2016). Social hierarchy modulates neural responses of empathy for pain. *Social Cognitive and Affective Neuroscience, 11*, 485–95.

Fonagy, P., & Adshead, G. (2012). How mentalisation changes the mind. *Advances in Psychiatric Treatment, 18*, 353–62. https://doi.org/10.1192/apt.bp.108.005876

Genders, E., & Player, E. (1995). *Grendon: A study of a therapeutic prison.* Oxford: Clarendon Press.

Gilmore, D. D. (1990). *Manhood in the making: Cultural concepts of masculinity.* New Haven, CT: Yale University Press.

Haigh, R. (1999). The quintessence of a therapeutic community. In P. Campling & R. Haigh (Eds.). *Therapeutic communities: Past, present and future* (pp.246–57). London, UK: Jessica Kingsley.

Haney, C., Banks, C., & Zimbardo, P. (1973). Interpersonal dynamics in a simulated prison. *International Journal of Criminology and Penology, 1*, 69–97.

Haslam, A. (2018). Unlocking the social cure, *The Psychologist, 31*, 28–31.

Haslam, C., Jetten, J., Cruwys, T., Dingle, G. & Haslam, S. A. (2018). *The new psychology of health: Unlocking the social cure.* Abingdon: Routledge.

Hawksley, L. C., Burleson, M. H., Berntson, G. G., & Cacioppo, J. T. (2003). Loneliness in everyday life: Cardiovascular activity, psychosocial context, and health behaviors. *Journal of Personality and Social Psychology, 85*, 105–20.

Holt-Lunstad, J., Smith, T. B., & Layton, J. B.(2010). Social relationships and mortality risk: A meta-analytic review. *PLOS Medicine, 7,* 2–20.

Hubble, M., Duncan, B., Miller, S., & Wampold, B. (2010), 'Introduction'. In B. Duncan, S. Miller, B. Wampold, and M. Hubble (Eds.). *The Heart and Soul of Change: Delivering What Works in Therapy* (2nd ed.). American Psychological Association, Washington, DC, pp.23–46.

Johnstone, L., & Boyle, M., with Cromby, J., Dillon, J., Harper, D., Kinderman, P., Longden, E., Pilgrim, D., & Read, J. (2018). *The Power Threat Meaning Framework: Towards the identification of patterns in emotional distress, unusual experiences and troubled or troubling behaviour, as an alternative to functional psychiatric diagnosis.* Leicester: British Psychological Society.

Jones, L. F. (2015) The Peaks unit: from a pilot for 'untreatable' psychopaths to trauma informed milieu therapy. *Prison Service Journal, 218,* 17–23.

Layard, R., & Clark, D. M. (2014). *Thrive: The power of evidence-based psychological therapies.* London, UK: Allen Lane.

Leamy, M., Bird, V., Le Boutillier, C., Williams, J., & Slade, M. (2011). Conceptual framework for personal recovery in mental health: systematic review and narrative synthesis. *British Journal of Psychiatry, 199,* 445–52.

Leibling, A., Laws, B., Lieber, E., Auty, K., Schimidt, B. E., Crewe, B., Gardon, J., Kant, D., & Morey, M. (2019). Are hope and possibility achievable in prison? *The Howard Journal of Crime and Justice, 58,* 104–26.

McNeill, F. (2006). A desistance paradigm for offender management. *Criminology and Criminal Justice, 6,* 39–62.

Mews, A., Di Bella, L., & Purver, M. (2017), *Impact evaluation of the prison-based core sex offender treatment programme.* Ministry of Justice Analytical Series. London, Author.

Moloney, P., & Kelly, P. (2008). Beck never lived in Birmingham: Why cognitive behaviour therapy may be a less helpful treatment for psychological distress than is often supposed. In R. House & D. Loewenthal (Eds.). *Against and for CBT: Towards a constructive dialogue?* (pp.278–88). Ross-on-Wye: PCCS Books.

Moos, R. H. (2008). Active ingredients of substance use focussed self help groups. *Addiction, 103,* 387–96.

Needs, A., & Stantiall, A. (2018). The social context of transition and rehabilitation. In G. Akerman, A. Needs, & C. Bainbridge. (Eds.). *Transforming environments and rehabilitation. A guide for practitioners in forensic and criminal justice* (pp.31–62). Taylor & Francis.

Newberry, M. (2010). A synthesis of outcome research at Grendon therapeutic community prison. *Therapeutic Communities, 31*(4), 357–373.

Newton, M. (2010). Changes in prison offending among residents of a prison-based therapeutic community. In R. Shuker & E. Sullivan (Eds.). *Grendon and the emergence of forensic therapeutic communities: Developments in research and practice* (pp.281–91).Chichester: Wiley-Blackwell.

Oakes, P. J., Haslam, S. A., & Turner, J. C. (1994). *Stereotyping and social reality.* Oxford, UK: Blackwell.

Oyserman, D., & Lee, S. W. S. (2008). Does culture influence what and how we think? Effects of priming individualism and collectivism. *Psychological Bulletin, 134*(2), 311–42.

Oyserman, D., Coon, H., & Kemmelmeier, M. (2002). Rethinking individualism and collectivism: Evaluation of theoretical assumptions and meta-analyses. *Psychological Bulletin, 128,* 3–72.

Pearce, S., & Haigh, R. (2017). *The theory and practice of democratic therapeutic community treatment*. London, UK: Jessica Kingsley.

Pearce, S., & Pickard, H. (2013). How therapeutic communities work: Specific factors related to positive outcome. *International Journal of Social Psychiatry, 59*, 636–45. https://doi.org/ 10.1177/ 0020764012450992

Platow, M. J., & Hunter, J. A. (2014). Necessarily collectivistic. *The Psychologist, 27*, 838–41.

Reicher, S. (2017). The rules of unlawliness. *The Psychologist, 30*, 38–45.

Reicher, S., & Hopkins, N. *Self and nation. Categorisation, contestation and mobilisation*. London, UK: SAGE.

Rhodes, L. A. (2010). 'This can't be real': Continuity at HMP Grendon. In R. Shuker & E. Sullivan (Eds.). *Grendon and the emergence of forensic therapeutic communities* (pp.203–6). John Wiley & Sons.

Richins, M. T., Barreto, M., Karl, A., & Lawrence, N. (2018). Empathic responses are reduced to competitive but not non-competitive outgroups. *Social Neuroscience, 14*(3), 345–58. https:// doi.org/10.1080/17470919.2018.1463927

Sampson, E. E. (1988). The debate on individualism: Indigenous psychologies of the individual and their role in personal and societal functioning. *American Psychologist, 43*, 15–22.

Scott, D. (2015). Eating your insides out: Cultural, physical and institutionally-structured violence in the prison place. *Prison Service Journal, 221*, 55–62.

Sherif, M., & Sherif, C. W. (1969). *Social psychology*. New York, NY: Harper & Row.

Shine, J., & Newton, M. (2000) Damaged, disturbed and dangerous: a profile of receptions to Grendon therapeutic prison 1995–2000. In J. Shine (Ed.). *A compilation of Grendon research* (pp.23–36). Leyhill: Leyhill Press, HMP Grendon.

Sofsky, W. (1993). *The order of terror*. Princeton, NJ: Princeton University Press.

Stevens, A. (2013). *Offender rehabilitation and therapeutic communities: Enabling change the TC way*. Abingdon: Routledge.

Summerfield, D. (2012). Afterword: Against 'global mental health'. *Transcultural Psychiatry, 49*(3), 1–12.

Sykes, G. (1958). *The society of captives: A study of maximum security prison*. Princeton, NJ: Princeton University Press.

Tajfel, H.(1972). La categorisation sociale (English trans.). In S. Moscovici (Ed.). *Introduction à la psychologie sociale* (Vol. 1, pp.272–302). Paris: Larousse.

Turner, J. C., Hogg, M., Oakes, P., Reicher, S., &Wetherell, M. (1987). *Rediscovering the social group: A self-categorization theory*. Oxford, UK: Basil Blackwell.

Todorov, T. (2001). *The fragility of goodness: Why Bulgaria's Jews survived the Holocaust*. London, UK: Weidenfeld & Nicolson.

Veale, D., Gilbert, P., Wheatley, J., & Naismith, I. (2014). A new therapeutic community: Development of a compassion-focussed and contextual behavioural environment. *Clinical Psychology & Psychotherapy, 22*(4), 285–303. https://doi.org/10.1002/cpp.1897

Wacquant, L. (2002). The curious eclipse of prison ethnography in the age of mass incarceration. *Ethnography, 3*(4), 371–97.

Ward, T., & Maruna, S. (2007). *Rehabilitation: Beyond the risk assessment paradigm*. London, UK: Routledge.

Warner, R. (2004). *Recovery from schizophrenia: Psychiatry and political economy* (3rd ed.). Hove and New York: Brunner-Routledge.

Weaver, B. (2016). *Offending and desistance: The importance of social relations*. London, UK: Routledge.

Woodward, R. (2011). The director's tale|: A search engine for meaning. In E. Cullen & J. Mackenzie (Eds.). *Dovegate: A therapeutic community in a private prison and developments in therapeutic work with personality disordered offenders* (pp.127–54). Hampshire, UK: Waterside Press.

Yalom, I. (1985). *The theory and practice of group psychotherapy* (3rd ed.). New York, NY: Basic Books.

Index

For Product Safety Concerns and Information please contact our EU
representative GPSR@taylorandfrancis.com
Taylor & Francis Verlag GmbH, Kaufingerstraße 24, 80331 München, Germany